Therapeutic Nutrition

A Guide to Patient Education

EILEEN BEHAN, RD, LD
Nutritionist
Exeter Health
Exeter, New Hampshire

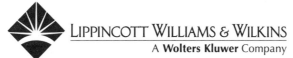

LIPPINCOTT WILLIAMS & WILKINS
A **Wolters Kluwer** Company

Philadelphia • Baltimore • New York • London
Buenos Aires • Hong Kong • Sydney • Tokyo

Acquisitions Editor: Patricia Casey
Editorial Assistant: Katherine Rothwell
Senior Production Manager: Helen Ewan
Senior Managing Editor / Production: Erika Kors
Production Project Manager: Cynthia Rudy
Creative Director: Doug Smock
Senior Manufacturing Manager: William Alberti
Production Services / Compositor: Aptara, Inc.
Printer: Courier–Kendallville

9 8 7 6 5 4 3 2

Library of Congress Cataloging-in-Publication Data

Behan, Eileen.
    Therapeutic nutrition : a guide to patient education / Eileen Behan.
        p. ; cm.
    Includes bibliographical references and index.
    ISBN 13: 978-1-58255-380-1
    ISBN 10: 1-58255-380-7 (alk. paper)
    1. Diet therapy—Study and teaching—Handbooks, manuals, etc.   2. Nutrition—Study and teaching—Handbooks, manuals, etc.   3. Patient education—Handbooks, manuals, etc.   I. Title.
    [DNLM: 1. Nutrition. 2. Diet. 3. Food. 4. Patient Education—methods. QU 145 B419t 2006]
RM218.B44 2006 615.8'54—dc22
                            2005015566

LWW.com

To Sarah and Emily

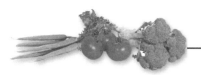

John W. Distler, FNP
Clinical Instructor, FNP Program
University of Maryland
Baltimore, Maryland

Margaret A. Dow, RNC, BA, CMA
Nurse Manager
Danvers, Massachusetts

Melinda Jenkins, PhD, APRN-BC
Assistant Professor of Clinical Nursing
Columbia University School of Nursing
New York, New York

Marilee Murphy Jensen, MN, ARNP
Nurse Practitioner and Lecturer
University of Washington School of Nursing
Seattle, Washington

Kara A. Lauze, RN, MS, ARNP
Critical Care Nurse Practitioner
UMASS Memorial Hospital
Worcester, Massachusetts

Patricia B. Lisk, RN, BSN
Department Chairperson and Instructor
Augusta Technical College
Augusta, Georgia

Carolyn Mason, RN, MS
Assistant Professor of Nursing
Miami University
Oxford, Ohio

Mary Beth Modic, MSN, RN, CNS
Clinical Nurse Specialist, Diabetes, Patient
    Education
The Cleveland Clinic Foundation
Cleveland, Ohio

Whitney B. Nowak, RN, MS
Adult Nurse Practitioner
Core Physicians Services Inc.
Exeter, New Hampshire

Rhonda J. Reed, RN, MSN, CRRN
Instructor, Technology Coordinator, and PRN Staff
    Nurse
Indiana State University College of Nursing
Union Hospital Medical Rehabilitation Unit
Bloomington, Indiana
Terre Haute, Indiana

Kate Willcutts, MS, RD, CNSD
Lead Nutrition Support Nutritionist and Instructor,
    School of Nursing
University of Virginia
Charlottesville, Virginia

The idea for this manual developed over the last twenty-five years as I worked within a variety of healthcare settings. As a consulting nutritionist, I am asked almost daily about diet, food, cookbooks, safe vitamins, and the latest food trends. This book has evolved from these questions.

The book is written for non-nutrition healthcare professionals, the people in the position of answering many of the public's questions about food and diet. The content has been culled from textbooks, peer-reviewed articles, and nonprofit and government-funded nutrition education programs into one practical manual for easy reference and reproduction. Each handout provides basic nutrition guidance until a patient can make an appointment with a nutrition professional for information about food choices that will prevent disease and appropriate diets to treat or manage illness.

Each section begins with a discussion, followed by patient education handouts that providers can refer to and reproduce single copies of to give to patients. Section 1—Integrating Nutrition Into Your Practice—deals with how and why nutrition education needs to be integrated into healthcare practice. Section 2—Guiding Patients Toward a Healthy Diet—provides guidelines for understanding and implementing recommendations for healthy eating. This is not a cookbook, but it would be incomplete without a few recipes to put the principles of good nutrition into action; therefore, Section 2 also includes recipes that can answer the very real question, "What should I cook?".

Section 3—Supplements and Dietary Reference Intakes: Vitamins, Minerals, and Macronutrients—provides a practical guide to the use of common supplements and the new "Dietary Reference Intakes for Individuals" for vitamins, minerals, carbohydrates, fats, and protein. Section 4—Therapeutic Nutrition—begins with a general discussion of the medical conditions that are most affected by food choices, followed by patient education handouts that providers can use to guide individuals toward the diet that is indicated for their condition. In most cases, a referral to a dietitian is encouraged, and resources for finding one are provided. In Section 5—Family Nutrition—lifecycle nutrition issues are addressed, including foods for infants, toddlers, and adolescents; pregnancy and lactation; and vegetarianism. The complex issue of obesity and weight control is addressed in Section 6—Weight Control, Obesity Treatment and Prevention. This will be particularly useful for the provider in the position of providing weight counseling. Section 7—Calories, Fast Food, and Caffeine—includes data on calories, fast food restaurants, and the caffeine content of food. The purpose of each of these sections is to get accurate, effective information and resources about food and nutrition into the hands of healthcare providers so that they can pass it on to their patients. Any comments, suggestions, or recommendations will be welcomed.

Eileen Behan, RD, LD

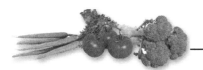

Acknowledgments

Special thanks to the following individuals who helped in the creation of this book: Madeleine Walsh, RD; Judith Paige, RD; Marilyn DeSimone, RD; Vicki Irwin, RD; Jane Hackett, MA, RD; Melissa Snow, RD; Patricia Murray Derr, RD; Whitney Nowak, ARNP; Robert Murray, MD; Mary McGowan, MD; and at Lippincott Williams & Wilkins, Katherine Rothwell and Patricia Casey.

Credits

Nutrition Facts Panel (Nutrition Label) on Handout 1-3 is reprinted from the Center for Food Safety and Applied Nutrition, United States Food and Drug Administration (FDA).

USDA Food Pyramid on Figure 2-1 is reprinted from the U.S. Department of Agriculture and the U.S. Department of Health and Human Services.

USDA MyPyramid Food Guide on Handout 2-1 is reprinted from the U.S. Department of Agriculture and the U.S. Department of Health and Human Services.

U.S. Dietary Guidelines for Americans, 2000, 5th edition, on Handouts 2-6 through 2-15 are reprinted from the U.S. Department of Agriculture Center for Nutrition Policy and Promotion.

Thrifty Recipes on Handouts 2-16 through 2-29 are reprinted from the U.S. Department of Agriculture Center for Nutrition Policy and Promotion, Recipes and Tips for Healthy, Thrifty Meals.

Dietary Approach to Stop Hypertension (DASH) on Handout 4-1 is reprinted from the National Heart, Lung and Blood Institute, the Department of Health and Human Services, and the National Institutes of Health (NIH).

Diabetes: What I Need to Know About Eating and Diabetes on Handout 4-6, *Warning Signs of a Diabetic Low Blood Sugar* on Handout 4-7, *Hypoglycemia for People Who Do Not Have Diabetes* on Handout 4-9, and *What I Need to Know About Gestational Diabetes* on Handout 5-6 are reprinted from the National Diabetes Information Clearinghouse (NDIC), a service of the National Institute of Diabetes and Digestive and Kidney Disease (NIDDK), and the NIH.

Do You Have Pre-diabetes? on Handout 4-8 is reprinted from the National Diabetes Education Program (NDEP), a partnership of the NIH, the Centers for Disease Control (CDC) and Prevention, and more than 200 public and private organizations.

Gluten-free Diet for Celiac Disease on Handout 4-18, *Diet for Heartburn and Gastroesophageal Reflux Disease* on Handout 4-20, *Diet and Constipation* on Handout 4-22, and *Constipation in Children* on Handout 5-8 are reprinted from National Digestive Diseases Information Clearinghouse (NDDIC), a service of the NIDDK, and the NIH.

What to Eat While Pregnant on Handout 5-3 and *How Can I Help My Overweight Child?* on Handout 6-16 are reprinted from the National Institute of Diabetes and Digestive and Kidney Diseases of the National Institutes of Health Weight-Control Information Network (WIN).

Handouts 6-1 through 6-14 are reprinted from *Clinical Guidelines on the Identification, Evaluation and Treatment of Overweight and Obesity in Adults*, a report from the Obesity Education Initiative from the National Heart, Lung, and Blood Institute (NHLBI) of the NIH.

Glycemic Index—What Is It? on Handout 6-17 is reprinted from the International Food Information Council (IFIC) Foundation.

Emergency Health Care Plan for Food Allergies on Handout 5-11 is from Manifestations of food allergy: Evaluation and treatment. *American Family Physician*, available at http://aafp.org/afp/990115ap/415.html, accessed 12/9/03.

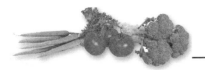

SECTION 4   *Therapeutic Nutrition*   151

PATIENT EDUCATION HANDOUTS

SECTION 5   *Family Nutrition*   221

PATIENT EDUCATION HANDOUTS

SECTION 6   **Weight Control, Obesity Treatment and Prevention   287**

PATIENT EDUCATION HANDOUTS

SECTION 7   **Calories, Fast Food, and Caffeine   335**

PATIENT EDUCATION HANDOUTS

Integrating Nutrition Into Your Practice

The association between nutrition and health is increasingly recognized as an important aspect of primary health care. More than half of Americans are either overweight or obese. The total U.S. medical expenditures attributed to excessive weight may be as great as $78.5 billion per year (or an additional $395 for each overweight adult) (Finkelstein, 2003). Medicare and Medicaid pay half of these costs. Primary care providers continually ask for advice on how to address the issue of proper diet in an efficient and effective manner. Individuals with a complicating medical condition (e.g., diabetes, dyslipidemia, and hypertension) may eventually find their way to a registered dietitian through a referral from their primary care provider. Obesity often leads to complicating medical issues but reimbursement for obesity alone is problematic without reimbursable comorbidity (Cook, 2002). In an ideal world all patients would have access to a registered dietitian for personal nutrition advice. Because the medical cost of treating obesity-related illness continues to increase, such referrals might be seen as cost-effective. Currently, however, patients turn to their primary care provider for accurate advice. Are you ready?

WHY NUTRITION NEEDS TO BE INTEGRATED INTO PRIMARY CARE

Obesity is a visible characteristic of poor diet; less obvious is the accompanying rise in diabetes and heart disease. According to the United States Surgeon General's 2001 report, being overweight or obese contributes to the increased risk of coronary heart disease; type 2 diabetes; endometrial, colon, and postmenopausal breast cancers; and other cancers (Surgeon General, 2001). Type 2 diabetes is becoming more common among Native American, African American, and Hispanic and Latino children and adolescents. Almost 9% of Americans age 20 years or older have diabetes and in those more than 60 years of age the number exceeds 18% of the population (National Diabetes Fact Sheet, 2004).

Recognizing the rise in obesity among children with its eventual accompanying health consequences, the American Academy of Pediatrics has called on pediatricians to address nutrition in well-child visits and to offer anticipatory guidance to parents, intervening before the problem becomes severe (American Academy of Pediatrics Committee on Nutrition, 2003). Although data are lacking on physician-directed education, doing nothing to influence positive eating habits will frustrate healthcare providers and be potentially dangerous to their patients.

The nonacute care visit, particularly the adult and well-child visit, and the examination room provide an ideal opportunity and setting in which to give advice about proper nutrition. Primary care providers must integrate nutrition messages into routine health care to balance the messages heard from the American food industry. In 1997, Coca-Cola spent $277 million to advertise its soda; Pepsi spent almost $200 million. The largest public education nutrition program, the National Cancer Institute's "5 A Day" campaign that encourages people to eat more fruits and vegetables, involved a budget of less than $1 million (CSPI, 2000). Most Americans visit their doctor, or are in contact with their doctor, at least once in any year (Surgeon General, 2001), yet less than half of obese adults report being advised to lose weight by their healthcare provider (Galuska, 1999).

The U.S. Department of Agriculture (USDA) reports only 3% of Americans surveyed meet four of the five recommendations for the intake of grains, vegetables, dairy products, and meats. And though the U.S. Dietary Guidelines for Americans recommends 30 minutes of activity, on most days less than one-third of Americans surveyed met this target and 40% were not active at all. Only 65% of adolescents reported vigorous activity. Healthcare providers can influence their patients' behavior related to diet. In a survey of adults receiving routine healthcare, those patients who were asked by their doctor about diet were more likely to have changed their fat or fiber intake and somewhat more likely to have lost weight than those who were not asked about diet (Nawaz, Adams, and Katz, 2000).

Diet choices and activity patterns can be altered by addressing nutrition and dietary issues during clinical visits using a simple nutrition history form and having readily available patient education handouts to answer questions and provide resources about healthy eating. The goal should be to optimize health by promoting a nutritionally adequate diet, with moderate food intake.

HOW TO INTEGRATE NUTRITION INTO PRIMARY CARE

Much nutrition information could be integrated into patient care, but repeating just a few simple messages clearly and frequently is an effective way to improve diet and thus reduce obesity, heart disease, diabetes, and cancer. An example of a clear, effective, specific health message can be found in recommendations made to reduce sudden infant death syndrome (SIDS). In 1992, 70% of parents were putting their infants to bed face down. When the prone sleeping position was identified as a risk factor for SIDS, pediatric health care providers changed their sleep advice to include the clear and specific message: "Do not put your baby to sleep face down." By 1996, the prevalence of prone sleeping decreased to 24% and the number of deaths attributed to SIDS decreased by 30% (Information on Sudden Infant Death Syndrome, 2004). It would not have been adequate to advise parents to "put your child to bed safely" just as it is not adequate to tell individuals to "eat a little better." Individuals, both adults and children, need clear, specific advice about fruit and vegetable consumption, eating regular meals, avoiding saturated fats, and including exercise in their daily activity.

A brief nutrition history form completed in the waiting room and discussed within the context of a routine clinical visit can effectively address nutrition issues within primary care. Hark and Deen (1999) suggest that a nutrition history be part of routine health care. A nutrition history form, with survey questions and recommendations, is shown in Handout 1-1. Suggested "talking points" or anticipatory guidance on nutrition, using the history form, are included in Box 1-1.

HOW TO INTEGRATE NUTRITION INTO PEDIATRIC CARE AND WHAT MESSAGES TO SHARE

Convincing evidence shows that overweight and inactivity are increasing among children. These factors are associated with comorbidities that are likely to continue into adulthood (National Diabetes Fact Sheet, 2004). Coronary artery disease is the leading cause of death in the United States. Data show atherosclerosis begins in childhood; therefore healthy lifestyle practices promoting good cardiovascular health must be initiated in childhood (Williams, Hayman, Daniels, et al., 2002).

In a presentation at the American Academy of Pediatrics National Conference and Exhibition in Boston, Massachusetts, on October 20, 2000, Robert Murray, MD, FAAP, director of the Center for Nutrition and Wellness at Columbus Children's Hospital, suggested that the 12 well-child visits provide an ideal opportunity to counsel families about nutrition and impact routine family eating practices (Columbus Children's Hospital, 2002). Imparting nutrition advice and anticipatory guidance at these visits, before problems become severe, is likely to be more effective than waiting to talk about nutrition once eating habits are established.

The well-child nutrition messages suggested in Box 1-2 are culled from Dr. Murray's presentation, peer-reviewed journals, and personal experience. The messages promote the Healthy People 2010 goals, a U.S. Department of Health and Human Services program that challenges individuals and professionals to take specific steps to promote fitness to prevent obesity and health problems, and to achieve wellness. These messages are only a guide; the goal is to encourage positive eating habits and educate parents about unhealthy eating styles **before** they are established and entrenched. Healthy eating habits that encourage a balanced diet, regular meals, and thoughtful snacks should be introduced at well-child visits from birth to age two and reinforced into the adolescent years.

FIVE WAYS TO INTEGRATE NUTRITION INTO YOUR PRACTICE

1. At each physical examination, ask your patients to complete the Nutrition History Form (use Patient Education Handout 1-1), review results, and identify areas to change. Include the history and targeted changes to be reviewed at the next physical examination or revise the existing physical examination form to include specific questions about red meat consumption, saturated fat intake, quantity of fruits and vegetables consumed

BOX 1-1 ■ *Anticipatory Guidance and Nutrition During Primary Care Well Examinations: Suggested Topics to Discuss or Reinforce*

How many meals do you eat on a typical day?

This question can identify irregular eating habits and individuals who skip breakfast, a habit associated with weight gain. The National Weight Control Registry at the University of Colorado Health Sciences in Denver, Colorado includes a registry of 3,000 members who have lost more than 60 pounds and kept it off for more than 5 years. Eating five small meals and never skipping breakfast are two of the most common characteristics of this group of "successful losers" (Wyatt and Jortberg, 2004).

How many meals are eaten away from home?

Generally, meals eaten away from home include more calories. Research shows when children ate at a fast food restaurant they consumed more calories, more sugar, less fiber, and fewer fruits and vegetables when compared with children who did not eat at fast food restaurants (Bowman, Gortmaker, Ebbeling, et al., 2004). Restaurant meals are often higher in sodium and fat. Healthcare providers can encourage "brown bag" lunches or suggest selecting from menus that indicate low fat or heart healthy choices.

How often are whole grains, fruits, and vegetables consumed?

The recommended daily intake of fruits and vegetables is five for children, seven for women, and nine for men. See Handout 2-9 (Fruits and Vegetables) for serving sizes. Fruits and vegetables are rich in phytochemicals, which may explain their protective effect against some forms of cancer. Fruits, vegetables, and whole grains contain soluble fiber—a substance that lowers serum cholesterol and low-density lipoprotein. They also affect homocysteine levels by providing folate and vitamins B_6 and B_{12}, which help to keep homocysteine levels normal. A low homocysteine level is an independent risk factor for mortality (Anderson, Jensen, Carlquist, et al., 2004). In addition to the recommended number of fruits and vegetables for age and gender, individuals should eat most grains and cereals in their whole grain form. See Handout 2-8 for how to choose whole grains.

How often is red meat, poultry, or seafood consumed?

"A general rule of thumb is that patients who consume red meat more than four times per week are least likely to be following a low-fat diet." (Hark, Deen, 1999) Encourage patients to eat skinless poultry, fish, and nonmeat protein sources, including vegetarian burgers and legumes, rather than red meat whenever possible. The 2000 American Heart Association guidelines recommend the consumption of fish at least twice per week (AHA Dietary Guidelines, 2000). The omega-3 fatty acid content in fish is identified as reducing the risk of cardiovascular disease. All protein sources, including red meat, fish, and poultry, should be served grilled, baked, or broiled and limited to a total of 6 ounces per day. Discourage fried food.

How many hours of television are watched and is snacking part of TV viewing?

Television viewing is associated with obesity in children. The American Academy of Pediatrics recommends a limit of 2 hours per day (American Academy of Pediatrics, 2003–2004).

Is calcium intake adequate?

Children require two to four servings of calcium-rich food daily to meet their needs; adults require three to four servings. Good calcium sources include low-fat or nonfat dairy products that provide 30% calcium per serving and nondairy foods, such as green leafy vegetables, almonds, and soy milk. See Handout 6-5 for a list of calcium-rich foods.

How often do you eat desserts and on what do you snack?

Encourage patients to read calorie content on prepared foods; caution them about the use of diet or low-fat products that may be consumed in excess because of their perceived low calorie status. Encourage them to choose fruit, vegetables, and low fat calcium foods for desserts and snacks.

(continued)

BOX 1-1 ■ *Continued*

What beverages do you drink on most days?

Sweetened drinks, including juice drinks, soda, or ice tea, can provide hundreds of calories. Real fruit juice, although nutritious, has the same calorie content as soda and, in most cases, should be limited to one 6 ounce serving per day (encourage consumption of whole fruit—fresh, canned, or frozen—as the optimal way to consume fruit) without sacrificing nutrition.

Alcoholic beverages can be a significant source of calories (see Handout 2-14 for the calorie content in alcoholic beverages). The current recommendation for moderate alcohol consumption is one drink per day for women and two for men.

BOX 1-2 ■ *Nutrition Talking Points at Well-Child Visits: Anticipatory Guidance and Nutrition*

Newborn or First Visit

- Support a mother's decision to breastfeed (breastfeeding is associated with obesity prevention [Agras, 1990 and Gilman, 2001]).
- Recommend iron-based formula (if the infant is formula fed).
- Discuss hunger and satiety cues.
- Encourage baby to self-regulate feeding.
- Discuss expected volumes of intake per feed per day.
- Discourage solids; nothing in bottle.

Age 1 to 2 Months

- Discuss expected amounts per feeding and per day.
- Avoid juices and solids.

Age 4 Months

- Discuss indicators for the addition of solid foods.
- Start with a single grain, iron-fortified cereal (if solids are introduced).
- Serve cereal with a spoon; never in a bottle.
- Water is ok; minimize juice consumption.
- Encourage juice from a cup (when offered), not in a bottle.

Age 6 Months

- Discuss when to expand the list of foods and what to offer.
- Avoid combo dinners that are high in starch and desserts.
- Encourage variety. Introducing a variety of flavors in the first two years can lead to a better acceptance of new and more varied foods (Butte et al., 2004).
- Inform parents it takes five to ten exposures to establish familiarity with a new food (Birch, 1998) and do not assume a child is a picky eater or does not like a food after one refusal. Try, try again!
- Inform parents that parental eating influences a child's choices.
- Encourage parents to eat with child, including all food groups.

Age 9 Months

- Introduce finger foods and table foods.
- Avoid unsafe textures (hard, round foods can promote choking).

BOX 1-2 ■ *Continued*

- Transition child toward cup.
- Avoid soda, Kool-aid, fruit drinks, and sweetened tea. Explain that the purpose of a beverage is to quench thirst or provide nutrients.
- Do not control food portions; control type of food served, including when and where food is eaten.
- Reassure parents it is not their responsibility to make their child eat; it is to offer good food in a secure comfortable manner. The child is to decide what and how much is to be eaten. The parent who is over-controlling in the area of food may teach a child self-doubt; children who are trusted learn responsibility and increase their self-esteem (Satter, 1996).
- The too strict parent can create a preference for the food being controlled.

Age 12 Months

- Introduce the parents to label reading. Sodium intake can increase when children move to table food.
- Wean child to regular milk—whole not skim milk.
- Avoid sweetened drinks; encourage consumption of water.
- Emphasize consumption of fruits and vegetables. Suggested serving size is 1 to 3 tablespoons for each year of life.
- Continue to try new foods (reinforce the need to offer a new food five to ten times).
- Provide a list of healthful, age-appropriate snacks.
- Encourage the patient to eat at least one whole grain food, such as whole wheat bread, brown rice, whole wheat pasta, or whole grain cereal, such as oatmeal, per day.
- Have a Nutrition Facts Label posted in your office for a quick reference.

Age 15 to 18 Months

- Discourage bottle; continue with whole milk in a cup.
- Reinforce a predictable meal pattern, including three meals, plus healthy snacks.
- Discourage "highly advertised" food; review a list of appropriate snacks.
- Encourage variety, (remember the need to offer new foods five to ten times).
- Adults set the example of healthy eating patterns. Eat in one location and discourage TV watching during meals.
- Meals are social time; children who eat with their families tend to have a better vocabulary and better social skills and, when older, are less likely to be involved in high risk behavior than their peers who do not eat with the family.
- Make dessert a part of the family meals.
- Try the "Rule of One" to reduce food struggles. If children are clamoring for junk food, suggest parents allow one serving a day of a food that is fun but not very nutritious (candy, desserts, soda, or novelty foods). That is one per day, not one per meal.
- Discuss control issues. Review with parents their responsibility to offer wholesome food in a predictable, secure setting, not to control how much of good, wholesome food their child eats. Young children have an innate ability to determine what they need (Rolls et al.,2000). Parents who serve too much food or make a child "clean the plate" may teach their child to overeat.
- Discourage using "good" and "bad" labels for food.
- Do not control food; instead, offer good food at predictable times (three meals and snacks).
- Help parents choose wholesome snacks; review a written list. General rule of thumb: snack foods that are highly advertised tend to be less nutritious and often over consumed.
- Encourage supper as the last eating event of the day.
- Encourage active play daily. For more active 5 and 15-year-olds, it is necessary to encourage active play at this young age.

(continued)

BOX 1-2 ■ *Continued*

Age 2 Years

- Switch from whole to 2% milk.
- Limit TV; no TV in bedroom (introduce this message early before it is a problem). TV watching encourages isolation and is linked with being overweight (American Academy of Pediatrics, 2001).
- Review juice choices; encourage orange, pineapple, grapefruit, and apple juice with vitamin C. The American Academy of Pediatrics suggests only 2 to 6 ounces of juice daily.
- Encourage parents to control the quality, not portions, of food.
- Offer five servings of fruits and vegetables daily; 1 to 3 tablespoons per year of life is a suggested portion at this age.
- Review label reading with parents. Post a label for easy reference.

Age 3 to 4 Years

- Encourage regular meals. Family meals develop vocabulary.
- Avoid TV at meals; limit TV at other times.
- Encourage parents to avoid critiquing eating habits or being the "food police" at mealtimes. Save discussions about healthy eating for later when they will be more effective and not ruin the family meal.
- Encourage all family members to eat in one location (preferably dining table).
- Do not use food as the exclusive response or reward for good behavior or accomplishment. Encourage non–food-related activity such as crafts, reading, or a walk.
- Review list of appropriate snacks.
- Continue offering five fruits and vegetables each day.
- Review the "Rule of One" as a solution to foods over which parents and child struggle.
- Relocate the bathroom scale to an out-of-the-way location now. Many young children are on diets because they see and hear their mothers are on a "diet" (Schreiber, 1996).
- Review the use of food labels.
- Reinforce regular mealtimes; eat in one location and avoid TV at meals.
- Limit TV to 2 hours or less per day.
- Limit novelty foods (foods that are highly advertised and low in nutrient density). Suggest a child select only one package per week and make it last the week or keep the Rule of One in place.
- Offer five fruits and vegetables daily; serve them as snack foods when not consumed as part of meals.
- Create the opportunity for physical activity everyday.

Age 5 Years

- Review the need for a nutritious breakfast.
- Discuss school lunch and school snacks.
- Encourage a good calcium choice at most meals.
- Fruits and vegetables are to be consumed daily.
- Review healthy snacks.
- Limit soft drinks and fruit drinks.
- Encourage daily physical activity: Limit "screens." (TV, computers, video games).

daily, and whether whole grain foods and adequate calcium are part of the family diet. Ask about snack and beverage choices.

2. At well-child visits, provide parents with a copy of *Healthy Eating Habits for Infants, Toddlers, and Young Children* (Patient Education Handout 1-2); discuss and suggest appropriate changes for the child and family.

3. Post a Nutrition Facts Label in each examination room (see Patient Education Handout 1-3 for a copy). It will be useful in answering questions on the *Nutrition History Form* (Patient Education Handout 1-1). Point out the Daily Values for saturated fat and fiber at the bottom of the label. Check to see if patients understand how to read serving size and servings per con-

tainer. Encourage them to choose foods with a low percentage of saturated fat and sodium and a high percentage of fiber, vitamins A and C, calcium, and iron.

4. Post a Food Guide Pyramid in each examination room. Use Patient Education Handouts 2-1 through 2-5. Encourage the recommended intake of fruits, vegetables, and whole grains.

5. Develop a nutrition library and be familiar with nutrition referral resources that you can recommend to your patients, when needed. Refer to Patient Education Handout 5-23 (Recommended Resources: Cookbooks, Newsletters and Web Pages). To find a local dietitian, contact the American Dietetics Association at www.eatright.org.

PATIENT EDUCATION HANDOUTS: TOOLS TO INTEGRATE NUTRITION EDUCATION INTO YOUR PRACTICE

1-1	Nutrition History Form
1-2	Healthy Eating for Infants, Toddlers, and Young Children
1-3	Nutrition Facts Panel (Nutrition Label)

Name_____

_____

Date_____

DOB_____

Please answer the questions below.

1. How many pieces of fruit or glasses of juice do you drink or eat on most days? _____

2. How many servings of vegetables do you eat on most days? _____

3. How often do you eat whole grain foods such as whole grain breakfast cereal (shredded wheat, oatmeal), whole grain bread, whole grain pasta, brown rice, or other whole grain food? _____

4. How many times do you eat red meat (beef, lamb, veal) or pork in a week? _____

5. How many times do you eat chicken or turkey in a week? _____

6. How many times do you eat fish or shellfish in a week? _____

7. How many hours of television do you watch most days? _____

8. What do you snack on while you watch TV? _____

9. Do you read food labels? _____

10. Do you know how many grams of saturated fat you should eat in a day? _____

11. Do you know how many grams of fiber you should eat in a day? _____

12. How many calories do you think you need each day? _____

13. What type of beverage do you drink each day and how much?

Water ____	Milk (what type?)____
Juice ____	Beer ____
Soda ____	Wine ____
Diet soda ____	Hard liquor ____
Sports drink ____	Iced tea ____

NUTRITION HISTORY FORM ANSWERS

1. Suggested number of fruits you should try to eat each day:

Children[1]	2 or more servings of fruit
Women	3 or more servings of fruit
Men	4 or more servings of fruit

2. Suggested number of vegetables you should try to eat each day:

Children[1]	3 or more servings
Women	4 or more servings
Men	5 or more servings

3. Whole grain foods include brown rice, oatmeal, barley, and any cereal or bread made with whole wheat. Try to include some every day.

4, 5, 6. According to the *American Family Physician Journal* (1999), people consuming red meat more than four times per week are least likely to be eating a low fat diet. The white meat of turkey and chicken

_____

[1]A serving for young children is 1–3 tablespoons for each year of age. A serving for adults is ½ to 1 cup.

should be substituted for red meat whenever possible and skin should be removed before eating. Eating fish at least once per week is associated with a decrease in heart disease.

7, 8. Snacking while watching TV and watching more than 2 hours of TV per day can contribute to obesity. Aim to accumulate 30 minutes (adults) or 60 minutes (children) of moderate physical activity most days of the week, preferably daily. An example of moderate activity is walking 2 miles in 30 minutes.

9, 10, 11. Information on saturated fat and fiber can be found on the bottom of most food labels. Most American need less than 20 to 25 grams of saturated fat and more than 25 to 35 grams of fiber. Children need 5 grams of fiber plus 1 gram for each year of life.

12. Depending on age and activity, calorie needs can range from 1,600 to 2,800 for most Americans.

13. Regular soda, sweetened ice tea, juices, whole milk, and alcohol contain significant calories; choose beverages wisely.

Healthy Eating Habits for Infants, Toddlers, and Young Children

ENCOURAGE A WIDE VARIETY OF FOODS

It takes 5 to 10 tries before a child becomes familiar with a new food. Do not assume your child does not like a food because he/she refused it once. Offer it again until it becomes familiar to the child.

Serve lots of differently colored foods and offer five servings of fruit and vegetables every day. A serving size is 1 to 3 tablespoons for each year of age. Let your child see you eating fruits and vegetables, too!

CHOOSE JUICE CAREFULLY

Most children do not need juice for good nutrition. Fruit (pureed, cut up, whole, or cooked) has more fiber, is more filling, and makes a great snack or dessert. When juice is served, use a cup, not a bottle. Six ounces of 100% fruit juice is enough juice for most children to drink in a day.

To quench thirst, offer water or water flavored with a very small amount of juice.

AVOID HIGHLY ADVERTISED SNACKS

The best snacks are simple ones, including cut-up fruit, vegetable slices, simple crackers, and plain cookies (graham crackers and animal crackers). Protect your child from highly advertised snacks (fruit roll-ups, cereal bars, yogurt-covered candies, sweetened cereal, snack cakes, fruit drinks, and soda). The clever packaging and high salt or sugar content can be irresistible to children, leading to overeating.

TRY THE "RULE OF ONE"

Parents often wonder how often they should serve dessert or "junk food." No child needs these foods but eliminating them completely may make a child crave them more. One solution is the "rule of one": allow one dessert (cake, cookie, pie), one novelty food (foods that are fun but not so nutritious, such as neon-colored gelatin), or one serving of fries or chips per day. Use this rule, starting at 15 to 18 months of age.

The child served three balanced meals and snacks (aim for five fruits and vegetables in those meals and snacks) will learn there is room for everything in moderation.

LIMIT TELEVISION

Children with a TV in their room report being less happy and less active, and are more likely to be overweight than children who do not have a TV in their bedroom. Eating family meals or snacks while watching TV often leads to overeating and less nutritious food choices. Children who eat meals while watching TV miss out on vocabulary-building conversations that should occur at mealtime.

SCHEDULE FAMILY MEALTIME

Do not underestimate the power of the family meal. Children who eat family meals do better in school, have a better diet and, when older, are less likely to engage in high-risk behavior. At age 15 to 18 months, a child should be on a three-meal-per-day schedule, with appropriate snacks. Serve most meals in the same location, such as at the dining table.

BE ACTIVE TOGETHER

Infants and young children do not need structured exercise; they just need the opportunity to move often. Examples include playing with push and pull toys, animals on wheels, or simple cars, or playing clapping games, tossing bean bags, or rolling a ball. Get in the habit of a daily walk, with your child in a backpack or stroller. When older, your child will need 60 minutes of active play to become stronger. Adults need 30 minutes of activity to keep healthy. Make daily activity a goal for the whole family.

Sample Label for Macaroni and Cheese

Nutrition Facts Panel
(Nutrition Label)

Nutrition Facts

Start Here

Serving Size 1 cup (228g)
Servings Per Container 2

Amount Per Serving

Calories 250   Calories from Fat 110

% Daily Value*

Limit These
Nutrients

	% Daily Value*
Total Fat 12g	18%
Saturated Fat 3g	15%
Trans Fat 1.5g	
Cholesterol 30mg	10%
Sodium 470mg	20%
Total Carbohydrate 31g	10%
Dietary Fiber 0g	0%
Sugars 5g	
Protein 5g	

Quick Guide
to % DV:

5% or less
is low;
20% or more
is high

Get Enough
of These
Nutrients

Vitamin A	4%
Vitamin C	2%
Calcium	20%
Iron	4%

Footnote

* Percent Daily Values are based on a 2,000 calorie diet.
Your Daily Values may be higher or lower depending on
your calorie needs.

	Calories:	2,000	2,500
Total Fat	Less than	65g	80g
Sat Fat	Less than	20g	25g
Cholesterol	Less than	300mg	300mg
Sodium	Less than	2,400mg	2,400mg
Total Carbohydrate		300g	375g
Dietary Fiber		25g	30g

REFERENCES

Agras, S. W. (1990). Influence of early feeding style on adiposity at 6 years of age. *Journal of Pediatrics, 116*(5), 805–809.

American Hospital Association. (2000). Scientific statement AHA Dietary Guidelines: Revision 2000: a statement for healthcare professionals from the Nutrition Committee of the American Heart Association, 2000. *Circulation, 102*(18), 2284–2299.

American Academy of Pediatrics. (2001). Committee on Public Education. Children, Adolescents, and Television. *Pediatrics, 107*(2), 423–426.

American Academy of Pediatrics. (2003). Committee on Nutrition, Policy Statement Prevention of Pediatric Overweight and Obesity, 2003. *Pediatrics, 112*(2), 424–430.

American Academy of Pediatrics. (2003–2004). Committee on Nutrition. *Pediatric Nutrition Handbook* (5th ed.) (p. 579). American Academy of Pediatrics Elkgrove Village, IL.

Anderson, J. L., Jensen, K. R., Carlquist, J. F., Bair T. L., Horne, B. D., & Muhlestein, J. B. 2004. Effect of folic acid fortification on homocysteine-related mortality. *American Journal of Medicine, 116*,(3), 158–164.

Birch, L. (1998). Development of eating behaviors among children and adolescents. *Pediatrics, 101*(3 pt 2), 539–549.

Bowman, S. A., Gortmaker, S. L., Ebbeling, C. A., Pereira, M. A., & Ludwig, D. S. (2004). Effects of fast-food consumption on energy intake and diet quality in a national household survey. *Pediatrics, 113*(1), 112–118.

Butte, N., Cobb, K., Dwyer, J., Graney, L., Heird, W., & Rickard, K. (2004). The start healthy feeding guidelines for infants and toddlers. *Journal of the American Dietetic Association, 104*(3), 442–454.

Cook, D. (2002) Coverage of obesity problematic for most health plans. *Managed Care , 11*(7), 41–44, 46.

Center for Science in the Public Interest. (2000). CSPI Year 2000 Report. Center for Science in the Public Interest. Washington, DC: Author.

Columbus Children's Hospital (2002). Childhood obesity expert recommends simple intraventions. Retrieved October 27, 2002 from http://www.newswise.com/articles/2002/10/OBESITY. COH.html

Finkelstein, E. 2003. National medical spending attributable to overweight and obesity: How much, and who's paying. *Health Affairs*, Web exclusive. Retrieved on May 15, 2005 from www.healthaffairs.org.

Gilman, M. W. (2001). Risk of overweight among adolescents who were breastfed as infants. (2001). *Journal American Medical Association, 285*(19), 2461–2467.

Galuska, D. (1999). Are health care professionals advising obese patients to lose weight? *Journal of the American Medical Association, 282*(16), 1576–1578.

Hark, L., & Deen, D. (1999). Taking a nutrition history: A practical approach for family physicians. *American Family Physician, 59*(6), 1521–1528.

Information on Sudden Death Syndrome: What is SIDS? http://www.angelfire.com/tx2/angelbecca/sidsinformation.html. Accessed February 12, 2003.

National Diabetes Fact Sheet. (2004). www.diabetes.org/diabetes-statistics/national-diabetes-fact-sheet.jsp. Accessed December 1, 2003.

Nawaz, H., Adams, M. L., & Katz, D. (2000). Physician-patient interactions regarding diet, exercise and smoking. *Preventive Medicine, 31*(6), 652–657.

Rolls, B. J., Engell, D., & Birch, L. (2000). Serving portion size influences 5-year-old but not 3-year-old children's food intakes. *Journal American Dietetic Association, 100*(2), 232–234.

Satter, E. M. (1996). Internal regulation and the evolution of normal growth as the basis for prevention of obesity in children. *Journal American Dietetic Association, 96*(9), 860–864.

Schreiber, G. B. (1996). Weight modification efforts reported by Black and White preadolescent girls: National Heart, Lung, and Blood Institute Growth and Health Study. *Pediatrics, 98*(1), 63–70.

US DHHS Public Health Service, Office of the Surgeon General. 2001. *The Surgeon General's call to action to prevent and decrease overweight and obesity*. Retrieved May 15, 2005 from www.surgeongeneral.gov/library.

Wyatt, H., & Jortberg, B. (2004). National weight control registry. www.uchsc.edu/nutrition/WyattJortberg/nwcr.htm. Accessed August 27, 2004.

Williams, C. L., Hayman, L. L., Daniels, S. R., Robinson, T. N., Steinberger, J., Paridon, S., et al. (2002). American Heart Association Scientific Statement Cardiovascular Health in Childhood. *Circulation, 106*(1), 143–160.

Guiding Patients Toward a Healthy Diet

Individuals eating a diet rich in foods that prevent disease are the exception and not the rule in most medical practices. The United States Department of Agriculture's (USDA) Economic Research Services report (Putnam, Kantor, & Allshouse, 2004) on American food trends for the year 2000 found the average American diet to be high in fat and sugar and low in fruit and dairy products (Putnam, Kantor, and Allshouse, 2004). Americans underconsume fruit, dark green vegetables, and deep yellow vegetables, and do not eat the recommended amounts of fish, dry beans, nuts, or low-fat dairy products. Cheese accounted for two-fifths of total dairy servings, and more than half the dairy servings in 1999 came from cheese or whole milk (foods naturally high in fat). When consumers do eat vegetables, they choose from a very limited selection; iceberg lettuce, frozen potatoes, fresh potatoes, potato chips, and canned tomatoes account for 52% of all vegetable servings, despite the evidence that more colorful produce can protect against disease. For example, the American Cancer Society states that 35% of cancer deaths could be avoided by altering the typical American diet to include more fruits and vegetables, less animal fat and meat, and reduced total calories (Ressel, 2002). Americans eat plenty of refined breads and cereals, and commercially prepared baked goods, but not enough of the whole grain choices known to reduce disease.

The state of the current American diet provides even more reasons for health care providers to integrate nutrition questions or nutrition histories into well examinations. Inclusion of nutrition in such examinations will inevitably lead patients to ask their own questions about nutrition and diet. This section offers practical patient education tools about food and cooking. It includes a discussion of the controversy surrounding the USDA Food Guide Pyramid, the government's most recognizable nutrition education tool.

DEFINING A HEALTHFUL DIET FOR PATIENTS

Clearly, a link exists between diet and disease prevention, but what specific, accurate and effective guidance should be given to patients? More than a decade ago, the USDA developed a tool to help answer the question: What is a healthy diet? That tool is the Food Guide Pyramid (USDA, 1993), a symbol used today in schools, nutrition brochures, food labels, and various media. However, it has just been revised in part because of criticism for its bias in promoting American agriculture (the meat, dairy, and grain industries) more than health.

On April 28, 1992, U.S. Secretary of Agriculture Edward Madigan introduced the Food Guide Pyramid at a widely-covered press conference. Designed to replace the Four Food Groups, it was to communicate through graphics (and some text) the Dietary Guidelines for Americans, which in 1990 included the following:

- Eat a variety of foods.
- Maintain a healthy weight.
- Choose a diet low in fat, saturated fat, and cholesterol.
- Choose a diet with plenty of vegetables, fruits, and grain products.
- Use sugars only in moderation.
- Use salt and sodium only in moderation.
- If you drink alcoholic beverages, do so in moderation.

Although these seven dietary guidelines imparted reasonable advice, critics felt the message from the graphic was misleading. The USDA Food Guide Pyramid (Figure 2-1) places bread, cereal, rice, and pasta at the base of the pyramid. The pyramid does not emphasize the health benefits of whole grain (brown rice, whole wheat bread, and whole wheat pasta) products over refined or processed foods (white rice, white bread, and white pasta) and it ignores the effect these foods can have on blood sugar and weight.

The goal for fruits and vegetables is set at five a day, an amount critics cite as a goal for children, but a target of seven servings daily for women and nine for men is thought to be more beneficial. Potatoes are included in the pyramid's vegetable group, but, unlike their more colorful cousins—carrots, beets, and green beans—they do not carry the nutrients that are likely to reduce the risk of heart disease and stroke. Research also suggests that potatoes should not be an everyday vegetable choice for Americans because of their undesirable effect on blood sugar levels.

In the calcium group, nondairy calcium sources (broccoli, spinach, tofu, and fortified foods) are not included, and the harmful saturated fat content of full-fat dairy food (whole milk and cheese) is not identified.

In the protein group, meat, poultry, fish, dry beans, eggs, and nuts are grouped together without distinguishing those high in saturated fat (beef, bacon, and bologna) from the heart-healthy protein choices (fish, nuts, and dry beans).

The greatest criticism probably comes from labeling all fats as bad. Butter is in the same group as olive oil, but butter has saturated fat that contributes to heart disease, whereas olive oil, a heart-healthy unsaturated fat, may help prevent heart disease. Critics say that placing all fats in the same "use sparingly" group led to the wave of no-fat foods produced in the 1990s that replaced fat with sugar and probably fueled the obesity epidemic we have today.

In addition to the USDA Food Guide Pyramid, there are many other food guide pyramids. Two groups with respected food pyramid alternatives include the Harvard School of Public Health's Healthy Eating Pyramid and the Oldways Preservation and Exchange Trust of Cambridge, Massachusetts' Mediterranean, Asian, Latin American, and Vegetarian Diet Pyramids. Oldways is a nonprofit "food issues think tank" with the goal of translating complex nutrition science into consumer-friendly tools for consumers, health professionals, and the food industry. The Oldways food pyramids are particularly useful because they represent cultural eating patterns. (Copies of the Mediterranean, Asian, Latin American and Vegetarian Food Pyramids are found in Patient Education Handouts 2-2, 2-3, 2-4, and 2-5, or at their Web site www.oldwayspt.org.)

The New Food Pyramid

The United States Department of Agriculture has released the MyPyramid food guidance system. Along with the new pyramid symbol, the system provides many options to help Americans make healthy food choices and to be active every day. Patients can be referred to the USDA web page and learn what and how much an individual can eat for health. The amounts are

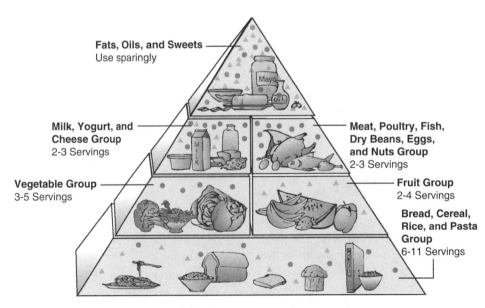

Fats, Oils, and Sweets
Use sparingly

Milk, Yogurt, and Cheese Group
2-3 Servings

Meat, Poultry, Fish, Dry Beans, Eggs, and Nuts Group
2-3 Servings

Vegetable Group
3-5 Servings

Fruit Group
2-4 Servings

Bread, Cereal, Rice, and Pasta Group
6-11 Servings

Figure 2-1 Redrawn from USDA Food Guide Pyramid. Source: www.usda.gov/cnpp.

BOX 2-1 ■ *The Harvard School of Public Health's (HSPH) Healthy Eating Pyramid*

- Daily exercise and weight control should be the foundation of health and food recommendations.
- Whole grain choices, such as oatmeal, whole-wheat bread, and brown rice are to be encouraged over refined flour products. These foods carry unique nutrients and may help control blood sugar and hunger.
- Instead of limiting all fat, plant oils, including olive, canola, soy, corn, sunflower, peanut, and other vegetable oils, are to be encouraged.
- Vegetables are to be consumed "in abundance" and 2 to 3 servings of fruit are advised daily.
- Fish, poultry, and eggs (0 to 2 times per day) are encouraged as protein sources. Fish can reduce the risk of heart disease; chicken and turkey are low in saturated fat. Eggs, although rich in cholesterol, are not very high in saturated fat and are not associated with an increased risk for heart disease as was once thought.
- Nuts and legumes (1 to 3 times per day) are recommended. These foods are rich sources of protein, fiber, vitamins, and minerals and may protect against heart disease.
- Dairy (1 to 2 servings daily) or a calcium supplement is to be included to meet calcium needs.
- Red meat and butter are to be used "sparingly" because of their high saturated fat content.
- White rice, white bread, potatoes, pasta, and sweets are to be used "sparingly." These foods raise blood sugar, and contribute weight gain, diabetes, and heart disease. Their whole grain counterparts are preferred.
- Multiple vitamins: A daily multivitamin, multimineral supplement is encouraged for "nutritional back-up."
- Alcohol (in moderation) unless contraindicated

Source: Willett, W. & Stampfer, M. (2003). The Harvard School of Public Health's alternative to the USDA Food Pyramid called the "Healthy Eating Pyramid" can be accessed at http://www.hsph.harvard.edu/nutritionsource/.

based on person's sex, age, and activity level. The new graphic can be found in Patient Education Handout 2-1 and at the USDA website (www.mypyramid.gov).

No matter what food pyramid or future USDA graphic becomes available, the important food messages remain the same: eat enough fruits and vegetables, eat more unprocessed carbohydrate foods (whole grains), and eat less saturated fats (red meat and butter). Questions about weight control, exercise, whole grains, and what counts as a serving of fruit and vegetable are likely to be common questions from patients. The USDA has provided good direction on these subjects in its publication *Nutrition and Your Health: Dietary Guidelines for Americans, 2000* (USDA, 2000). These guidelines can serve as a good resource and are available as Patient Education Handouts 2-6 through 2-15. Government information is particularly useful when working with individuals who learn best with simple, basic messages. More in-depth information on these topics as they relate to medical conditions and therapeutic nutrition can be found in Sections Three through Six. The most recent Dietary Guidelines can be found at www.health.gov/dietaryguidelines/dga 2005/document/

Questions About the Safety of Fish

Many nutrition education tools promote fish as a healthy alternative to red meat. Patients will ask about the health risks from mercury and other pollutants in fish. Read more about this in Section Five, Handout 5-4.

Many patients will ask for very practical guidance in the area of nutrition, which means answering the question: "What do I cook?" To answer the challenge of implementing a healthy diet, the USDA, Center for Nutrition Policy and Promotion (CNPP) and Food, and Nutrition and Consumer Services created *Recipes and Tips for Healthy, Thrifty Meals* (USDA, CNPP, 2000). This booklet can be accessed at their Web site (http://www.usda.gov/cnpp/Pubs/Cookbook/thriftym .pdf.)

This publication includes shopping lists, menus, and 40 recipes, 23 of which are included in the patient education handouts. Use these handouts to educate individuals about increasing their consumption of fruits, vegetables, and whole grains, and to introduce them to methods of food preparation that are healthful. Handout 2-39, *Cooking with Flaxseed*, and Handout 2-40,

Cooking with Whole Grains, can answer patients' questions about these foods, which are often promoted for their nutritional benefits.

PATIENT EDUCATION HANDOUTS

Use the patient education handouts that follow to effectively answer your patient's questions about salt, sugar, fat, fruits and vegetables, calcium choices, and more. If your patient has in-depth questions about nutrition, a referral to a registered dietitian is to be encouraged.

The handouts are as follows:

2-1	USDA MyPyramid Food Guide
2-2	Traditional Healthy Mediterranean Diet Pyramid
2-3	Traditional Healthy Latin American Diet Pyramid
2-4	Traditional Healthy Vegetarian Diet Pyramid
2-5	Traditional Healthy Asian Diet Pyramid
2-6	Healthy Weight
2-7	Exercise
2-8	Whole Grains
2-9	Fruits and Vegetables
2-10	Fat and Cholesterol
2-11	Sugar
2-12	Calcium and Iron
2-13	Salt
2-14	Alcohol
2-15	Keep Food Safe to Eat
2-16	Baked Meatballs
2-17	Southwestern Salad
2-18	Stir-fried Pork and Vegetables with Rice
2-19	Baked Spicy Fish
2-20	Spanish Baked Fish
2-21	Tuna Pasta Salad
2-22	Baked Chicken Nuggets
2-23	Chicken and Vegetables
2-24	Oven Crispy Chicken
2-25	Turkey-Cabbage Casserole
2-26	Turkey Chili
2-27	Turkey Stir-fry
2-28	Turkey Patties
2-29	Chicken Noodle Soup
2-30	Baked Beans
2-31	Baked Crispy Potatoes
2-32	Potato Cakes
2-33	Ranch Beans
2-34	Shoestring Potatoes
2-35	Chickpea Dip
2-36	Oatmeal Cookies
2-37	Peach-apple Crisp
2-38	Peach Cake
2-39	Cooking with Flaxseed
2-40	Cooking with Whole Grains

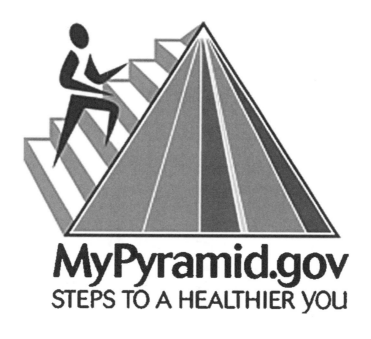

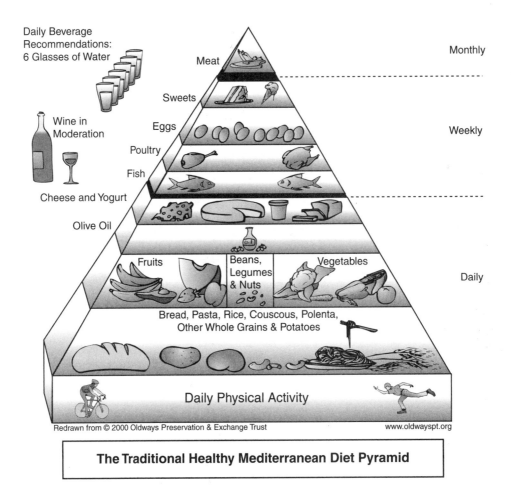

Daily Beverage Recommendations: 6 Glasses of Water

Meat — Monthly

Wine in Moderation

Sweets

Eggs — Weekly

Poultry

Fish

Cheese and Yogurt

Olive Oil

Fruits — Beans, Legumes & Nuts — Vegetables — Daily

Bread, Pasta, Rice, Couscous, Polenta, Other Whole Grains & Potatoes

Daily Physical Activity

Redrawn from © 2000 Oldways Preservation & Exchange Trust   www.oldwayspt.org

The Traditional Healthy Mediterranean Diet Pyramid

The Traditional Healthy Latin American Diet Pyramid

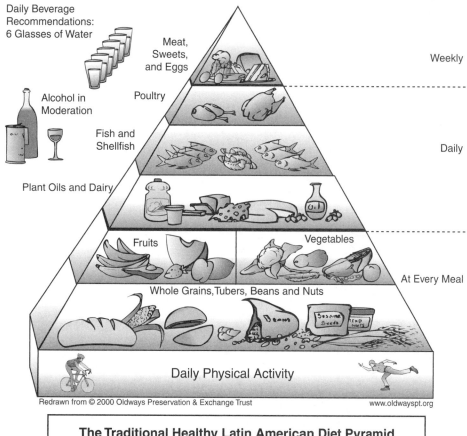

Daily Beverage Recommendations: 6 Glasses of Water

Meat, Sweets, and Eggs

Weekly

Alcohol in Moderation

Poultry

Fish and Shellfish

Daily

Plant Oils and Dairy

Fruits

Vegetables

At Every Meal

Whole Grains, Tubers, Beans and Nuts

Daily Physical Activity

Redrawn from © 2000 Oldways Preservation & Exchange Trust

www.oldwayspt.org

The Traditional Healthy Latin American Diet Pyramid

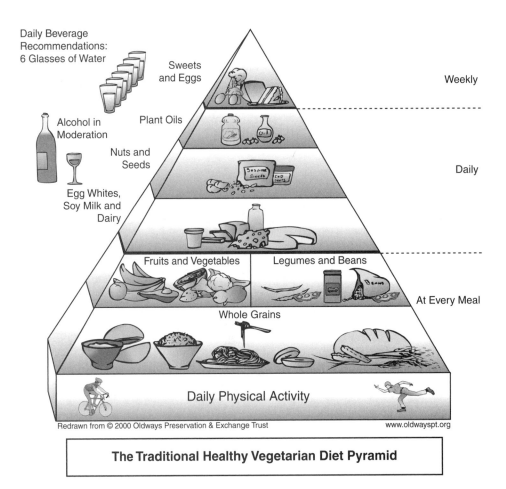

Daily Beverage Recommendations: 6 Glasses of Water

Sweets and Eggs

Weekly

Alcohol in Moderation

Plant Oils

Nuts and Seeds

Daily

Egg Whites, Soy Milk and Dairy

Fruits and Vegetables

Legumes and Beans

At Every Meal

Whole Grains

Daily Physical Activity

Redrawn from © 2000 Oldways Preservation & Exchange Trust

www.oldwayspt.org

The Traditional Healthy Vegetarian Diet Pyramid

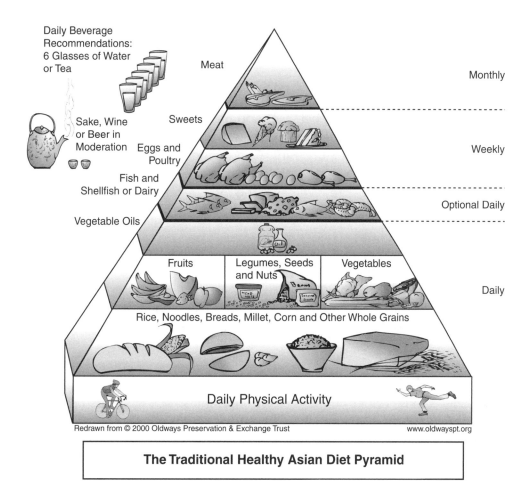

The Traditional Healthy Asian Diet Pyramid

Our genes affect our tendency to gain weight, but plentiful food and labor-saving devices can make it very difficult to avoid weight gain. It is possible to manage your weight through smart food and activity choices.

FOR PERMANENT WEIGHT CONTROL

Make long-term changes in your eating behavior and physical activity. To do this, choose a healthful assortment of foods that includes vegetables, fruits, grains (especially whole grains), skim milk, and fish, lean meat, poultry, or beans. Choose foods that are low in fat and added sugars most of the time. Eating mainly vegetables, fruits, and grains helps you feel full, achieve good health, and manage your weight. Whatever the food, eat a sensible portion size.

Activity Counts

Try to be more active throughout the day. To maintain a healthy weight after weight loss, it helps for adults to do at least 45 minutes of moderate physical activity daily (at least 60 minutes daily for children). Over time, even a small decrease in calories eaten and a small increase in physical activity can keep you from gaining weight or help you lose weight.

Choose Healthy Foods

High-fat foods contain more calories than the same amount of other foods, so they can make it difficult for you to avoid excess calories. However *low-fat* does not always mean low calorie. Sometimes extra sugars are added to low-fat muffins or desserts, for example, and they may be very high in calories. Be aware of the calorie content in low-fat and "diet" foods.

When and Where Do You Eat?

Your pattern of eating may be important. Snacks and meals eaten away from home provide a large part of daily calories for many people. Choose them wisely. Try fruits, vegetables, whole grain foods, or a cup of low-fat milk or yogurt for a snack. When eating out, choose small portions of foods. If you choose fish, poultry, or lean meat, ask that it be grilled rather than fried.

A Healthy Weight at Every Age

Like younger adults, overweight and obese older adults can improve their health by losing weight. The guidance of a health professional is recommended for obese children and older adults. Since older people tend to lose muscle and replace it with fat, regular weight-bearing physical activity is a valuable part of a weight-loss plan. Building or maintaining muscle helps keep older adults active and reduces their risk of falls and fractures. Staying active throughout your adult years helps maintain muscle mass and bone strength for your later years.

Lose Weight Gradually

If you are overweight, a loss of 5 to 15% of your body weight is likely to improve your health, ability to function, and quality of life. Aim to lose about 10% of your weight over 6 months. This would be 20 pounds of weight loss for someone who weighs 200 pounds. Loss of ½ to 2 pounds per week is usually safe. Even if you have regained weight in the past, it is worthwhile to try again. Your health is more likely to improve over the long term if you achieve and maintain a healthy weight rather than lose and regain many times. Staying at a healthy weight requires healthy eating habits and physical activity as a regular part of your life.

Encourage Healthy Weight in Children

Children need enough food for proper growth, but too many calories and too little physical activity lead to obesity. The number of overweight U.S. children has risen dramatically in recent years. Encourage healthy weight by offering children whole grain products, vegetables and fruits, low-fat dairy products, fish, or nuts—and let them see you enjoying the same foods. Let the child decide how much of these foods to eat. Offer only small amounts of foods high in fat or sugars. Encourage children to take part in vigorous activities (and join them whenever possible). Limit the time they spend in sedentary activities like watching television or playing computer or video games.

Take care when helping overweight children to develop healthy eating habits. Make small changes. For example, serve low-fat milk rather than whole milk and offer one cookie instead of two. Since children still need to grow, weight loss is not recommended unless guided by a healthcare professional.

Serious Eating Disorders

Frequent binge eating, with or without periods of food restriction, may be a sign of a serious eating disorder. Other sign of eating disorders include preoccupation with body weight or food (or both), regardless of body weight; dramatic weight loss, excessive exercise, self-induced vomiting, and the abuse of laxatives. Seek help from a healthcare professional if any of these apply to you, a family member, or a friend.

ADVICE FOR TODAY

- If you are at a healthy weight, aim to avoid weight gain. If you are overweight, first aim to prevent further weight gain, then lose weight to improve health.
- Build a healthy diet by eating vegetables, fruits, and grains (especially whole grains). If you eat these foods with little added fat or sugar, they will help you feel comfortably full without a lot of calories. Select sensible portion sizes.
- In addition, get moving. That is, make sure you get regular physical activity.

- Set a good example for children by practicing healthy eating habits and enjoying regular physical activities together.
- Keep in mind, that even though heredity and the environment are important influences, your behaviors help to determine body weight.

Where Can I Get More Information?

The American Dietetic Association: www.eatright.org. To find a registered dietitian in your area, click Find a Nutrition Professional.

This report was reprinted from the "Report of the Dietary Guidelines for Americans 2000." The full report is available at www.usda.gov/cnpp/DietGd.pdf, page 10–11.

2-7 Exercise

Compared with being sedentary, being physically active for at least 30 minutes on most days of the week reduces the risk of developing or dying of heart disease. It has other health benefits as well. No one is too young or too old to enjoy the benefits of regular physical activity. Physical activity can

- Increase physical fitness
- Help build and maintain healthy bones, muscles, and joints
- Build endurance and muscular strength
- Help manage weight
- Lower risk factors for cardiovascular disease, colon cancer, and type 2 diabetes
- Help control blood pressure
- Promote psychological well-being and self-esteem
- Reduce feelings of depression and anxiety

To get these health benefits, adults need a moderate amount of physical activity for a total of at least 30 minutes most days of the week, and children need at least 60 minutes per day. A moderate physical activity is any activity that requires about as much energy as walking 2 miles in 30 minutes.

Aim to accumulate at least 30 minutes of physical activity daily, instead of doing it all at once you can take three, 10-minute walks. If you already get 30 minutes of physical activity daily, you can gain even more health benefits by increasing the amount of time you are physically active or by taking part in more vigorous activities. No matter what activity you choose, you can do it all at once, or spread it out over two or three times during the day.

Two types of physical activity are beneficial

- Aerobic activities. These are activities that speed your heart rate and breathing. They help cardiovascular fitness.
- Activities for strength and flexibility.
- Developing strength may help build and maintain bones. Carrying groceries and lifting weights are two strength-building activities. Gentle stretching, dancing, or yoga can increase flexibility.

MAKE PHYSICAL ACTIVITY A REGULAR PART OF YOUR ROUTINE

Choose activities that you enjoy and that you can do regularly. If you are planning to start a vigorous activity plan and have one or more of the following conditions consult your health care professional:

- Chronic health problem such as heart disease, hypertension, diabetes, or obesity

- High risk for heart disease
- Over age 40 for men or 50 for women

EXAMPLES OF PHYSICAL ACTIVITY FOR ADULTS

For at least 30 minutes most days of the week, do any one of the activities listed below or combine activities. Look for additional opportunities among other activities that you enjoy.

As part of your routine activities

- Walk or bike ride more, drive less.
- Walk upstairs instead of taking an elevator.
- Get off the bus a few stops early and walk the remaining distance.
- Mow the lawn with a manual mower.
- Rake leaves.
- Garden.
- Wheel self in wheelchair (if wheelchair bound).
- Push a stroller.
- Clean the house.
- Do exercises or pedal a stationary bike while watching television.
- Play actively with children.
- Take a brisk 10-minute walk in the morning, at lunch, and after dinner.

As part of your exercise or recreational routine

- Walk, bicycle, swim, or do water aerobics; play racket sports, golf (pull or carry clubs), canoe, play basketball, dance; take part in an exercise program at work, home, school, or gym.

HELP CHILDREN BE PHYSICALLY ACTIVE

Children and adolescents benefit from physical activity in many ways. They need at least 60 minutes of physical activity daily. Parents can help:

- Set a good example. For example, arrange active family events in which everyone takes part. Join your children in physical activities.
- Encourage your children to be physically active at home, at school, and with friends by jumping rope, playing tag, riding a bike.
- Limit television watching, computer games, and other inactive forms of playing by alternating with periods of physical activity.

PHYSICAL ACTIVITIES FOR CHILDREN AND TEENS

Aim for at least 60 minutes total per day:

- Be spontaneously active.

- Play tag.
- Jump rope.
- Ride a bicycle or a tricycle.
- Play actively during school recess.
- Roller skate or blade.
- Take part in physical education activity class during school.
- Join after-school or community physical activity programs.
- Dance.

OLDER PEOPLE NEED TO BE PHYSICALLY ACTIVE TOO

Older persons can engage in moderate physical activity for at least 30 minutes a day, and take part in activities to strengthen muscles and improve flexibility. Staying strong and flexible can reduce your risk of falling and of breaking bones, preserve muscle, and improve your ability to live independently. Lifting small weights and carrying groceries are two ways to include strength building into your routine.

Where Can I Get More Information?

The American Dietetic Association: www.eatright.org. To find a registered dietitian in your area, click Find a Nutrition Professional.

This report was reprinted from the "Report of the Dietary Guidelines for Americans 2000." The full report is available at www.usda.gov/cnpp/DietGd.pdf, page 12–14.

2-8 Whole Grains

Foods made from grains (like wheat, rice, and oats) are the foundation of a nutritious diet. They provide vitamins, minerals, carbohydrates (starch and dietary fiber), and other substances that are important for good health. Grain products are low in fat, unless fat is added in processing, in preparation, or at the table.

HOW DO WHOLE GRAINS DIFFER FROM REFINED GRAINS?

Whole grains differ from refined grains in the amount of fiber and nutrients they provide, and different whole grain foods differ in nutrient content, so choose a variety. If you eat plenty of whole grains, such as whole wheat bread or oatmeal, you may reduce your risk of coronary heart disease, bowel diseases, and possibly some types of cancer. Aim for at least 6 servings per day—more if you are very active—and include several servings of whole grains.

WHY CHOOSE WHOLE GRAIN FOODS?

Vitamins, minerals, fiber, and other protective substance in whole grain foods contribute to the health benefits of whole grains. Refined grains are low in fiber and in the protective substances that accompany fiber. Eating plenty of fiber-containing foods such as whole grains (and also many fruits and vegetables) promotes proper bowel function. The high fiber content of many whole grains may also help you to feel full with fewer calories.

SHOULD I TAKE FIBER SUPPLEMENTS?

Fiber is best obtained from foods like whole grains, fruits, and vegetables rather than from fiber supplements for several reasons: there are many types of fiber, the composition of fiber is poorly understood, and other protective substances accompany fiber in food.

HOW TO INCREASE YOUR INTAKE OF WHOLE GRAINS

Choose foods that name one of the following ingredients *first* on the labels ingredient list.

Brown rice, bulgur, cracked wheat, graham flour, oatmeal, popcorn, whole barley, whole cornmeal, whole oats, whole rye, whole wheat

Try some of these whole grain foods:

Whole wheat bread, whole grain ready-to-eat cereal, low-fat whole wheat crackers, oatmeal, corn tortillas, whole wheat pasta, whole barley in soup, tabouli salad.

Sample Ingredient List for a Whole Grain Food

Ingredients: Whole wheat flour, water, high fructose corn syrup, wheat gluten, soybean and/or canola oil, yeast, salt, honey.

Use the nutrition facts label to help choose grains that are rich in fiber and low in saturated fat and sodium.

Note: "wheat flour," "enriched flour," and "degerminated corn meal" are not whole grains.

Enriched grains are a new source of folic acid.

Folate, also called folic acid, is a B vitamin that reduces the risk of serious types of birth defects and may help protect against coronary heart disease and possibly certain cancers. Folic acid is now added to all enriched grain products (thiamin, riboflavin, niacin, and iron have been added to enriched grains for many years). Whole grain foods naturally contain some folate, but only a few (mainly ready-to-eat breakfast cereals) contain added folic acid as well. Read the ingredient label to find out if folic acid has been added, and check Nutrition Facts to compare nutrient content of foods like breakfast cereals.

Where Can I Get More Information?

The American Dietetic Association: www.eatright.org. To find a registered dietitian in your area, click Find a Nutrition Professional.

This report was reprinted from the "Report of the Dietary Guidelines for Americans 2000." The full report is available at www.usda.gov/cnpp/DietGd.pdf, page 22–23.

YOU NEED FIVE A DAY

Fruits and vegetables are key parts of your daily diet. Eating plenty of fruits and vegetables of different kinds may help protect you against heart disease, stroke, and some types of cancer. It also promotes healthy bowel function. Fruits and vegetables provide essential vitamins and minerals, fiber, and other substances that are important for good health. Most people, including children, eat fewer servings of fruits and vegetables than are recommended. To promote your health eat a variety of fruits and vegetables—at least 2 servings of fruits and 3 servings of vegetables—each day.

Why Eat Plenty of Different Fruits and Vegetables?

Different fruits and vegetables are rich in different nutrients. Some fruits and vegetables are excellent sources of vitamin A (carotenoids), while others may be rich in vitamin C, folate, or potassium. They also contain fiber and other substances that are associated with good health. Dark green leafy vegetables, deeply colored fruits, and dried peas and beans are especially rich in nutrients. Most fruits and vegetables are low in calories and filling. Some are high in fiber, and many are quick to prepare and easy to eat. Eating plenty of fruits and vegetables makes it easier to avoid getting too many calories.

Which Fruits and Vegetables Provide the Most Nutrients?

Sources of vitamin A (carotenoids)

- Bright orange vegetables like carrots, sweet potatoes, pumpkin
- Dark-green leafy vegetables such as spinach, collards, turnip greens
- Bright orange fruits like mango, cantaloupe, apricots

Sources of Vitamin C

- Citrus fruits and juices, kiwi, strawberries, and cantaloupe
- Broccoli, peppers, tomatoes, cabbage, and potatoes
- Leafy greens such as romaine, turnip greens, and spinach

Sources of folate

- Cooked dried beans and peas
- Oranges, orange juice
- Deep green leaves like spinach and mustard greens

Sources of potassium

- Baked white or sweet potato, cooked greens (such as spinach), winter (orange) squash
- Bananas, plantains, many dried fruits, orange juice
- Cooked dried beans (such as baked beans) and lentils

What to Choose?

Choose whole or cut-up fruits and vegetables rather than juices most often. Juices contain little or no fiber. Often, the brighter the color, the higher the content of vitamins and minerals. Try many colors and kinds. Choose any form: fresh, frozen, canned, dried juices. But most of all, aim for 5 A Day!

Where Can I Get More Information?

The American Dietetic Association: www.eatright.org. To find a registered dietitian in your area, click Find a Nutrition Professional.

This report was reprinted from the "'Report of the Dietary Guidelines for Americans 2000." The full report is available at www.usda.gov/cnpp/DietGd.pdf, page 24–25.

You need some fat in the food you eat, but choose sensibly. Fat in food supplies energy, essential fatty acids, and helps absorb the fat-soluble vitamins A, D, E, and K. Some kinds of fat, especially saturated fats, increase the risk for coronary heart disease by raising the blood cholesterol. In contrast, unsaturated fat (found mainly in vegetable oils) do not increase blood cholesterol. Fat intake in the United States is lower than it was many years ago, but most people still eat too much saturated fat. Eating lots of any type can provide excess calories.

KNOW THE DIFFERENT TYPES OF FATS

Saturated Fats

Foods high in saturated fats tend to raise blood cholesterol. These foods include high-fat dairy products (like cheese, whole milk, cream, butter, and full-fat ice cream), fatty fresh and processed meats, the skin and fat of poultry, lard, palm oil, and coconut oil. Keep your intake of these foods low.

Dietary Cholesterol

Foods that are high in cholesterol also tend to raise blood cholesterol. These foods include liver, and other organ meats, egg yolks, and dairy fats.

Trans Fatty Acids

Foods high in trans fatty acids tend to raise blood cholesterol. These foods include those high in partially hydrogenated vegetable oils, such as many hard margarines and shortenings. Foods with high amounts of these ingredients include some commercially fried foods and some bakery goods.

Unsaturated Fats

All kinds of unsaturated fats (oils) help keep blood cholesterol low. Unsaturated fats occur in vegetable oils, most nuts, olives, avocados, and fatty fish like salmon. Unsaturated oils include both *monounsaturated* fats and *polyunsaturated* fats. Olive, canola, and peanut oils are some of the oils high in monounsaturated fats. Vegetable oils such as soybean oil, corn oil, and cottonseed oil and many kinds of nuts are good sources of polyunsaturated fats. Fatty ocean fish have a special type of polyunsaturated fat (omega-3 fatty acids) that may protect you against heart disease. Use moderate amounts of foods high in unsaturated fats, taking care to avoid excess calories.

FOOD CHOICES LOW IN SATURATED FAT AND CHOLESTEROL AND MODERATE IN TOTAL FAT

Get most of your calories from plant foods (grains, fruits, vegetables). If you eat foods high in saturated fat for a special occasion, return to foods that are low in saturated fat the next day.

Following the tips below will help keep your saturated fat intake at less than 10% of calories and your cholesterol intake less than 300 mg/day.

Fats and Oils

- Choose vegetable oils over butter, lard and shortening.
- If you need fewer calories, decrease the amount of fat you use in cooking and at the table.

Meat, Poultry, Fish, Shellfish, Eggs, Beans, and Nuts

- Choose 2 to 3 servings of fish, shellfish, lean poultry, other lean meats, beans, or nuts daily. Trim fat from meat and take skin off poultry—this removes about half the fat. Choose dried beans, peas or lentils often.
- Limit your intake of high-fat processed meats such as sausages, salami, bologna, and other cold cuts. Try the lower fat varieties.
- Limit your intake of liver and other organ meats. Use egg yolks and whole eggs in moderation. Use egg whites and egg substitutes freely when cooking since they contain no cholesterol.

Dairy Products

- Choose fat-free or low-fat milk, fat-free or low-fat yogurt, and low-fat cheese most often. Try switching from whole to fat-free or low-fat milk. This decreases the saturated fat and calories but keeps all other nutrients the same.

Prepared Foods

- Check the Nutrition Facts Label to see how much saturated fat and cholesterol are in a serving of prepared food. Choose foods lower in saturated fat and cholesterol.

Foods at Restaurants or Other Eating Establishments

- Try to order fish or lean meats as suggested above. Try to avoid or limit ground meat and fatty processed meats, marbled steaks, and cheese.
- Avoid foods with creamy sauces, and add little or no butter to your food.
- Choose fruit dessert most often.

What Is Your Upper Limit on Fat for the Calories You Consume?

Calories per day	Saturated fat (in grams)	Total fat (in grams)
1,600	18 or less	53
2,200	24 or less	73
2,800	31 or less	93

A COMPARISON OF SATURATED FAT IN SOME FOODS

Food	Portion	Saturated fat (in grams)
Cheese	1 oz	6
Low-fat cheese	1 oz	3
Regular ground beef	3 oz	8
Extra lean ground beef	3 oz	6
Whole milk	1 cup	5
1% milk	1 cup	1.5
Croissant	1 medium	7
Bagel	1 medium	0
Ice cream	½ cup	4.5
Frozen yogurt	½ cup	2

Advice for Children

The dietary advice included here about cholesterol and saturated fat applies to children who are 2 years of age or older. It does not apply to infants and toddlers below the age of 2 years. Beginning at age 2, children should get most of their calories from grain products; fruits; vegetables; low-fat dairy products; and beans, lean meat and poultry and fish, or nuts.

Reduce Your Intake of Saturated Fat and Cholesterol

- Limit use of animal fats, hard margarines, and partially hydrogenated shortenings. Use vegetable oils as a substitute.
- Eat plenty of grain products, vegetables, and fruit daily.
- Read labels carefully.

Where Can I Get More Information?

The American Dietetic Association: www.eatright.org. To find a registered dietitian in your area, click Find a Nutrition Professional.

This report was reprinted from the "Report of the Dietary Guidelines for Americans 2000." The full report is available at www.usda.gov/cnpp/DietGd.pdf, page 30–32.

INTAKE OF SUGARS IS INCREASING

Since the early 1990s, Americans have increased their calorie intake. This increase has come largely from an increased intake of carbohydrates, mainly in the form of added sugars. Added sugars are sugars and syrups added to foods in processing or preparation, not the naturally occurring sugars in foods like fruit and milk.

In the United States, the number one source of added sugars is non-diet soft drinks (soda or pop). Sweets and candies, cakes and cookies, and fruit drinks and fruitades are also major sources of added sugars. Intake of a lot of foods high in added sugars, like soft drinks, is of concern because children, adolescents, and women who consume these foods consume less of more nutritious foods like milk.

Some foods, like chocolate milk, presweetened cereals, and sweetened canned fruits are high in vitamins and minerals as well as in added sugars. These foods provide extra calories along with the nutrients. These foods are fine if you need the extra calories. However, if you eat lots of beverages and foods high in sugars, you may get less of the nutrients you need for good health. So choose sensibly to limit your intake of sugars. And brush your teeth or rinse your mouth with water after eating foods that contain sugars.

MAJOR SOURCES OF ADDED SUGARS IN THE UNITED STATES

- Soft drinks*
- Candy
- Cakes, cookies, pies
- Fruitades and drinks such as fruit punch and lemonade

READ LABELS

The Nutrition Facts Label gives the content of total sugars (naturally occurring sugars plus added sugars, if any). You need to look at the ingredient list to find out if sugars have been added. Use the sugar content on a label to compare like products such as different brands of peanut butter, ready-to-eat cereals, or snack crackers.

NAMES FOR ADDED SUGAR THAT APPEAR ON FOOD LABELS

A food that is likely to be high in sugars if one of these names appears first or second in the ingredient list, or if several of these names are listed.

---

*All kinds, except diet or sugar-free.

Brown sugar	Invert sugar
Corn sweetener	Lactose
Corn syrup	Maltose
Dextrose	Malt syrup
Fructose	Molasses
Fruit juice concentrate	Raw sugar
Glucose	Sucrose
Syrup	High-fructose corn syrup
Honey	Table sugar

SUGAR SUBSTITUTES

Sugar substitutes such as saccharin, aspartame, acesulfame potassium, and sucralose are extremely low in calories. Some people find them useful if they want a sweet taste without the calories. Some foods that contain sugar substitutes, however, still have calories. Unless you reduce the total calories you eat or increase your physical activity, using sugar substitutes will not by itself cause you to lose weight.

SUGARS AND OTHER HEALTH PROBLEMS

Behavior: Intake of sugars does not appear to affect children's behavior patterns or their ability to learn. Many scientific studies conclude that sugars do not cause hyperactivity in children.

Weight control: Children and adults have increased the amounts of sugars they consume. This has contributed to higher caloric intakes. Foods that are high in sugars are often high in calories but low in essential nutrients. When you take in extra calories and don't offset them by increasing your physical activity, you will gain weight. As you aim for a healthy weight and fitness, keep an eye on serving size for all foods and beverages, not only those high in sugars,

Sugar and teeth: Foods containing sugars and starches can promote tooth decay, especially if they stay in contact with your teeth for a long time. Eating or drinking sweet or starchy foods between meals is more likely to harm teeth than eating the same foods at meals and then brushing.

FOR HEALTHY TEETH AND GUMS

- Between meals, eat few foods or beverages containing sugars or starches. If you do eat them, rinse your mouth afterward to reduce risk of tooth decay.
- Rinse your mouth after eating dried fruit.
- Brush and floss teeth regularly. Use fluoride toothpaste.
- Ask your dentist or health care professional about the need for supplemental fluoride, especially for children if the water you drink is not fluoridated.

CHOOSE BEVERAGES AND FOODS THAT LIMIT YOUR INTAKE OF SUGARS

- Choose sensibly to limit your intake of beverages and foods that are high in sugars.

- Remember the simple tips to keep your teeth and gums healthy.
- Get most of your calories from grains (especially whole grains), fruits and vegetables, low-fat or non-fat dairy products, and lean meats or substitutes.
- Drink water often.
- Take care not to let soft drinks or other sweets crowd out other foods you need to maintain health, such as low-fat milk or other good sources of calcium.

Where Can I Get More Information?

The American Dietetic Association: www.eatright.org. To find a registered dietitian in your area, click Find a Nutrition Professional.

This report was reprinted from the "Report of the Dietary Guidelines for Americans 2000." The full report is available at www.usda.gov/cnpp/DietGd.pdf, page 34–35.

Growing children, teenagers, women, and older adults have higher needs for some nutrients. Adolescents and adults over age 50 have an especially high need for calcium, but most people need to eat plenty of good sources of calcium for healthy bones throughout life. When selecting dairy products to get enough calcium, choose those that are low in fat or fat-free to avoid getting too much saturated fat. Young children, teenage girls, and women of childbearing age need enough good sources of iron, such as lean meats and cereals with added nutrients, to keep up their iron stores (see *Some Sources of Iron*). Women who could become pregnant need extra folic acid, and older adults need extra vitamin D.

SOME SOURCES OF IRON*

- Shellfish, like shrimp, clams, mussels, and oysters
- Lean meats (especially beef), liver** and other organ meats**
- Ready-to-eat cereals with added nutrients (amount varies)
- Turkey dark meat without skin
- Sardines,*** anchovies***
- Cooked dry beans (such as kidney beans), peas (such as black-eyed peas), and lentils and spinach
- Enriched and whole grain breads

SOME SOURCES OF CALCIUM†

- Most foods in the dairy group‡

  Yogurt

  Milk

  Natural cheeses such as mozzarella, cheddar, Swiss, and parmesan

  Soy-based beverage with added calcium

- Tofu, if made with calcium sulfate (read the label)
- Breakfast cereal with added calcium (iron content varies)
- Canned fish with soft bones such as salmon*** and sardines***
- Fruit juice with added calcium

---

*Read food labels for brand-specific information. The foods at the top of this list are highest in iron per serving.
**Very high in cholesterol.
***High in salt.
†Read labels for brand-specific information. The foods at the top of this list are highest in calcium per serving.
‡Choose low-fat or fat-free.

■ Pudding made with milk[‡]

■ Soup made with milk[‡]

■ Dark-green leafy vegetables such as collards, turnip greens

LEARN HOW TO READ THE NUTRITION FACTS LABEL

Use the Nutrition Facts Label to see if a food is a good source of a nutrient or to compare different foods—for example to find which brands are higher in calcium or iron look at the % Daily Value (% DV) column to see whether a food is high (20% more) or low (5% or less) in nutrients.

Where Can I Get More Information?

The American Dietetic Association: www.eatright.org. To find a registered dietitian in your area, click Find a Nutrition Professional.

This report was reprinted from the "Report of the Dietary Guidelines for Americans 2000." The full report is available at www.usda.gov/cnpp/DietGd.pdf, page 19–21.

2-13 Salt

You can reduce your chances of developing high blood pressure by consuming less salt. You also can take several other steps to help keep blood pressure in the healthy range. In the body, sodium, which you get mainly from salt, plays an essential role in regulating fluids and blood pressure. Many studies in diverse populations have shown that a higher sodium intake is associated with higher blood pressure.

There is no way to tell who might develop high blood pressure from eating too much salt. However, consuming less salt or sodium is not harmful and can be recommended for the healthy, normal person.

At present, the firmest link between salt intake and health relates to blood pressure. High salt intake also increases the amount of calcium excreted in the urine. Eating less salt may decrease the loss of calcium from bone. Loss of too much calcium from bone increases the risk of osteoporosis and fractures.

STEPS THAT MAY HELP KEEP BLOOD PRESSURE IN A HEALTHY RANGE

- Choose and prepare foods with less salt.
- Aim for a healthy weight: Blood pressure increases with increases in body weight and decreases when excess weight is reduced.
- Increase physical activity: It helps lower blood pressure, reduce risk of other chronic diseases, and manage weight.
- Eat fruits and vegetables. They are naturally low in salt and calories. They are also rich in potassium, which may help decrease blood pressure.
- If you drink alcoholic beverages, do so in moderation. Excessive alcohol consumption has been associated with high blood pressure.

IS LOWERING SALT INTAKE SAFE?

- Eating too little salt is not generally a concern for healthy people. If you are being treated for a chronic health problem, ask your doctor about whether it is safe for you to reduce your salt intake.
- As a public health measure, some table salt is fortified with iodine. If you use table salt to meet your need for iodine, ½ teaspoon of iodized salt provides more than half the daily iodine requirement.
- Your body can adjust to prevent too much salt loss when you exercise heavily or when it is very hot. However, if you plan to reduce your salt intake and you exercise vigorously, it is sensible to decrease gradually the amount of salt you consume.

SALT IS FOUND MAINLY IN PROCESSED AND PREPARED FOODS

Salt (sodium chloride) is the main source of sodium in foods. Only small amounts of salt occur naturally in foods. Most of the salt you eat comes from processed food, restaurant meals or food prepared at home with salt added. Some recipes include table salt or a salty broth or sauce, and some cooking styles call for adding a very salty seasoning such as soy sauce. Not all foods with added salt taste salty. Some people add salt or a salty seasoning to their food at the table. Your preference for salt may weaken if you gradually add smaller amounts of salt or salty seasoning to your food.

SALT VERSUS SODIUM

- Salt contains sodium. Sodium is a substance that affects blood pressure.
- The best way to cut back on sodium is to cut back on salt and salty foods and seasonings.
- When reading a Nutrition Facts Label, look for the sodium content. Foods that are low in sodium (less than 5% of the Daily Value or DV) are low in salt.

AIM FOR A MODERATE SODIUM INTAKE

Most people consume too much salt, so moderate your salt intake. Healthy children and adults need to consume only small amounts of salt to meet their sodium needs, less than ¼ teaspoon of salt daily. The Nutrition Facts Label lists a Daily Value of 2,400 mg of sodium per day. This is the amount of sodium in 1 teaspoon of salt.

WAY TO DECREASE YOUR SALT INTAKE

At the Store

- Choose fresh, plain frozen, or canned vegetables without added salt most often. They are low in salt.
- Choose fresh or frozen fish, shellfish, poultry, and meat most often. They are lower in salt than most canned and processed forms.
- Read the Nutrition Facts Label to compare the amount of sodium in processed foods, such as frozen dinners, packaged mixes, cereals, cheese, breads, soups, salad dressings, and sauces. The amount in types and different brands varies widely.
- Look for labels that say "low-sodium." They contain 140 mg (about 5% of the Daily Value) or less of sodium per serving.
- Ask your grocer or supermarket to offer more low-sodium foods.

Cooking and Eating at Home

- If you salt foods in cooking or at the table, add small amounts. Learn to use spices and herbs, rather than salt, to enhance the flavor of food.
- Go easy on condiments such as soy sauce, ketchup, mustard, pickles, and olives—they can add a lot of salt to your food.
- Leave the salt shaker in a cupboard.

Eating Out

- Choose plain foods like grilled or roasted entrees, baked potatoes, and salad with oil and vinegar. Batter-fried foods tend to be high in salt, as do combination dishes like stews or pasta with sauce.
- Ask to have no salt added when food is prepared.

Any Time

- Choose fruits and vegetables often.
- Drink water freely. It is usually very low in sodium. Check the label on bottled water for sodium content.
- Use herbs, spices, and fruits to add flavor to food, and cut the amount of salty seasoning by half.

Where Can I Get More Information?

The American Dietetic Association: www.eatright.org. To find a registered dietitian in your area, click Find a Nutrition Professional.

This report was reprinted from the "Report of the Dietary Guidelines for Americans 2000." The full report is available at www.usda.gov/cnpp/DietGd.pdf, page 36–37.

If you drink alcoholic beverages, do so in moderation. Alcoholic beverages are harmful when consumed in excess. Excess alcohol alters judgment and can lead to dependency and a great many other serious health problems. Taking more than one drink per day for women or two drinks per day for men can raise the risk for auto accidents, other accidents, high blood pressure, stroke, violence, suicide, birth defects, and certain cancers. Even one drink per day can slightly raise the risk of breast cancer. Too much alcohol may cause social and psychological problems, cirrhosis of the liver, inflammation of the pancreas, and damage to the brain and heart. Heavy drinkers also are at risk of malnutrition because alcohol contains calories that may substitute for those in nutritious foods. If adults choose to drink alcoholic beverages, they should consume them only in moderation—and with meals to slow absorption.

WHAT IS DRINKING IN MODERATION?

Moderation is defined as no more than one drink per day for women and no more than two drinks per day for men. This limit is based on difference between the sexes in both weight and metabolism.

Drinking in moderation may lower risk for coronary heart disease mainly among men over age 45 and women over age 55. Moderate consumption provides little, if any, benefit for younger people. Risk of alcohol abuse increases when drinking starts at an early age.

Count as a Drink

12 oz of regular beer (150 calories)*

5 oz of wine (100 calories)

1.5 oz of 80-proof distilled spirits (100 calories)

WHO SHOULD NOT DRINK?

Some people should not drink alcoholic beverages at all. These include

- Children and adolescents.
- Individuals of any age who cannot restrict their drinking to moderate levels. This is a special concern for recovering alcoholics, problem drinkers, and people whose family members have alcohol problems.
- Women who have become pregnant or who are pregnant
- Individuals who plan to drive, operate machinery, or take part in other activities that require attention or skill.

---

*Note that even moderate drinking provides extra calories.

■ Individuals taking certain prescription or over-the-counter medications that can interact with alcohol.

If you chose to drink alcoholic beverages, do so sensibly. Limit intake to one drink per day for women or two per day for men, and take with meals to slow alcohol absorption. Avoid drinking before or when driving, or whenever it puts you or others at risk.

Where Can I Get More Information?

The American Dietetic Association: www.eatright.org. To find a registered dietitian in your area, click Find a Nutrition Professional.

This report was reprinted from the "Report of the Dietary Guidelines for Americans 2000." The full report is available at www.usda.gov/cnpp/DietGd.pdf, page 38.

2-15 Keep Food Safe to Eat

Farmers, food producers, markets, food service establishments, and other food preparers have a role to keep food as safe as possible. However, we also need to keep and prepare food safely in the home, and be alert when eating out.

WHAT IS FOOD BORNE ILLNESS?

Safe means that the food poses little risk of food borne illness. Food borne illness is caused by eating food that contains harmful bacteria, toxins, parasites, viruses, or chemical contaminants. Bacteria and viruses, especially Campylobacter, salmonella, and Norwalk-like viruses, are among the most common causes of food borne illness we know about today. Eating even a small portion of an unsafe food may make you sick. Signs and symptoms may appear within a half an hour of eating a contaminated food or may not develop for up to 3 weeks. Most food borne illness lasts a few hours or days. Some food borne illnesses have effects that go on for weeks, months, or even years. If you think you have become ill from eating a food, consult your health care provider.

TIPS FOR THOSE AT HIGH RISK OF FOOD BORNE ILLNESS

Who is at high risk of food borne illness?

- Pregnant women
- Young children
- Older persons
- People with weakened immune systems or certain chronic illnesses

Besides following the guidance in this guideline some of the extra precautions those at risk should take are:

- Do not eat or drink unpasteurized juices, raw sprouts, raw (unpasteurized) milk, and products made from unpasteurized milk.
- Do not eat raw or undercooked meat, poultry, eggs, fish, and shellfish (clams, oysters, scallops, and mussels).

CLEAN, SEPARATE, COOK, CHILL

Follow these steps to keep food safe. Be very careful with perishable foods such as eggs, meats, poultry, fish, shellfish, milk products, and fresh fruits and vegetables.

Clean: Wash hands and surfaces often.

Separate: Separate raw, cooked, and ready-to-eat foods while shopping, preparing, or storing.

Cook: Cook foods to a safe temperature.

Chill: Refrigerate perishable foods promptly.

Check: Follow the label for cooking and storage advice.

Serve safely: Keep hot foods hot and cold foods cold.

When in doubt throw it out.

New information on food safety is constantly emerging. If you are among those at high risk, you need to be aware of and follow the most current information on food safety.

For the latest information, call USDA's Meat and Poultry Hotline (1-800-535-4555) or FDA's Food Information Line (1-888-SAFEFOOD), or consult your healthcare provider. Or check the government's food safety website at www.foodsafety.gov.

Where Can I Get More Information?

The American Dietetic Association: www.eatright.org. To find a registered dietitian in your area, click Find a Nutrition Professional.

This report was reprinted from the "Report of the Dietary Guidelines for Americans 2000." The full report is available at www.usda.gov/cnpp/DietGd.pdf, page 26–28.

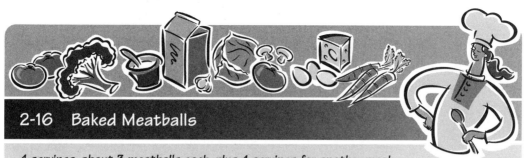

2-16   Baked Meatballs

4 servings, about 3 meatballs each, plus 4 servings for another meal

Onions, minced	¼ cup
Vegetable oil	1 tablespoon
Lean ground beef	2 pounds
Eggs	2
Bread crumbs	¾ cup
Whole milk*	½ cup
Salt	⅛ teaspoon
Pepper	½ teaspoon
Onion powder	2 teaspoons
Garlic powder	½ teaspoon

Preparation time; 15 minutes

Cooking time: 10 to 12 minutes

1. Preheat oven 400°F. Grease baking sheet lightly with oil.
2. Add 1 tablespoon oil and onions to small skillet. Cook over medium heat, until tender, about 3 minutes.
3. Mix remaining ingredients together in bowl; add onions. Mix until blended, using a large serving spoon.
4. Shape beef mixture into 1- to 2-inch meatballs; place on baking sheet.
5. Bake until thoroughly cooked about 10 to 12 minutes.

Note: Serve with spaghetti sauce and in a meatball sandwich.

Per serving:

Calories*	345
Total fat*	21 grams
Saturated fat*	7 grams
Cholesterol*	142 milligrams
Sodium	224 milligrams

---

* Replacing ½ cup whole milk with ½ cup non-fat milk will reduce the calorie, total fat, saturated fat, and cholesterol. Reprinted from USDA's *Recipes and Tips for Healthy, Thrifty Meals* at http://www.usda.gov/cnpp/Pubs/Cookbook/thriftym.pdf, page 20.

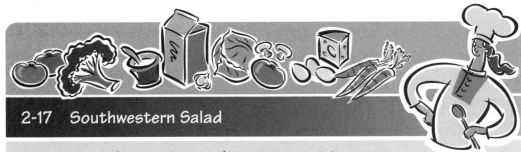

2-17   Southwestern Salad

4 servings about ½ cup beef mixture, ½ cup lettuce and cheese mixture each serving

Onions, chopped	½ cup
Lean ground beef	1 pound
Chili powder	1 tablespoon
Dry oregano	2 teaspoons
Ground cumin	½ teaspoon
Canned kidney beans, red drained	1 cup
Canned chick peas, drained	1 15-ounce can
Tomato, diced	1 medium
Lettuce	2 cups
Cheddar cheese	½ cup

Preparation time: 15 minutes

Cooking time: 10 to 15 minutes

1. Cook ground beef and onions in a large skillet until the beef no longer remains pink. Drain.
2. Stir chili powder, oregano, and cumin into beef mixture; cook for 1 minute.
3. Add beans, chickpeas, and tomatoes. Mix gently to combine.
4. Combine lettuce and cheese in large serving bowl. Portion lettuce and cheese onto 4 plates. Add 1 cup of beef mixture on top of lettuce and cheese.

Note: Garbanzo bean is another name for chickpea.

Per serving:

Calories	485
Total fat	22 grams
Saturated fat	9 grams
Cholesterol	98 milligrams
Sodium	411 milligrams

Reprinted from USDA's *Recipes and Tips for Healthy, Thrifty Meals* at http://www.usda.gov/cnpp/Pubs/Cookbook/thriftym.pdf, page 25.

2-18 Stir-fried Pork and Vegetables with Rice

4 servings of pork and vegetables, about ½ cup each. 4 servings of cooked rice, about 2 cups each.

Chicken broth, reduced sodium	2 cups
Hot water	2 cups
Rice, uncooked	2 cups
Vegetable oil	2 tablespoons
Broccoli cuts, frozen	2 cups
Carrots, cleaned, sliced thinly	1 cup
Onions, minced	¼ cup
Garlic powder	1 teaspoon
Canned mushrooms, drained	½ cup
Ground pork	1 pound + 7 ounces
Soy sauce	4 tablespoons

Preparation time: 20 minutes

Cooking time: 25 to 30 minutes

1. Heat broth and water to a boil in a saucepan; add rice and return to boil. Reduce heat to low and simmer until tender, about 15 minutes.
2. Heat 1 tablespoon of oil in skillet. Add broccoli, carrots, onions, and garlic powder. Cook until crisp-tender, about 5 minutes. Remove from skillet. Add mushrooms. Cook for 1 minute and set aside.
3. Heat second tablespoon of oil in skillet. Add pork; cook until pork no longer remains pink. Drain liquid.
4. Add soy sauce and stir until mixed; add vegetables to pork mixture. Cook until heated, about 1 to 2 minutes.
5. Serve pork mixture over cooked rice.

Note: Sodium level can be reduced from 799 milligrams to 532 milligrams by reducing soy sauce from 4 to 2 tablespoons.

Per serving:
Calories	860
Total fat	33 grams
Saturated fat	10 grams
Cholesterol	108 milligrams
Sodium	799 milligrams

Reprinted from USDA's *Recipes and Tips for Healthy, Thrifty Meals* at http://www.usda.gov/cnpp/Pubs/Cookbook/thriftym.pdf, page 26.

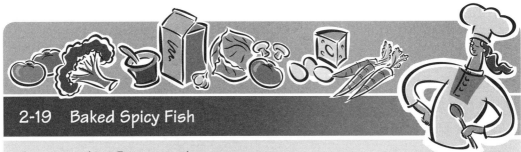

2-19   Baked Spicy Fish

4 servings, about 3 ounces each

Cod fillets, frozen	1 pound
Paprika	¼ teaspoon
Garlic powder	¼ teaspoon
Onion powder	¼ teaspoon
Pepper	⅛ teaspoon
Ground oregano	⅛ teaspoon
Ground thyme	⅛ teaspoon
Lemon juice	1 tablespoon
Margarine, melted	1½ tablespoons

Preparation time: 15 minutes

Cooking time: 25 minutes

1. Thaw frozen fish according to package directions.
2. Preheat oven to 350°F.
3. Separate fish into four fillets or pieces. Place fish in ungreased 13-x 9-x 2-inch baking pan.
4. Combine paprika, garlic and onion powder, pepper, oregano, and thyme in small bowl. Sprinkle seasoning mixture and lemon juice evenly over fish. Drizzle margarine evenly over fish.
5. Bake until fish flakes easily with a fork, about 20 to 25 minutes.

Per serving:

Calories	140
Total fat	5 grams
Saturated fat	1 gram
Cholesterol	51 milligrams
Sodium	123 milligrams

Reprinted from USDA's *Recipes and Tips for Healthy, Thrifty Meals* at http://www.usda.gov/cnpp/Pubs/Cookbook/thriftym.pdf, page 29.

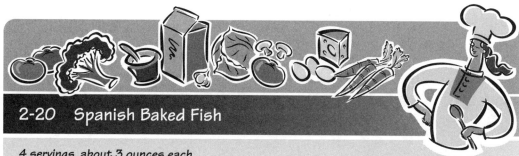

2-20 Spanish Baked Fish

4 servings, about 3 ounces each

Perch fillets, fresh or frozen	1 pound
Tomato sauce	1 cup
Onions, sliced	½ cup
Garlic powder	½ teaspoon
Chili powder	2 teaspoons
Dried oregano flakes	1 teaspoon
Ground cumin	⅛ teaspoon

Preparation time: 15 minutes

Cooking time: about 10 to 20 minutes

1. Thaw frozen fish according to package directions.
2. Preheat oven to 350°F. Lightly grease baking dish.
3. Separate fish into four fillets or pieces. Arrange fish in baking dish.
4. Mix remaining ingredients together and pour over fish.
5. Bake until fish flakes easily with fork, about 10 to 20 minutes.

Per serving:
Calories	135
Total fat	1 gram
Saturated fat	trace
Cholesterol	104 milligrams
Sodium	448 milligrams

Reprinted from USDA's *Recipes and Tips for Healthy, Thrifty Meals* at http://www.usda.gov/cnpp/Pubs/Cookbook/thriftym.pdf, page 30.

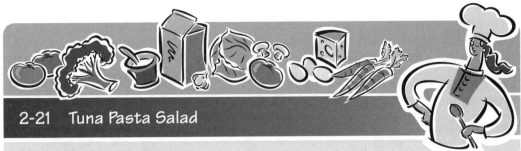

2-21   Tuna Pasta Salad

4 servings, about 1½ cups each

Macaroni, uncooked	2 cups
Tuna, canned, water-pack	2 6- to 12-ounce cans
Zucchini, chopped	½ cup
Carrots, sliced	¼ cup
Onions, diced	⅓ cup
Salad dressing, mayonnaise-type	¼ cup

Preparation time: 25 minutes

Cooking time: 8 minutes

1. Cook macaroni according to package directions. Drain.
2. Drain tuna.
3. Wash vegetables. Chop zucchini; slice carrots into thin slices; dice onions.
4. Mix macaroni, tuna, and vegetables together in mixing bowl. Stir in salad dressing.
5. Chill until ready to serve.

Per serving:
Calories	405
Total fat	13 grams
Saturated fat	2 grams
Cholesterol	25 milligrams
Sodium	360 milligrams

Reprinted from USDA's *Recipes and Tips for Healthy, Thrifty Meals* at http://www.usda.gov/cnpp/Pubs/Cookbook/thriftym.pdf, page 32.

2-22 Baked Chicken Nuggets

4 servings, about 3 ounces each

Chicken thighs, boneless, skinless	1½ pounds
Ready-to-eat cereal, cornflakes, crumbs	1 cup
Paprika	1 teaspoon
Italian herb seasoning	½ teaspoon
Garlic powder	¼ teaspoon
Onion powder	¼ teaspoon

Preparation time: 15 minutes

Conventional cooking time: 12 to 14 minutes

Microwave cooking time: 6 to 8 minutes

1. Remove skin and bone; cut thighs into bite-sized pieces.
2. Place cornflakes in plastic bag and crush by using a rolling pin.
3. Add remaining ingredients to crushed cornflakes. Close bag tightly and shake until blended.
4. Add a few chicken pieces at a time to crumb mixture. Shake to coat evenly.

Conventional Method

1. Preheat oven to 400°F. Lightly grease a cooking sheet.
2. Place chicken pieces on cooking sheet so they are not touching.
3. Bake until golden brown, about 12 to 14 minutes.

Microwave Method

1. Lightly grease an 8- × 12-inch baking dish.
2. Place chicken pieces on baking dish so they are not touching. Cover with waxed paper and cook on high.
3. Rotate chicken every 2 to 3 minutes. Cook until tender, about 6 to 8 minutes.

Note: To remove bone from chicken thighs

1. Place chicken on cutting board. Remove skin from thighs.
2. Turn chicken thighs over.
3. Cut around bone and remove it.

Per serving:

Calories	175
Total fat	8 grams
Saturated fat	2 grams
Cholesterol	67 milligrams
Sodium	127 milligrams

Reprinted from USDA's *Recipes and Tips for Healthy, Thrifty Meals* at http://www.usda.gov/cnpp/Pubs/Cookbook/thriftym.pdf, page 34.

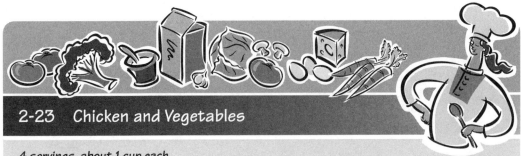

2-23 Chicken and Vegetables

4 servings, about 1 cup each

Margarine	1½ tablespoons
Garlic powder	1 teaspoon
Onions, chopped	½ cup
Chicken thighs, boneless, skinless	1 pound + 4 ounces
Cut green beans, frozen	10-ounce package
Pepper	¼ teaspoon

Preparation time: 6 minutes

Cooking time: 25 minutes

1. Melt margarine in heavy skillet. Add garlic and onions; stir until blended. Cook over medium heat, until tender, about 5 minutes. Remove from skillet.
2. Place chicken in the skillet. Cook over medium heat, until chicken is thoroughly done and no longer pink in color, about 12 minutes. Remove chicken from skillet; keep warm.
3. Place frozen green beans, pepper, and cooked onions in same skillet. Cover and cook over medium-low heat until beans are tender, about 5 minutes.
4. Add chicken to vegetable mixture. Continue cooking, stirring occasionally, until heated through, about 3 minutes.

Note: To remove bone from chicken thighs

1. Place chicken on cutting board. Remove skin from thighs.
2. Turn chicken thighs over.
3. Cut around bone and remove it.

Per serving:
Calories	190
Total fat	11 grams
Saturated fat	3 grams
Cholesterol	57 grams
Sodium	109 milligrams

Reprinted from USDA's *Recipes and Tips for Healthy, Thrifty Meals* at http://www.usda.gov/cnpp/Pubs/Cookbook/thriftym.pdf, page 36.

2-24   Oven Crispy Chicken

4 servings, about 4 ounces each

Broiler fryer chicken, cut-up	1½ pounds
Whole milk	¼ cup
Flour	½ cup
Paprika	1 teaspoon
Pepper	½ teaspoon
Ready-to-eat flake cereal, slightly crushed	1 cup
Vegetable oil	4 tablespoons

Preparation time: 15 minutes

Cooking time: 30 minutes

1. Remove skin and all visible fat from chicken. Place milk in large bowl. Add chicken pieces; turn to coat.
2. Combine flour, paprika, and pepper on a plate.
3. Lift chicken pieces from milk and reserve milk. Coat chicken thoroughly with seasoned flour and place on a wire rack until all pieces have been coated, redip chicken pieces into reserved milk.
4. Place crushed cereal on plate. Place chicken pieces on crushed cereal. Using 2 forks, turn chicken pieces in crushed cereal to coat.
5. Place chicken on a foil-lined baking tray; drizzle oil over chicken.
6. Bake at 400°F for 15 minutes. Turn chicken pieces over; continue to bake until chicken is thoroughly cooked and crust is crisp, about 15 more minutes.

Per serving:

Calories	350
Total fat	15 grams
Saturated fat	4 grams
Cholesterol	93 milligrams
Sodium	503 milligrams

Reprinted from USDA's *Recipes and Tips for Healthy, Thrifty Meals* at http://www.usda.gov/cnpp/Pubs/Cookbook/thriftym.pdf, page 37.

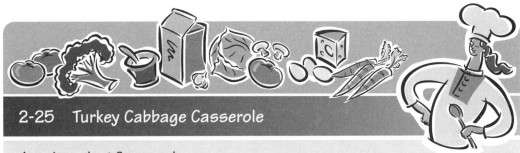

2-25   Turkey Cabbage Casserole

4 servings, about 2 cups each

Cabbage, shredded	1 cup
Ground turkey	1 pound
Onions, chopped	½ cup
White rice, uncooked	1 cup
Tomato sauce	2 cups
Garlic powder	½ teaspoon
Ground oregano	½ teaspoon
Preparation time:	10 minutes
Cooking time:	60 minutes

1. Place shredded cabbage in a lightly greased 2-quart casserole dish.
2. In skillet cook turkey until browned and no longer pink in color. Add chopped onions; stir occasionally and cook 3 minutes. Add uncooked rice to cooked turkey.
3. Place turkey-rice mixture over cabbage in casserole dish.
4. Combine tomato sauce, garlic, and oregano. Pour over cooked turkey.
5. Cover and bake at 350°F about 1 hour.

Per serving:
Calories   380
Total fat   11 grams
Saturated fat   3 grams
Cholesterol   77 milligrams
Sodium   829 milligrams

Reprinted from USDA's *Recipes and Tips for Healthy, Thrifty Meals* at http://www.usda.gov/cnpp/Pubs/Cookbook/thriftym.pdf, page 38.

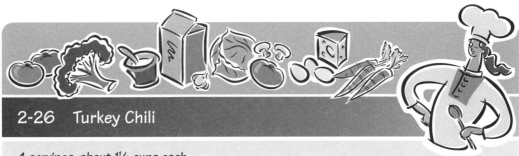

2-26   Turkey Chili

4 servings, about 1½ cups each

Ground turkey	1 pound
Onion, minced	¾ cup
Margarine	2 tablespoons
Water	3 cups
Garlic powder	½ teaspoon
Chili powder	1 tablespoon
Dry parsley flakes	1 tablespoon
Paprika	1 teaspoon
Dry mustard	2 teaspoons
Canned red kidney beans, drained	1 15½-ounce can
Tomato paste	1 6-ounce can
Pearl barley	½ cup
Cheddar cheese, shredded	¾ cup

Preparation time: 30 minutes

Cooking time: 70 minutes

1. In large saucepan, cook turkey and onions in margarine until turkey is browned and no longer pink in color, about 9 minutes. Drain; return turkey and onions to pan.
2. Add remaining ingredients except the cheese to turkey mixture; bring to boil, stirring frequently. Cover, reduce heat, and simmer 30 minutes, stirring occasionally.
3. Uncover and simmer 30 minutes, stirring occasionally.
4. Serve over cooked macaroni.
5. Sprinkle 3 tablespoons of cheese over each serving of chili.

Per serving:

Calories	540
Total fat	26 grams
Saturated fat	9 grams
Cholesterol	104 milligrams
Sodium	579 milligrams

Reprinted from USDA's *Recipes and Tips for Healthy, Thrifty Meals* at http://www.usda.gov/cnpp/Pubs/Cookbook/thriftym.pdf, page 39.

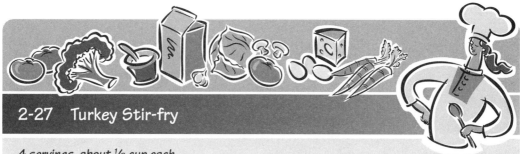

2-27   Turkey Stir-fry

4 servings, about ½ cup each

Chicken bouillon cube	1
Hot water	½ cup
Soy sauce	2 tablespoons
Cornstarch	1 tablespoon
Vegetable oil	2 tablespoons
Garlic powder	½ teaspoon
Turkey, cubed	1 pound
Carrots, thinly sliced	1¾ cups
Zucchini, sliced	1 cup
Onions, thinly sliced	½ cup
Hot water	¼ cup

Preparation time: 15 minutes

Cooking time: 10 minutes

1. Combine chicken bouillon cube and hot water to make broth; stir until dissolved.
2. Combine broth, soy sauce, and cornstarch in small bowl, set aside.
3. Heat oil in skillet over high heat. Add garlic and turkey. Cook, stirring, until turkey is thoroughly cooked and no longer pink in color.
4. Add carrots, zucchini, onion, and water to cooked turkey. Cover and cook, stirring occasionally, until vegetables are tender-crisp, about 5 minutes. Uncover, bring turkey mixture to boil. Cook until almost all liquid has evaporated.
5. Stir in cornstarch mixture. Bring to boil, stirring constantly until thickened.

Note: Serve over steamed rice.

Per serving:
Calories	195
Total fat	9 grams
Saturated fat	2 grams
Cholesterol	44 milligrams
Sodium	506 milligrams

Reprinted from USDA's _Recipes and Tips for Healthy, Thrifty Meals_ at http://www.usda.gov/cnpp/Pubs/Cookbook/thriftym.pdf, page 40.

2-28 Turkey Patties

4 servings, 1 patty each

Ground turkey	1 pound + 4 ounces
Bread crumbs	1 cup
Egg	1
Green onions, chopped	¼ cup
Prepared mustard	1 tablespoon
Margarine	1½ tablespoons
Chicken broth	½ cup

Preparation: 15 minutes

Cooking time: 10 minutes

1. Mix ground turkey, bread crumbs, egg, onions, and mustard in large bowl. Shape into 4 patties, about ½-inch thick.
2. Melt margarine in large skillet over low heat. Add patties and cook, turning once to brown other side. Cook until golden brown outside and white inside, about 10 minutes. Remove from skillet and place onto plate.
3. Add chicken broth to skillet, and boil over high heat until slightly thickened, about 1 to 2 minutes. Pour sauce over patties.
4. Serve on buns.

Per serving:

Calories	305
Total fat	18 grams
Saturated fat	5 grams
Cholesterol	149 milligrams
Sodium	636 milligrams

Reprinted from USDA's *Recipes and Tips for Healthy, Thrifty Meals* at http://www.usda.gov/cnpp/Pubs/Cookbook/thriftym.pdf page, 41.

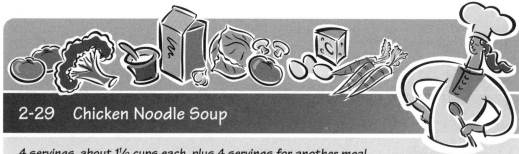

2-29   Chicken Noodle Soup

4 servings, about 1½ cups each, plus 4 servings for another meal

Vegetable oil	1 teaspoon
Onion, minced	½ cup
Carrots, diced	½ cup
Celery, sliced	½ cup
Garlic powder	½ teaspoon
Flour	⅛ cup
Dried oregano flakes	¼ teaspoon
Chicken broth, reduced sodium	3 cups
Potatoes, peeled, diced	2 cups
Chicken, cooked chopped	¼ cup
Whole milk*	½ cup
Noodles, yolk-free, enriched, uncooked	1 cup

Preparation time: 25 minutes

Cooking time: 35 to 40 minutes

1. Heat oil over medium heat in large saucepan. Add minced onions, carrots, celery, and garlic powder. Cook until onions are tender, about 3 to 5 minutes.
2. Sprinkle flour and oregano over vegetables; cook about 1 minute.
3. Stir in chicken broth and potatoes. Cover and cook until tender, about 20 minutes.
4. Add chicken, milk, and noodles. Cover and simmer until noodles are tender, about 10 minutes.

Per serving:

Calories	205
Total fat	4 grams
Saturated fat	1 grams
Cholesterol	8 milligrams
Sodium	107 milligrams

---

*Total fat and calorie content can be reduced by substituting skim milk.

Reprinted from USDA's Recipes and Tips for Healthy, Thrifty Meals at http://www.usda.gov/cnpp/Pubs/Cookbook/thriftym.pdf, page 45.

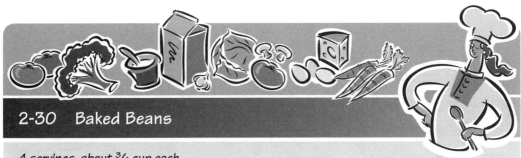

2-30   Baked Beans

4 servings, about ¾ cup each

Canned vegetarian beans	3 cups
Catsup	¼ cup
Brown sugar	2 tablespoons

Preparation time: 5 minutes

Cooking time: 30 minutes

1. In small (1 quart) casserole dish, combine beans, catsup, and brown sugar.
2. Cover and bake at 350°F until bubbly, about 30 minutes.

Per serving:

Calories	220
Total fat	1 gram
Saturated fat	trace
Cholesterol	0
Sodium	937 milligrams

Reprinted from USDA's *Recipes and Tips for Healthy, Thrifty Meals* at http://www.usda.gov/cnpp/Pubs/Cookbook/thriftym.pdf, page 48.

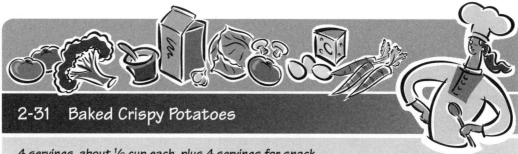

2-31   Baked Crispy Potatoes

4 servings, about ½ cup each, plus 4 servings for snack

Potatoes	4 pounds
Vegetable oil	4 tablespoons
Ground cumin	1 teaspoon
Red pepper	¼ teaspoon

Preparation time: 10 minutes

Cooking time: 20 minutes

1. Lightly coat a 7- × 12- × 1- inch pan with oil.
2. Wash potatoes; cut in half lengthwise.
3. Place cut sides of potatoes on the oiled pan; turn potatoes so that cut sides are facing up.
4. Mix cumin and red pepper together; sprinkle over potatoes.
5. Bake at 400°F until potatoes are golden brown and tender, about 20 minutes.

Per serving:
Calories	170
Total fat	5 grams
Saturated fat	1 gram
Cholesterol	0
Sodium	10 milligrams

Reprinted from USDA's *Recipes and Tips for Healthy, Thrifty Meals* at http://www.usda.gov/cnpp/Pubs/Cookbook/thriftym.pdf, page 49.

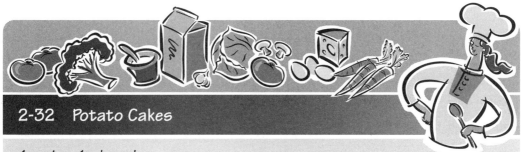

2-32 Potato Cakes

4 servings, 1 cake each

New potatoes, cooked, peeled, mashed	2 cups
Egg	1
Flour	1 tablespoon
Whole milk	2 tablespoons
Vegetable oil	¼ cup

Preparation time: 10 minutes

Cooking time: 5 minutes

1. Mix mashed potatoes, egg, flour, and milk thoroughly.
2. Shape into flat cakes, about ½ inch thick.
3. Heat oil in skillet.
4. Add potato cakes to hot skillet. Cook until golden brown and thoroughly heated.

Per serving:

Calories	210
Total fat	15 grams
Saturated fat	3 grams
Cholesterol	54 milligrams
Sodium	222 milligrams

Reprinted from USDA's *Recipes and Tips for Healthy, Thrifty Meals* at http://www.usda.gov/cnpp/Pubs/Cookbook/thriftym.pdf, page 50.

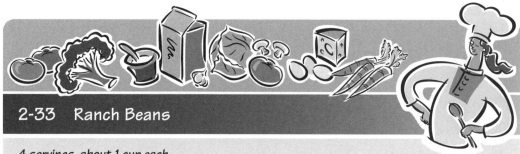

2-33   Ranch Beans

4 servings, about 1 cup each

Green pepper, chopped	¼ cup
Canned vegetarian beans	1¾ cups
Canned kidney beans, red, drained	1¾ cups
Catsup	2 tablespoons
Molasses	2 tablespoons
Dried onion	½ teaspoon

Preparation time: 5 minutes

Cooking time: 5 to 10 minutes

Conventional Method

1. Place all ingredients in sauce pan and heat thoroughly, about 10 minutes

Microwave Method

1. Place all ingredients in microwave–safe bowl. Cover with waxed paper. Cook on high; stirring every 2 minutes; cook about 5 minutes

Per serving:
Calories	240
Total fat	1 gram
Saturated fat	trace
Cholesterol	0
Sodium	916 milligrams

Reprinted from USDA's *Recipes and Tips for Healthy, Thrifty Meals* at http://www.usda.gov/cnpp/Pubs/Cookbook/thriftym.pdf, page 51.

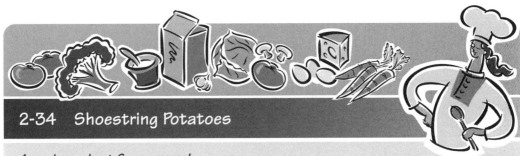

2-34   Shoestring Potatoes

4 servings, about 6 ounces each

Potatoes	1½ pounds
Vegetable oil	3 tablespoons
Salt	¼ teaspoon
Pepper	¼ teaspoon

Preparation time: 15 minutes

Cooking time: 30 minutes

1. Preheat oven to 450°F.
2. Wash potatoes; cut lengthwise into thin strips.
3. Combine remaining ingredients in plastic bag. Put potatoes in single layer on baking sleet.
4. Bake until crisp and golden, about 30 minutes.

Per serving:

Calories	255
Total fat	14 grams
Saturated fat	2 grams
Cholesterol	0
Sodium	156 milligrams

Reprinted from USDA's *Recipes and Tips for Healthy, Thrifty Meals* at http://www.usda.gov/cnpp/Pubs/Cookbook/thriftym.pdf, page 53.

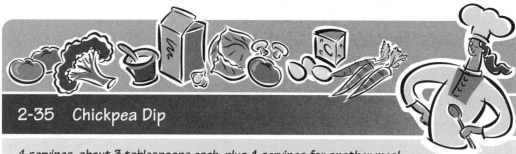

2-35   Chickpea Dip

4 servings, about 3 tablespoons each, plus 4 servings for another meal or snack

Canned chickpeas, drained	1 can (12½ oz)
Vegetable oil	2 tablespoons
Lemon juice	1 tablespoon
Onions, chopped	2 tablespoons
Salt	½ teaspoon

Preparation time: 10 minutes

1. Mash chickpeas in a small bowl until they are smooth.
2. Add oil and lemon juice; stir to combine.
3. Add chopped onions and salt.
4. Serve on bread or crackers.

Note: *Garbanzo bean is another name for chickpea.*

Per serving:
Calories   90
Total fat   4 grams
Saturated fat   trace
Cholesterol   0
Sodium   148 milligrams

Reprinted from USDA's *Recipes and Tips for Healthy, Thrifty Meals* at http://www.usda.gov/cnpp/Pubs/Cookbook/thriftym.pdf, page 54.

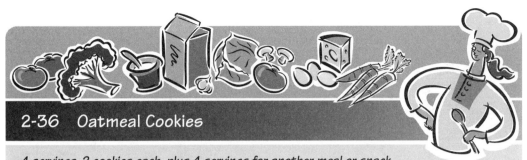

2-36   Oatmeal Cookies

4 servings, 2 cookies each, plus 4 servings for another meal or snack

Sugar	³⁄₄ cup
Margarine	2 tablespoons
Egg	1
Canned applesauce	¼ cup
Low-fat (1%) milk	2 tablespoons
Flour	1 cup
Baking soda	¼ teaspoon
Ground cinnamon	½ teaspoon
Quick rolled oats	1 cup + 2 tablespoons

Preparation time: 20 minutes

Cooking time: 13 to 15 minutes each batch

1. Preheat oven to 350°F and lightly grease cookie sheets.
2. In a large bowl, use an electric mixer on medium speed to mix sugar and margarine. Mix until well blended, about 3 minutes.
3. Slowly add egg; mix on medium speed 1 minute. Gradually add applesauce and milk; mix on medium speed, 1 minute. Scrape sides of bowl.
4. In another bowl, combine flour, baking soda, and cinnamon. Slowly add to applesauce mixture; mix on low speed until blended, about 2 minutes. Add rolled oats and blend 30 seconds on low speed. Scrape sides of bowl.
5. Drop by teaspoonfuls onto cookie sheet, about 2 inches apart.
6. Bake until lightly browned, about 13 to 15 minutes. Remove from baking sheet while still warm. Cool on wire rack.

Per serving:

Calories	215
Total fat	4 grams
Saturated fat	1 gram
Cholesterol	27 milligrams
Sodium	84 milligrams

Reprinted from USDA's *Recipes and Tips for Healthy, Thrifty Meals* at http://www.usda.gov/cnpp/Pubs/Cookbook/thriftym.pdf, page 64.

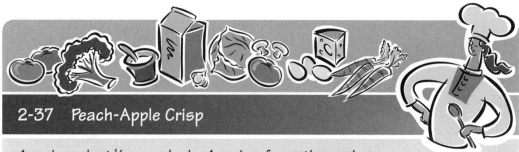

2-37   Peach-Apple Crisp

4 servings, about ½ cup each, plus 4 servings for another meal

Canned sliced peaches, light syrup pack, drained	20 ounces
Apples, tart, peeled, sliced	2 medium
Vanilla	½ teaspoon
Ground cinnamon	¼ teaspoon
Flour	¾ cup + 3 tablespoons
Brown sugar, packed	¼ cup
Margarine, chilled	3 tablespoons

Preparation time: 20 minutes

Cooking time: 20 minutes

1. Preheat oven to 350°F. Lightly grease 9- × 9- × 2-inch casserole dish.
2. Combine peaches, apples, vanilla, and cinnamon in a bowl. Toss well and spread evenly in greased casserole dish.
3. Combine flour and sugar in small bowl. Cut in margarine with two knives until the mixture resembles coarse meal.
4. Sprinkle flour mixture evenly over fruit.
5. Bake until lightly browned and bubbly, about 20 minutes.

Per serving:
Calories	175
Total fat	5 grams
Saturated fat	1 gram
Cholesterol	0
Sodium	57

Reprinted from USDA's *Recipes and Tips for Healthy, Thrifty Meals* at http://www.usda.gov/cnpp/Pubs/Cookbook/thriftym.pdf, page 65.

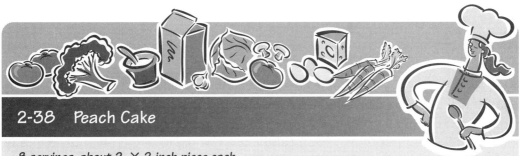

2-38   Peach Cake

8 servings, about 2- × 2-inch piece each

Canned peaches, light syrup pack, drained and chopped	2¼ cup (29 ounce)
Sugar	½ cup
Flour	1 cup
Egg	1
Baking soda	1 teaspoon
Vegetable oil	2 tablespoons
Vanilla	1 teaspoon
Brown sugar, firmly packed	2 tablespoons
Whole milk	2 teaspoons

Preparation time: 20 minutes

Cooking time: 30 to 35 minutes

1. Preheat oven to 350°F. Lightly grease 8- × 8-inch pan.
2. Spread peaches in baking pan. Mix remaining ingredients, except brown sugar and milk, together in mixing bowl; spread over top of peaches.
3. Bake until toothpick inserted into cake comes out clean, about 30 to 35 minutes.
4. For topping, combine brown sugar and milk in small bowl. Drizzle mixture on top of cake; return cake to oven, and bake 2 to 3 minutes.
5. Cut into 8 pieces.

Per serving:

Calories	205
Total fat	4 grams
Saturated fat	1 gram
Cholesterol	27 milligrams
Sodium	171 milligrams

Reprinted from USDA's *Recipes and Tips for Healthy, Thrifty Meals* at http://www.usda.gov/cnpp/Pubs/Cookbook/thriftym.pdf, page 66.

Flaxseeds are a rich source of alpha-linolenic acid, the precursor to omega-3 fatty acids, a fat the body cannot make. Cooking with flaxseed is one way to get more of these potentially healthful oils. Flaxseed, a small, reddish-brown seed, can be used whole to add crunch to recipes or ground and blended with flour in baked goods. Flaxseed oil can be used to replace other oils in baked goods. Most bakers reduce the total oil called for when switching vegetable oil for flaxseed.

Safety: Flaxseed is a source of fiber that can have a laxative effect when consumed in large doses. For more information about flaxseed go to these two reputable sites: webMD at www.webmd.com or The Mayo Clinic at www.mayoclinic.com.

Walnut Oatmeal Flaxseed Cookies

Soft margarine	1 cup
Granulated sugar	½ cup
Brown sugar	1 cup
Eggs	2 or 1 egg and three egg whites
Vanilla	1 teaspoon
Ground flaxseed	½ cup
All-purpose flour	1 cup
King Arthur White Whole Wheat Flour or whole wheat pastry flour*	1 cup
Baking powder	1½ teaspoon
Oatmeal	1 cup
Walnuts, chopped	1½ cup

1. Preheat oven to 350°F.
2. Cream together the margarine and sugars until light and fluffy.
3. Beat in eggs (or egg whites) and vanilla.
4. Mix together dry ingredients and add to egg mixture. Stir until blended.
5. Drop by spoonfuls (about 2 tablespoons) on an ungreased baking sheet, 2 inches apart. Bake 10 to 12 minutes.

* King Arthur White Whole Wheat Flour is available at most markets. If whole wheat flour is not available use a total of 2 cups of all purpose flour and omit the whole wheat flour.

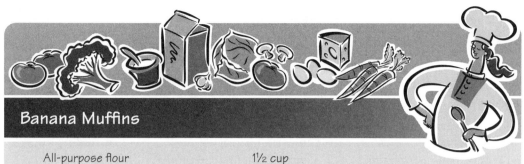

Banana Muffins

All-purpose flour	1½ cup
Wheat germ	¼ cup
Ground flaxseed	¾ cup
Sugar	¾ cup
Baking powder	1½ teaspoon
Salt	¼ teaspoon
Eggs	2 or 1 egg and 3 egg whites
Canola oil	2 tablespoons
Mashed ripe banana (at least two)	1 cup

1. Preheat oven to 350°F and lightly oil 12 muffin tins or line with muffin liners.
2. Mix together flour, ground flaxseed, sugar, baking powder, baking soda, and salt in a bowl.
3. Beat together eggs and oil, blend in mashed banana; mix until smooth.
4. Stir egg mixture into dry mixture blend until all ingredients are wet but do not over mix.
5. Pour into muffin pans and bake until done 15 to 18 minutes.

Whole grains are the tiny seeds of tall grasses. Barley, oats, rye, brown rice, and corn are the most familiar grains, but a much broader and delicious selection is available from which to choose. The term "whole grain" means the kernel is not refined; it has not had its outside layer removed. This outside protective coating carries the fiber, B vitamins, and antioxidants nutritionists find so beneficial. Whole grains can be consumed as a ready-to-eat whole grain cereal, whole grain bread or pasta, or as brown rice. They can also be used in soups and casseroles, and mixed in with vegetables or can be served as a substitute for potato, white rice, or plain white pasta. Below are cooking suggestions for a few popular grains.

BARLEY

Terrific in soups or as a replacement for rice in risotto, barley may help lower cholesterol.

To cook: Combine ½ cup barley in 2½ cups water or broth. Bring to a boil, stir, cover, and simmer for 45 minutes until tender. Add more liquid if it starts to look dry.

BULGUR (KASHA)

Nutty flavor, delicious mixed with soups, bulgur can even replace meat in chili.

To cook: Combine 1 cup of bulgur with 2 cups water and salt to taste. Bring to a boil, stir, cover, and cook for 20 minutes or until tender.

CORNMEAL

A sweet, bland tasting grain, cornmeal is delicious when topped with tomato sauce or roasted vegetables and herbs.

To cook: Bring 4 cups salted water to a boil, slowly add 1 cup of cornmeal, stir constantly. Reduce heat and cook for 25 minutes until all water is absorbed and the cornmeal is soft, smooth, and creamy.

COUSCOUS

A small grain–shaped pasta, couscous cooks quickly and is delicious topped with sauces or cooked vegetables.

To cook: Bring 2 cups water or broth to a boil. Stir in ¾ cup of couscous. Remove from heat, cover, and let stand for 5 minutes until liquid is absorbed. Top with soft margarine before serving.

QUINOA (PRONOUNCED KEENWA)

A nutty tasting grain originally from South America.

To cook: Bring 2 cups water or broth to a boil and stir in 1 cup of quinoa and 1 teaspoon canola oil. Cover, reduce heat, and cook for 20 minutes until tender. Some people toast the grain before cooking to bring out more flavors.

BROWN RICE

Brown rice maintains its color because the outside bran layer is intact; the bran layer is the reason brown rice takes longer to cook than white rice.

To cook: Combine 1 cup of brown rice in 2½ cups water or broth with 1 teaspoon canola or olive oil. Bring to a boil, stir, cover, reduce heat to low, and cook for 45 minutes until soft and tender. Add more liquid if it starts to look dry.

WHEAT BERRY

Wheat berries are whole wheat kernels that have a chewy, nutty texture.

To cook: Combine 1 cup of rinsed wheat berries in 2½ cups water or broth, 1 teaspoon canola or olive oil. Bring to a boil, stir, cover, reduce heat to low, and cook for 45 minutes until soft and tender. Add more liquid if it starts to look dry.

REFERENCES

Putnam, J., Kantor, L. S., Allhouse, J. (2004). Per capita food supply trends: Progress toward dietary guidelines. *Food Review, 23*(3), 2–14.

Ressel, G. V. (2002). American Cancer Society releases guidelines on nutrition and physical activity for cancer prevention. *American Family Physician, 66* (8), 1555, 1559–1560,1562.

United States Department of Agriculture. (1993). U.S. Department of Agriculture and Human Nutrition Information Service: *Food guide background and development.* Miscellaneous publication no. 1514. Washington, DC: U.S. Government Printing Office.

United States Department of Agriculture. (2000). U.S. Department of Agriculture and US Department of Health and Human Services. *Nutrition and your health: Dietary guidelines for Americans* (5th ed.). Washington, DC: U.S. Government Printing Office.

United States Department of Agriculture. CNPP (2000). U.S. Department of Agriculture, Center for Nutrition Policy and Promotion. *Recipes and tips for healthy, thrifty meals.* www.usda.gov/cnpp/Pubs/Cookbook/thriftym.pdf. Accessed May 18, 2004.

Willett, W., Stampfer, M. (2003). Rebuilding the food pyramid. *Scientific American, 288*(1), 64–71.

Supplements and Dietary Reference Intakes: Vitamins, Minerals, and Macronutrients

SUPPLEMENTS: HOW TO GUIDE PATIENTS

The number of adults using vitamin or mineral supplements increased from 23.2% in 1987 to 33.9% in 2000 (Millen, Dodd, & Subar, 2004). In addition, approximately 25% of adults reported using an herb within the past 12 months to treat a medical condition. Retail sales increased from $1 billion in 1994 to $4 billion in 1998 (Bent, & Ko, 2004). The popularity of herbs and vitamin supplements is clearly on the rise and health care providers need up-to-date information to answer questions about their use.

Herbs

Providing patients with accurate answers about the safe and effective use of medicinal herbs is not easy. "Of the top ten herbs sold in the United States, only four—garlic, ginkgo biloba, saw palmetto, and St. John's Wort—are likely to be effective, based on systematic reviews of randomized controlled trials" (Bent et al. p. 483). In addition to the lack of sound evidence on safety and efficacy, consumers incorrectly assume that the government is required to approve the safety of an herb before it can be sold. Since the Dietary Supplement Health and Education Act was passed in 1994, dietary supplements have been classified neither as drugs nor as food additives, but labeled "dietary supplements" (DSHEA 1994). Unlike pharmaceutical companies, which must convince the U.S. Food and Drug Administration (FDA) that their drugs are safe and effective before they go to market, and that their benefits justify their risk, manufacturers of dietary supplements do not need to prove that they are either safe or effective.

One source of reliable information about herbs is the compendium of herbal monographs developed by

The German Commission E (Blumenthal, Goldberg, Gruenwald, Hall, et al., 2000). Another is the non-profit trade organization, American Herbal Products Association (www.ahpa.org). This association has developed a safety rating scale for herbal products ranging from a source of 1 to 4. Clinicians can ask patients to look for a product's safety rating before they use it (Box 3-1). A list of herbs with the potential to cause harm is shown in Box 3-2. The FDA keeps a list of supplements that consumers are advised not to use at their Web site (www.cfsan.fda.gov/%7Edms/ds-warn.html) and Fact Sheets on Dietary Supplements can be found at http://dietary-supplements.info.nih.gov/

In addition, a list of web pages providing reliable information about herbs can be found in Box 3-3 and a list of the 11 most popular herbs, including comments about their safety and efficacy, can be found in Box 3-4.

As a result of the increasing interest in alternative treatments (including herbs) the National Institutes of Health (NIH) created the Alternative Medicine Center, now called the National Center for Complementary and Alternative Medicine (NCCAM). The center explores many therapies, including naturopathy, chiropractic, homeopathy, traditional Oriental medicine, and phytotherapy (the use of botanicals as medicine). The center can be accessed at http://www.nccam.nih.gov. It is a good source for patient education materials and it provides access to ongoing studies.

Advising Patients About the Use of Supplements

The following guidelines can be useful when working with clients who use herbs and vitamin or mineral supplements. Clinicians must keep in mind that, unlike medications, dietary supplements are presumed to be safe until the U.S. FDA receives reports

---

BOX 3-1 ■ *American Herbal Products Association's Botanical Safety Rating Classification*

Classification	Class definition
Class 1	Herbs that can be safely consumed when used appropriately
Class 2	Herbs for which the following use restrictions apply, unless otherwise directed by an expert qualified in the use of the described substance: (2a) For external use only (2b) Not to be used during pregnancy (2c) Not to be used while nursing (2d) Other specific use restrictions as noted
Class 3	Herbs for which significant data exist to recommend the following labeling: "To be used only under the supervision of expert qualified in the appropriate use of this substance." Labeling must include proper use information: dosage, contraindications, potential adverse effects and drug interactions, and any other relevant information related to safe use of the substance.
Class 4	Herbs for which insufficient data are available for classification.

Reprinted with permission from McGuffin, M., Hobbs, C., & Goldberg, A. (eds). (1995). American Herbal Product Association's Botanical Safety Handbook. Boca Raton: CRC Press.

BOX 3-2 ■ *Herbs to Avoid*

The Center for Science in the Public Interest listed the following eight products to be avoided because of serious health problems.
1. Aristolochic acid. Can be found in traditional Chinese medicines and herbs. Herbs that may contain aristolochic acid include bragantia, wallichii, asarum spp., cocculus spp., menispernum, dauricum, sinomenium, acutum, vladimiria, souyliei, akebia spp., clematis spp., diploclisia spp., saussurea lappa, AND stephania spp.
2. Chaparral
3. Comfrey
4. Ephedra
5. Kava
6. PC SPES and SPES
7. Tiratricol
8. Usnic acid

Sources: Schardt, D. (2003). Are your supplements safe? *Nutrition Action Healthletter, 30(9)*, 5.
Mahan, L. K., & Escott-Stump, S. (2004). *Krause's food, nutrition, & diet therapy* (11th ed., p. 1227). Philadelphia: W.B. Saunders.

BOX 3-3 ■ *Recommended Web Sites*

American Botanical Council	www.herbalgram.org
American Herbal Pharmacopeia	www.herbal-ahp.org
American Herbal Products Association	www.ahpa.org
Consumer Laboratories	www.consumerlab.com
The Natural Pharmacist	www.iherb.com
U.S. Food and Drug Administration Med Watch (for reporting dietary supplement adverse events)	www.fda.gov/medwatch

BOX 3-4 ■ *Commonly Used Herbal Medicines*

Aloe

Common use: dermatitis and wound healing.
Efficacy and comments: Limited evidence on efficacy; two studies found no effect; one found faster healing, another found it delayed wound healing (Bent and Ko, 2004).

Black Cohosh

Common use: to relieve symptoms of menopause.
Efficacy and comments: Efficacy unknown. The consumer group Center for Science in the Public Interest (CSPI) has asked the FDA to warn women that black cohosh may increase the risk of breast cancer metastasis and liver failure (Schardt, 2003).

Cranberry

Common use: to prevent or treat urinary tract infection.
Efficacy and comments: Recent research suggests cranberry juice may be beneficial in the treatment on urinary tract infection. Cranberry in excess may increase the risk of kidney stones and interfere with painkillers and antidepressants; caution susceptible patients. (Schardt, 2003).

Echinacea

Common use: to prevent or treat colds and boost the immune system.
Efficacy and comments: Not for people with autoimmune disorders (multiple sclerosis, lupus, rheumatoid arthritis). (Schardt, 2003). Not to exceed 8 weeks of continuous use. Six of eight studies reported a positive result. Two studies (one for treatment, one for prevention) found no benefit (Bent and Ko, 2004).

Garlic

Common use: lowers cholesterol. Also said to lower blood pressure, improve circulation, provide an anticancer effect, and act as an antibiotic.
Efficacy and comments: Not found to be efficacious in lowering cholesterol. Large quantities can cause stomachaches. Garlic may prolong bleeding. Caution the following patients about using garlic supplements: people who will or have had surgery, pregnant women before or after delivery, and individuals on blood thinning drugs or supplements (Schardt, 2003).

Ginkgo Biloba

Common use: to improve memory, improve circulation and to act as an antioxidant.
Efficacy and comments: Patients improved approximately 3% on the Alzheimer's Disease Assessment Scale (Bent and Ko, 2004). Because it may increase bleeding, avoid taking before surgery; monitor if patient is on anticoagulant medication. May interact with the antidepressant, trazodone, antidiabetes drugs, or thiazide diuretics (Schardt, 2003).

Ginseng

Common use: enhances energy and physical performance.
Efficacy and comments: Found not to be effective. Of seven studies, the four most recent found no improvement (Bent and Ko, 2004). Can cause insomnia, menstrual abnormalities, and breast tenderness. Women with breast cancer should be especially careful; in test tubes, ginseng increased breast cancer cell growth. May interact with the monoamine oxidase (MAO) inhibitor drugs, digitalis, insulin, oral hypoglycemics, warfarin (Coumadin) and ticlopidine (Ticlid), and any drug metabolized by the enzyme CYP 3A4, MAO (ask the pharmacist) (Schardt, 2003). "Not to be combined with phenelzine sulfate, estrogen therapy or corticosteroids or digoxin" (Sarubin, 2000, p. 427).

(continued)

BOX 3-4 ■ *Continued*

Saw Palmetto

Common use: to treat symptoms of enlarged prostrate.
Efficacy and comments: Improvement in self-rating of urinary tract symptoms (Bent and Ko, 2004). A large study is ongoing. Rarely causes gastrointestinal complaints. Long-term studies needed to fully evaluate safety. Patients with bleeding disorders or those about to have surgery should be particularly careful. May interact with aspirin, warfarin (Coumadin), heparin, or high doses of vitamin E and the supplement Ginkgo biloba (Schardt, 2003).

Soy Protein, Soy Isoflavone

Common use: to lower cholesterol, reduce risk of prostrate cancer, breast cancer and the risk of osteoporosis.
Efficacy and comments: soy protein (25 g) will decrease total cholesterol 5% to 9 %, and LDL-cholesterol 13%. Women with breast cancer should not use soy isoflavone supplements. Soy isoflavone may increase cell proliferation. No drug interactions have been reported (Sarubin, 2000).

St. John's Wort

Common use: to treat depression.
Efficacy and comments: Two trials found no benefit for patients with major depression. The herb may only be effective in cases of mild depression (Bent and Ko, 2004)."Not to be combined with antidepressant medications to prevent possible dangerous addictive effects" (Sarubin, 2000, p. 432). People sensitive to sunlight should be particularly cautious, especially fair skinned people, and those on sulfa drugs. May interact with methylphenidate (Ritalin), ephedrine, and caffeine. May increase the activity of protease inhibitors, digitalis, statin drugs, warfarin, chemotherapy drugs, oral contraceptives, tricyclic antidepressants, olanzapine and clozapine, theophylline, piroxicam (Feldene), omeprazole (Prilosec), or lansoprazole (Prevacid).

Valerian

Common use: enhances sleep, acts as antistress, antianxiety agent.
Efficacy and comments: Preliminary evidence comes from a few controlled human trials, but more research is needed. Not to be combined with sleep medications and not for individuals with liver disease (Sarubin, 2000). May cause morning drowsiness or impair attention for a few hours. Not to be used by people operating heavy equipment. May increase the activity of central nervous system depressants (Schardt, 2003).

Sources: Bent, S., & Ko, R. (2004). Commonly used herbal medicines in the United States: A review. *The American Journal of Medicine, 116,* 478–485.
Morelli, V., & Zoorob, R. J. (2000). Alternative therapies: Part II. Congestive heart failure and hypercholesterolemia. *American Family Physician, 62*(6),1325–1330.
Sarubin, A. (2000). *The Health Professional's Guide to Popular Dietary Supplements.* Chicago: The American Dietetic Association.
Schardt, D. (2003). Are your supplements safe? *Nutrition Action Health Letter, 30*(9), 1, 3–7.

of adverse effects. At particular risk for side effects are the elderly, children, individuals taking prescription and over-the-counter medications; those who are pregnant or breastfeeding; the chronically ill, and those with liver and kidney disease. It is important to note that little research has been done on the appropriate dosage of herbs and supplements for children.

1. Have clients bring all their supplements with them to their appointments.
2. Determine why each product is being taken.
3. Ask about dosage; try to determine if the dosage is both safe and effective by consulting the resources listed above.
4. Encourage patients to avoid combining products that have similar actions.
5. Encourage patients to keep within the recommended dosages on the label.
6. Encourage the use of products tested by Consumer Laboratories.

7. Check with a pharmacist for expected adverse reactions to prescription or over-the-counter medications.
8. Keep informed about dietary supplements.
9. Provide reliable resources to patients about supplements.
10. Consult the tolerable upper intake levels (UL) for specific nutrients listed in Box 3-7.

SUPPLEMENTS IN THE TREATMENT OF OSTEOARTHRITIS AND HYPERLIPIDEMIA

Osteoarthritis is the leading medical condition for which Americans seek alternative therapy. It accounts for more than 7 million physician visits per year (Arthritis, 2004). Box 3-5 provides an overview of supplements used in the treatment of osteoarthritis. The management of cholesterol through the use of alterna-tive therapies is also a common inquiry from patients. In the United States, an estimated 42 million people have total cholesterol greater than 240 mg/dL (Cholesterol, 2004). Natural supplements for the management of hypercholesterolemia abound, but not all are created equal. Despite initial positive findings, supplements including garlic, vitamin E, and guggulipid have failed to live up to their promise. Box 3-6 includes a list of products that may be beneficial in the treatment of patients with hyperlipidemia.

TOLERABLE UPPER INTAKE LEVELS OF VITAMINS AND MINERALS

Tolerable upper intake levels have been established for some nutrients for which adequate data are available. The Food and Nutrition Board of the Institute of Medicine, National Academy of Sciences has set these

---

BOX 3-5 ■ *Supplements Used in the Treatment of Osteoarthritis*

Glucosamine Sulfate

Derived from oyster and crab shells. Has mild anti-inflammatory effects, but may be more effective than placebo in relieving painful symptoms.

Usual dosage: 1,500 mg/d in three divided doses. Gastrointestinal discomfort is a possible side effect. Nonhuman studies suggest it may raise blood glucose levels. Must be taken for a month before any symptom relief is reported.

Chondroitin Sulfate

Derived from shark and cow cartilage. Studies suggest that chondroitin relieves symptoms of osteoarthritis. Usual dosage: 1,200 mg/d in three doses. Well tolerated. Patients with osteoarthritis report fewer gastrointestinal side effects than with nonsteroidal anti-inflammatory drugs (NSAID). Must be taken for a month or more before symptoms improve.

Glucosamine–Chondroitin Combinations

This combination has become extremely popular, but little evidence indicates that the combination is more effective than individual doses. Currently, the National Institutes of Health's Glucosamine/ Chondroitin Arthritis Intervention Trial (GAIT) is underway to compare efficacy of this combination. For more information contact http://altmed.od.nih.gov/news/ and search GAIT.

S-Adenosylmethionine (SAMe)

A naturally occurring compound obtained commercially from yeast-cell cultures, some evidence that it is more effective than placebo in treating pain and may be as effective as NSAID with fewer side effects. Reported dosage: 400 to 1,200 mg/d. Very costly. Side effects can include gastrointestinal discomfort, mainly as diarrhea.

Cetyl Myristoleate

Synthesized from cetyl alcohol and myristoleic acid. Some suggest that health-care providers not recommend this product until better clinical evidence is available (Morrelli, et al., 2003).

(*continued*)

BOX 3-5 ■ *Continued*

Ginger

Obtained from the root of the ginger plant. A recent comparison with ibuprofen showed the greater efficacy of ibuprofen. No side effects reported.

Dimethyl Sulfoxide (DMSO)

A sulfur-containing product obtained from wood pulp, used topically. Daily use of a DMSO gel for 3 weeks provided pain relief. Usual dosage: a daily application of 25% topical gel. Available as gel, liquid, or roll-on. Skin rash and pruritus have been reported. Drug interactions unknown.

Boron

An element found in bones and joints. In areas of the world where boron intake is low, the incidence of osteoarthritis is 20% to 70%. In populations where intake is high (3 to 10 mg), the incidence of osteoarthritis is zero to 10%. No dietary reference intake (DRI) has been established for boron, but the tolerable upper limit (UL) is 20 mg for adults. Boron is considered potentially dangerous and pregnant and lactating women are discouraged from using it (Sarubin, 2000).

Avocado/Soybean Unsaponifiables

A daily dose of 300 mg reduced NSAID use and provided long-term symptomatic relief of pain. Appears to be particularly useful in patients with hip osteoarthritis. No side effects known.

Sources: Morelli, V., Naquin, C., Weaver, V. (2003). Alternative therapies for traditional disease states: Osteoarthritis. *American Family Physician, 15,* 235–241. Can be accessed at www.aafp.org/afp/20030115/339.html.)
Sarubin, A. (2000). *The Health Professionals Guide to Popular Dietary Supplements.* Chicago: American Dietetic Association.

---

levels. Values are gauged to protect the most sensitive persons in the population and, unless stated otherwise, the upper level represents total intake from food, drinks, and supplements. More information can be found at the Institute of Medicine of the National Academy of Sciences (http://www.iom.edu/report) (Box 3-7 and Box 3-8).

DIETARY REFERENCE INTAKES

The first Recommended Dietary Allowances (RDA) were published in 1941 and have been updated ten times by the National Academy of Sciences. In 1995, the Food and Nutrition Board began a comprehensive review of the RDA and replaced them with the Dietary Reference Intakes (DRI).

The DRI include four separate reference values: RDA, adequate intakes (AI), UL, and estimated average requirements (EAR). RDA is the average daily dietary intake of a nutrient that will meet the requirement of nearly all healthy persons.

AI is determined when an RDA cannot be established. The AI is based on observed intakes of the nutrient in a healthy group of persons.

Tolerable UL is the highest daily intake of a nutrient that is not likely to pose a health risk. See Section 7 for more information on tolerable UL.

EAR is the amount of a nutrient that is estimated to meet the nutrition needs of half of all individuals in a population. EAR are for use with groups or populations and are not included in this text.

This section is designed to be a quick and easy reference to use when patients ask about a specific nutrient. Information is included on vitamins, minerals, and the macronutrients, including carbohydrate, fat, and protein. Under each nutrient heading, a brief description of the nutrient's function is given, followed by the DRI for individuals by age and a list of the nutrient content in selected foods.

Foods selected in these lists are included either because they are a good source of the nutrient or because they demonstrate how processing or cooking affects nutrient content. Individuals should use the information in these tables as approximations. They can provide an overview but should not be used as a sole resource. Anyone told to follow a diet modified in one particular nutrient should seek individual nutrition counseling. The recommendations made are for groups of people and are not to be used for individual medical treatment. Those individuals on a restricted

BOX 3-6 ■ *Supplements to Lower Cholesterol*

Cholestin (Red Rice Yeast)

Cholestin can provide a cost-effective alternative to lowering lipids; it lowers LDL cholesterol by 22% (Schardt, 2004; Morrelli and Zoorob, 2000). Used for centuries in china, Cholestin is made from rice fermented with red yeast. In 1998, the FDA redefined Cholestin as an unapproved drug because it contained lovastatin, the same active ingredient found in the prescription drug Mevacor (FDA, 1998). Cholestin has been reformulated to meet FDA guidelines, causing some concern that the Cholestin sold today may not be as effective at lowering LDL cholesterol as the original. Patients taking Cholestin should monitor liver function as well as creatine kinase as do statin users.

Stanols /Sterols

Plant sterols (also called phytosterols), which occur naturally, are isolated from soybean oil. Plant sterols are poorly absorbed and compete with cholesterol for absorption in the intestine, resulting in lower levels of LDL cholesterol. Intakes of 2 g/d lowered LDL by 9% to 20%. These phytosterols can be obtained in margarinelike "cholesterol-lowering" spreads sold as Benecol, Take Control, and Smart Balance Omega Plus. Advise patients to choose a spread that has the most phytosterols with the fewest calories. Heart-wise, fortified orange juice contains 1g phytosterol per 8 ounces. Patients will need to take the dose recommended on each product label to obtain therapeutic results. A plant sterol supplement called Beta Sitosterol or Cholest-off is available in pharmacies and easy to use. Plant sterols can be taken with statins, because they work in different ways.

Flaxseed

Whole or ground flaxseed (not oil*) can lower LDL cholesterol by 15%. Flaxseed contains both fiber and omega-3 fatty acids. A dose of 3 to 4 tablespoons contains 160 calories. Patients on a low-cholesterol diet, consuming 20 g of flaxseed fiber, reduced total cholesterol by 4.6% and LDL by 7.6%. Direct patients to Handout 2-39, *Cooking with Flaxseed*.

Walnuts

The addition of eight walnuts per day may lower cholesterol by 4%. Alert patients to the calorie content of walnuts (200 calories in eight whole nuts). Recommend they substitute the calories in nuts by reducing calories from cooking fats. Test lipids after 6 weeks.

Soy Protein

An intake of 25 g/d of soy protein can reduce LDL cholesterol 13% and total cholesterol by 5% to 9%. Soy protein may be most effective in people with the highest cholesterol levels. Encourage patients to use soy protein sources over animal sources, which will also reduce saturated fat intake. Encourage soy intake from soy foods, not soy isoflavone, extracted from soybeans.

Sources of Soy Protein

1 cup soy milk	3 to 10 g soy protein
4 ounces tofu	5 to 13 g soy protein
½ cup textured soy protein	6 to 11 g soy protein
½ cup soy flour	20 g soy protein

---

* Conflicting research exists on the role flaxseed oil may play in the progression of prostate cancer. The Center for Science in the Public Interest recommends flaxseed oil not be used by individuals at high risk for prostate cancer. Liebman, B. (2004). Prostate cancer: more questions than answers. *Nutrition Action Health Letter, 31*(6), 1, 3–6.

(continued)

BOX 3-6 ■ *Continued*

Fiber

Water-soluble fiber (legumes, rolled oats, oat bran) and pectin (apples, grapefruit, oranges) lowers cholesterol. Psyllium seeds found in Metamucil (2 teaspoons contain 7 g soluble fiber) may lower LDL cholesterol when used daily.

Fish Oil

The National Cholesterol Education Project recommends eating fish twice per week. The American Heart Association recommends a serving of fish daily for those with known coronary heart disease (Covington, 2004). If fish is not consumed regularly, encourage patients to consider a fish oil supplement. They should look for a supplement containing 1,000 mg omega-3 fatty acid. Add the EPA and DHA in the capsule to determine how much is needed to reach 1,000 mg. Fish oils have a blood thinning effect and should be stopped before surgery.

Folic Acid, Vitamin B_6, Vitamin B_{12}

The blood levels of folic acid, and vitamins B_6, and B_{12} correlate inversely with homocysteine levels. Lower levels of homocysteine are associated with a lower risk for coronary artery disease. Patients should be encouraged to eat foods rich in these nutrients or take a multivitamin to meet their needs. The dietary reference intake for adults is 1.5 mg B_6, 2.4 μg B_{12}, and 400 μg folic acid. Refer patients to Handouts 3-4, 3-5, and 3-6 for good food sources of these nutrients.

Niacin (Best for Increasing HDL)

The recommended intake for adults from food is 20 mg/d. The therapeutic dose to raise HDL and lower triglycerides may be as high as to 3,000 mg/day. At this dose, patients must be supervised by a health-care provider. Starting at a low dose and increasing slowly may reduce side effects, which can be severe.

Sources:

American Heart Association. (2000). Nutrition Committee of the American Heart Association. 2000 AHA Dietary Guidelines. *Circulation ,102,* 2284–2299.

Consumer Laboratories: Product Review: Cholesterol-Lowering Supplements www.consumerlab.com/results/cholest.asp. Covington, M. B. (2004). Omega-3 fatty acids. *American Family Physician 70*(1), 133-140.

Food and Drug Administration. (1998). FDA determines Cholestin to be an unapproved drug 5/20/98. Available at: www.fda.gov/bbs/topics/ANSWERS/ANS00871.html. Accessed 9/204.

Heber, D., Yip, I., Ashley, J. M., Elashoff, D. A. , Elashoff, R. M., & Go, V. L. (1999). Cholesterol-lowering effects of a proprietary Chinese red-yeast-rice dietary supplement. *American Journal Clinical Nutrition, 69*(2), 231–236.

McGowan, M. P., and Chopra, J. M. (2002). *50 Ways to Lower Your Cholesterol: Everything You Need To Know.* New York: McGraw-Hill.

Morelli, V., & Zoorob, R. J. (2000). Alternative therapies: Part II. Congestive heart failure and hypercholesterolemia. *American Family Physician, 62*(6), 1326.

Schardt, D. (2004). The heart of the matter. *Nutrition Action Health Letter, 31*(3), 8, 11.

BOX 3-7 ■ *Tolerable Upper Intake Levels for Nutrients*

Vitamin A: Tolerable Upper Intake Levels by Age (as Preformed Vitamin A, μg/d)

Vitamin A refers to three preformed compounds known as retinol, retinal, and retinoic acid. In addition to the preformed vitamin A found in animal products, vitamin A can be metabolized in the body from carotenoids. The most familiar of these is called beta carotene. Vitamin A can be measured several ways, depending on the form being measured. The DRI is in micrograms; the content in food is often measured in retinol equivalents (RE) or found on food labels as International Units (IU). The vitamin A content of foods is measured as retinol activity equivalents (RAE). One RAE equals the activity of 1 microgram of retinol. 1 RAE = 3.33 IU of vitamin A activity on a label. IU is an outdated term but still used on labels. To calculate RAE from RE of provitamin A carotenoids in foods, divide the RE by 2. For preformed vitamin A in foods or supplements and for provitamin A carotenoids in supplements, 1 RE = 1RAE.

Birth to 3 years	600
4–8 years	900
9–13 years	1,700
14–18 years	2,800
19–>70 years	3,000

Pregnancy and Lactation

≤18 years	2,800
19–50 years	3,000

Safety: Vitamin A at doses 10 times the RDA (not beta carotene) can be toxic.

Vitamin C: Tolerable Upper Intake Levels by Age (mg/d)

0–12 months	Not determined. Available data of adverse affects in this age group lacking and with concern exists of the ability to handle excess amounts. Source of intake should be from food only to prevent high levels of intake.
1–3 years	400
4–8 years	650
9–13 years	1,200
14–18 years	1,800
19–>70 years	2,000

Pregnancy and Lactation

≤18 years	1,800
19–50 years	2,000

Safety: Not to be used by individuals with hemachromatosis.
Individuals with recurrent kidney stones should stay under 100 mg/d.
May interfere with blood tests and diagnostic tests.

Vitamin D: Tolerable Upper Intake Levels by Age (μg/d)

0–12 months	25
All other ages	50

Safety: Usually safe at doses <UL
Vitamin D is measured in micrograms (μg) and international units (IU). One μg cholecalciferol = 40 IU vitamin D. Vitamin D fortified milk has 10 μg cholecalciferol or 400 IU/quart.

(continued)

BOX 3-7 ■ *Continued*

Vitamin E: Tolerable Upper Intake Levels by Age (as α-tocopherol, mg/d)

The upper limit applies to synthetic forms obtained from supplements, fortified foods, or a combination of the two.

0–2 months	Not determined
1–3 years	200
4–8 years	300
9–13 years	600
14–18 years	800
19 to >70 years	1,000

Pregnancy and Lactation

≤18 years	1,800
19–50 years	2,000

Safety: May increase bleeding, not to be used in patients with blood coagulation disorders.

Niacin: Tolerable Upper Intake Levels by Age (mg/d)

(The UL for niacin applies to synthetic forms obtained from supplements, fortified foods, or a combination of the two).

0–12 months	Not determined
1–3 years	10
4–8 years	15
9–13 years	20
14–18 years	30
19–>70 years	35

Pregnancy and Lactation

≤18 years	30
19–50 years	35

Safety: Usually safe at levels <UL. Pharmacologic doses to treat dyslipidemia should be monitored.

Vitamin B₆: Tolerable Upper Intake Levels by Age (mg/d)

0–12 months	Not determined
1–3 years	30
4–8 years	40
9–13 years	60
14–18 years	80
19–>70 years	100

Pregnancy and Lactation

≤18 years	80
19–50 years	100

Safety: Generally regarded as safe at levels <UL. Long-term use at levels in the range of 500 to 5,000 mg has caused nerve damage.

Folate: Tolerable Upper Intake Levels by Age (μg/d)

The upper limit applies to synthetic forms obtained from supplements, fortified foods, or a combination of the two.

0–12 months	Not determined
1–3 years	300
4–8 years	400
9–13 years	600
14–18 years	800
19–>70 years	1000

BOX 3-7 ■ *Continued*

Pregnancy and Lactation

≤18 years	800
19–50 years	1000

Safety: Usually safe at levels <UL. Doses above 400 μg/d may mask a vitamin B_{12} deficiency.

Choline: Tolerable Upper Intake Levels by Age (g/d)

0–12 months	Not determined
1–3 years	1.0
4–8 years	1.0
9–13 years	2.0
14–18 years	3.0
19–>70 years	3.5

Pregnancy and Lactation

≤18 years	3.0
19–50 years	3.5

Boron: Tolerable Upper Intake Levels by Age (mg/d)

0–12 months	Not determined
1–3 years	3
4–8 years	6
9–13 years	11
14–18 years	17
19–>70 years	20

Pregnancy and Lactation

≤18 years	17
19–50 years	20

Safety: Potentially dangerous; avoid during pregnancy and lactation

Calcium: Tolerable Upper Intake Levels by Age (g/d)

0–12 months	Not determined
All other ages	2.5

Safety: Usually safe at levels <UL. Not to be used in patients with absorptive hypercalciuria, primary hyperthyroidism, or sarcoidosis. May interfere with the absorption of atenolol, salicylates, biphosphates, fluoride, iron and tetracycline.

Copper: Tolerable Upper Intake Levels by Age (μg/d)

0–12 months	Not determined
1–3 years	1,000
4–8 years	3,000
9–13 years	5,000
14–18 years	8,000
19–>70 years	10,000

Pregnancy and Lactation

≤18 years	8,000
19 –50 years	10,000

(continued)

BOX 3-7 ■ *Continued*

Fluoride: Tolerable Upper Intake Levels by Age (mg/d)

0–6 months	0.7
7–12 months	0.9
1–3 years	1.3
4–8 years	2.2
9–>70 years	10
Pregnancy and Lactation	10

Iodine: Tolerable Upper Intake Levels by Age (μg/d)

0–12 months	Not determined
1–3 years	200
4–8 years	300
9–13 years	600
14–18 years	900
19–>70 years	1,100

Pregnancy and Lactation

≤18 years	900
19–50 years	1,100

Iron: Tolerable Upper Intake Levels by Age (mg/d)

0–12 months	40
1–13 years	40
14–>70 years	45
Pregnancy and Lactation	45

Magnesium: Tolerable Upper Intake Levels by Age (From Nonfood only, mg/d)

0–12 months	Not determined
1–3 years	65
4–8 years	110
9–70 years	350
Pregnancy and Lactation	350
Safety: usually safe at doses <UL.	

Manganese: Tolerable Upper Intake Levels by Age (mg/d)

0–12 months	Not determined
1–3 years	2
4–8 years	3
9–13 years	6
14–18 years	9
19–>70 years	11

Pregnancy and Lactation

≤18 years	9
19–50 years	11

Molybdenum: Tolerable Upper Intake Levels by Age (μg/d)

0–12 months	Not determined
1–3 years	300
4–8 years	600

BOX 3-7 ■ *Continued*

9–13 years	1,100
14–18 years	1,700
19–>70 years	2,000

Pregnancy and Lactation

≤18 years	1,700
19–50 years	2,000

Nickel: Tolerable Upper Intake Levels by Age (mg/d)

0–12 months	Not determined
1–3 years	0.2
4–8 years	0.3
9–13 years	0.6
14–>70 years	1.0
Pregnancy and Lactation	1.0

Phosphorus: Tolerable Upper Intake Levels by Age (g/d)

0–12 months	Not determined
1–8 years	3
9–70 years	4
70+ years	3
Pregnancy	3.5
Lactation	4

Selenium: Tolerable Upper Intake Levels by Age (μg/d)

0–6 months	45
7–12 months	60
1–3 years	90
4–8 years	150
9–13 years	280
14–>70 years	400
Pregnancy and Lactation	400

Safety: Doses ≥750 mg/d are associated with toxic effects.

Zinc: Tolerable Upper Intake Levels by Age (mg/d)

0–6 months	4
7–12 months	5
1–3 years	7
4–8 years	12
9–13 years	23
14–18 years	34
19 –>70 years	40

Pregnancy and Lactation

≤18 years	34
19–50 years	40

Safety: Chronic ingestion (100 to 300 mg) may impair immune function, induce copper deficiency, and negatively affect cholesterol levels. Can cause nausea and vomiting in acute doses.

(continued)

BOX 3-7 ■ Continued

Sodium: Tolerable Upper Intake Levels by Age (g/d)

0–12 months	Not determined
1–3 years	1.5
4–8 years	1.9
9–13 years	2.2
14–>70 years	2.3
Pregnancy and Lactation	2.3

Information about safety is adapted from Sarubin, A. (2000). *The Health Professionals Guide to Popular Dietary Supplements.* Chicago: American Dietetic Association.

Tolerable Upper Intake information is adapted from the following reports:
Dietary Reference Intake for Calcium, Phosphorous, Magnesium, Vitamin D, and Fluoride (1997). Dietary Reference Intakes for Calcium, Phosphorous, Magnesium, Vitamin D, and Fluoride (1997). Dietary Reference Intakes for Thiamin, Riboflavin, Niacin, Vitamin B_6, Folate, Vitamin B_{12}, Pantothenic Acid, Biotin, and Choline (1998). Dietary Reference Intakes for Vitamins A, Vitamin K, Arsenic, Boron, Chromium, Copper, Iodine, Iron, Manganese, Molybdenum, Nickel, Silicon, Vanadium, and Zinc (2000). Dietary Reference Intakes for Vitamin C, Vitamin E, Selenium, and Carotenoids (2000). Dietary Reference Intakes for Energy, Carbohydrate, Fiber, Fat, Fatty Acids, Cholesterol, Protein, and Amino Acids (Macronutrients) (2002). Dietary Reference Intakes for Water, Potassium, Sodium, Chloride, and Sulfate (2004).
Food and Nutrition Board, Institute of Medicine, National Academy of Sciences.
National Academics Press. The complete dietary reference intake report, including tolerable upper intake levels, can be accessed at www.nap.edu.

---

diet may need to contact the USDA for more in-depth nutrient data or contact the food company directly for specific nutrient content (www.nal.usda.gov/fnic/food-comp/). This information is not intended to substitute for the advise or services of a trained profesional. If a patient needs to follow a low-sodium diet, a list of foods that contain sodium is informative but not adequate. This material can help answer questions until the patient sees a dietitian but it cannot and should not replace a referral.

BOX 3-8 ■ How to Choose a Multivitamin

1. Look for a multivitamin that contains 100% of the daily value for thiamin (B_1), riboflavin (B_2), D, E, and folic acid and contains 90 mg of vitamin C (75 mg for women).
2. Limit vitamin A. Look for a multivitamin that does not exceed the tolerable upper intake level listed in Box 3-7.
3. Look for some vitamin K (at least 20 μg); the recommended intake for women is 90 μg/d (eat extra green leafy vegetables to get the vitamin K you need) and the upper limit (UL) for vitamin K has not been determined. Not recommended for use with warfarin (Coumadin).
4. Look for minerals, including chromium (20 to 35 μg), copper (900 μg), selenium (55 μg), and zinc (11 mg; 8 mg for women).
5. Calcium and magnesium. To get the recommended intake from a supplement alone would make the pill too large to fit in one multivitamin. Instead, look for lower percentages of these minerals and eat calcium-rich foods (e.g., milk) or take a calcium supplement. For magnesium, eat whole grain cereal, bread, and pasta.
6. Avoid excesses. Refer to the UL for nutrients and do not exceed those amounts.

Source: Spin the Bottle: How to Pick a Multivitamin. *Nutrition Action Healthletter* January/February 2003. The article can be accessed at www.cspinet.org/nah/01_03/spin.pdf.

PATIENT EDUCATION HANDOUTS ABOUT NUTRIENTS (ADAPTED FROM THE DRI FOR INDIVIDUALS)

3-1	Thiamin
3-2	Riboflavin
3-3	Niacin
3-4	Vitamin B_6
3-5	Vitamin B_{12}
3-6	Folic Acid
3-7	Vitamin C
3-8	Vitamin A
3-9	Vitamin D
3-10	Vitamin E
3-11	Vitamin K
3-12	Pantothenic Acid
3-13	Calcium
3-14	Copper
3-15	Iron
3-16	Potassium
3-17	Iodine
3-18	Magnesium
3-19	Manganese
3-20	Selenium
3-21	Phosphorus
3-22	Zinc
3-23	Protein
3-24	Carbohydrate
3-25	Fat
3-26	Omega-3 and Omega-6 Fatty Acids
3-27	Fiber
3-28	Additional nutrients for which limited data are available: Arsenic, biotin, boron, choline, chromium, fluoride, molybdenum, silicon, vanadium

Thiamin (Vitamin B₁)

Thiamin helps to metabolize energy, maintain appetite, and keep the nervous system functioning properly. Thiamin occurs in many foods in moderate amounts. A deficiency may be common with liver disease or among people eating a diet that includes a lot of empty calorie foods or alcohol. To obtain the thiamin you need, eat a variety of nutritious foods. Good sources include brewers yeast, pork liver, peas, beans, and whole or enriched grains.

Recommended Daily Dietary Reference Intake for Thiamin

This table presents Recommended Dietary Allowances (RDA) in **bold type** and Adequate Intakes (AI) in regular type, followed by an asterisk (*) (in milligrams [mg]). RDA and AI may both be used as goals for individual intake.

Infants			*Males*			*Females*		
Birth to 6 months	0.2*		9–13 years	**0.9**		9–13 years	**0.9**	
7–12 months	0.3*		14–70 years	**1.2**		14–18 years	**1.0**	
						19–70+ years	**1.1**	
Children						Lactating	**1.4**	
						Pregnant	**1.4**	
1–3 years	**0.5**							
4–8 years	**0.6**							

Approximate Thiamin Content of Selected Foods (mg)

Grain Group

White bread, 1 slice	0.12
Whole wheat bread, 1 slice	0.10
All-Bran, Kellogg's, ½ cup	0.38
Cornflakes, Kellogg's, 1 cup	0.38
Total, General Mills, ¾ cup	1.5
Shredded wheat, 1 biscuit	0.06
Brown rice, cooked, 1 cup	0.19
White rice, cooked, 1 cup	0.15

Vegetable Group

Celery, 1 stalk	0.02
Green peas, frozen, cooked, ½ cup	0.23
Potato, 1 baked	0.22
Spinach, frozen, cooked, ½ cup	0.06
Tofu, ½ cup	0.1

Fruit Group

Apple, 1 raw	0.02
Orange, 1 raw	0.11
Orange juice, 1 cup	0.2
Peach, 1 medium	0.01
Raisins, ⅔ cup	0.16
Watermelon, 1 cup	0.13

Protein Group

Beef, 3½ oz	0.07
Cod, 3 oz	0.07
Chicken, 3½ oz	0.06
Egg, 1	0.03
Pork liver, 3½ oz	0.26
Black beans, cooked, 1 cup	0.42
Kidney beans, cooked, 1 cup	0.28
Lentils, cooked, 1 cup	0.33

Calcium Group

American cheese, 1 oz	0.01
Cheddar cheese, 1oz	0.01
Cottage cheese, ½ cup	0.02
Milk, whole, 1 cup	0.09
Milk, skim, 1 cup	0.09

Miscellaneous

Brewers yeast, 1 oz	4.43
Peanuts, 1 oz	0.1
Sunflower seeds, dry roasted, 1 oz	0.03
Wheat germ, ¼ cup	0.48

Riboflavin (Vitamin B$_2$)

Riboflavin is a water-soluble vitamin, part of the B complex vitamins. It is essential to energy metabolism and it helps keep skin and eyes healthy. The best sources of riboflavin are found in milk, yogurt, cottage cheese, meat, leafy green vegetables, whole grains, and in enriched rice, grains, and cereal.

Recommended Daily Dietary Reference Intake for Riboflavin

This table presents Recommended Dietary Allowances (RDA) in **bold type** and Adequate Intakes (AI) in regular type followed by an asterisk (*) (in milligrams [mg]). RDA and AI may both be used as goals for individual intake.

Infants		Males		Females	
Birth to 6 months	0.3*	14–70+ years	**1.3**	14–18	**1.0**
7–12 months	0.4*			19–70+ years	**1.1**
				Pregnant	**1.4**
Children				Lactating	**1.6**
1–3 years	**0.5**				
4–8 years	**0.6**				
9–13 years	**0.9**				

Approximate Riboflavin Content of Selected Foods (mg)

Grain Group		Protein Group	
All-Bran, Kellogg's, ½ cup	0.43	Ground beef, 3½ oz	0.32
Cornflakes, General Mills, 1 cup	0.43	Pork, 3½ oz	0.30
Oatmeal, 1 packet instant	0.28	Egg, 1	0.26
Spaghetti, 1 cup	0.14	Chicken, 3½ oz	0.20
White bread, 1 slice	0.09	Fish sticks, 1 oz	0.05
Whole wheat bread, 1 slice	0.06	Haddock, 3 oz	0.04
Brown rice, cooked, 1 cup	0.05	Lentils, 1 cup	0.14
White rice, cooked, 1 cup	0.02	Kidney beans, 1 cup	0.10

Vegetable Group		Fruit Group	
Spinach, cooked, ½ cup	0.16	Strawberries, 1 cup	0.1
Kale, cooked, ½ cup	0.05	Peach, 1 medium	0.04
		Orange juice, 1 cup	0.04
		Apple, raw, 1 medium	0.02
		Grapefruit, ½	0.02

Calcium Group

Milk, 1 cup	0.40
Cottage cheese, 1 cup	0.40
Yogurt, 1 cup	0.30
American cheese, 1 oz	0.10
Cheddar cheese, 1 oz	0.11

Miscellaneous

Cashews, 1 oz	0.06
Peanut butter, 2 tablespoons	0.03

Niacin, also called nicotinic acid, nicotinamide, and niacinamide, helps release energy and helps keep skin, nervous system, and digestive system functioning properly. Niacin can be made in the body from tryptophan, an amino acid that can act as a niacin precursor. Large doses of supplemental niacin can produce an uncomfortable effect known as "niacin flush." Niacin is used to treat atherosclerosis. When taking a niacin supplement, follow your doctor's recommendation. Best food sources of niacin include meat, poultry, fish, whole grain and enriched bread and cereal, nuts, and all foods containing protein. Milk and egg are a good source of tryptophan, the niacin precursor.

Recommended Daily Dietary Reference Intake for Niacin†

This table presents Recommended Dietary Allowances (RDA) in **bold type** and Adequate Intakes (AI) in regular type followed by an asterisk (*) (in milligrams [mg]). RDA and AI may both be used as goals for individual intake.

Infants		Males		Females	
Birth to 6 months	2.0*	14–70+ years	**16.0**	14–70+ years	**14.0**
7–12 months	4.0*			Pregnant	**18.0**
				Lactating	**17.0**
Children					
1–3 years	**6.0**				
4–8 years	**8.0**				
9–13 years	**12.0**				

Approximate Niacin Content of Selected Foods (mg)

Grain Group

Oatmeal, 1 packet instant	5.5
All-Bran, Kellogg's, ½ cup	5.0
Cornflakes, Kellogg's, 1 cup	5.0
Rice, brown cooked, 1 cup	3.0
Rice, white enriched, cooked, 1 cup	2.3
Bagel, 3½ inches	2.4
Macaroni, enriched, cooked, 1 cup	2.3
English muffin	2.2
Waffle, frozen, 1–4 inch	1.5
Tortilla, flour, 7–8 inch	1.3
Whole wheat bread, 1 slice	1.1
White, enriched bread, 1 slice	1.0
Stuffing, Stove Top, ½ cup	0.8
Muffin, blueberry, 2 oz	0.6

Vegetable Group

Asparagus, ½ cup	1.0
Broccoli, ½ cup	0.4
Carrot, ½ cup	0.4

Fruit Group

Orange juice, 1 cup	0.5
Apple, 1 medium	0.1
Banana, 1 medium	0.6

Calcium Group

Goat's milk, 1 cup	0.7
Soy milk, 1 cup	0.4
Cow's milk, 1 cup	0.2
Cheese, 1 oz	0

Protein Group

Beef, ground, 3½ oz	5.8
Chicken, 3½ oz	9.2
Pork, 3½ oz	4.9
Haddock, 3 oz	3.9
Egg, 1	0
Peanut butter, 2 tablespoons	4.0
Lentils, 1 cup	2.1
Almonds, 1 oz	1.0
Chickpeas, 1 cup	0.9

†As niacin equivalent (NE): 1 mg niacin = 60 mg tryptophan; 0–6 months = preformed niacin (not niacin equivalent).

Pyridoxine (Vitamin B$_6$)

Vitamin B$_6$, also known as pyridoxine, is necessary for the metabolism of protein and the proper utilization of stored glycogen (a complex carbohydrate) as fuel for muscles. Vitamin B$_6$ can be lost during food processing; as much as 70% can be lost in freezing fruits and vegetables; 50% to 70% in processing luncheon meats; and up to 90% in milling cereal. The best sources of pyridoxine include chicken, fish, kidney, and liver. Good sources include egg, brown rice, soybeans, oats, whole wheat bread, peanuts, and walnuts.

Recommended Daily Dietary Reference Intake for Pyridoxine

This table presents Recommended Dietary Allowances (RDA) in **bold type** and Adequate Intakes (AI) in regular type followed by an asterisk (*) (in milligrams [mg]). RDA and AI may both be used as goals for individual intake.

Infants		Males		Females	
Birth to 6 months	0.1*	14–50 years	**1.3**	14–18 years	**1.2**
7–12 months	0.3*	51–70+ years	**1.7**	19–50 years	**1.3**
				51–70+ years	**1.5**
Children				Pregnant	**1.9**
1–3 years	**0.5**			Lactating	**2.0**
4–8 years	**0.6**				
9–13 years	**1.0**				

Approximate Pyridoxine Content of Selected Foods (mg)

Grain Group		Fruit Group	
Whole wheat bread, 1 slice	0.5	Apple, 1 raw	0.7
White bread, 1 slice	0.2	Banana, 1 medium	0.66
Wheat germ, 2 tablespoons	0.08	Cantaloupe, 1 cup	0.18
Cheerios, 1 cup	0.50	Orange, 1 raw	0.08
Cornflakes, 1 cup	0.50	Pear, 1 medium	0.03
Rice, brown, 1 cup	0.28	Peach, 1 medium	0.02
Rice, white, 1 cup	0.15		
Oatmeal, 1 packet instant	0.74	**Vegetable Group**	
		Kale, cooked, ½ cup	0.09
		Potato, 1 baked	0.70
		Spinach, cooked, ½ cup	0.22
		Sweet potato, 1 baked	0.27

Protein Group

Chicken, cooked, 3½ oz	0.60
Egg yolk	0.07
Egg white	0
Haddock, 3 oz	0.29
Kidney, beef, cooked, 3½ oz 0.52	
Liver, beef, cooked 3½ oz	0.91
Ground beef, cooked, 3½ oz	0.23
Black beans, 1 cup	0.12
Chickpeas, canned, 1 cup	1.14
Peanut butter, 2 tablespoons	0.14
Walnuts, 1 oz	.16

Calcium Group

Milk, 8 oz, 1%, 2%, whole	0.10
American cheese, 1 oz	0.02
Cheddar cheese 1 oz	0.02
Soy milk, 8 oz	0.10
Tofu, ½ cup	0.06

3-5 Vitamin B$_{12}$

Vitamin B$_{12}$, also know as cobalamin, is a water-soluble B vitamin. Vitamin B$_{12}$ is needed to make new cells and to keep nerve cells healthy. It is abundant in animal products. Vegetarians, consuming only plant-based foods (vegans), will require a B$_{12}$ supplement. Men and women over age 50 may lack the ability to separate B$_{12}$ from food and should obtain their B$_{12}$ in fortified food or a B$_{12}$ supplement. Ask your doctor about B$_{12}$ supplements if you are over age 50, or do not eat any animal products, including milk or eggs. Best food sources of vitamin B$_{12}$ include animal products, such as meat, fish, poultry, shellfish, milk, cheese, eggs; fortified cereal, meat analogs, and soy milk or other nondairy milks fortified with B$_{12}$.

Recommended Daily Dietary Reference Intake for Vitamin B$_{12}$

This table presents Recommended Dietary Allowances (RDA) in **bold type** and Adequate Intakes (AI) in regular type followed by an asterisk (*) (in micrograms [μg]). RDA and AI may both be used as goals for individual intake.

Infants		Males		Females	
Birth to 6 months	0.4*	14–70+ years	**2.4**	14–70+ years	**2.4**
7–12 months	0.5*			Pregnant	**2.6**
				Lactating	**2.8**

Children	
1–3 years	**0.9**
4–8 years	**1.2**
9–13 years	**1.8**

Approximate B$_{12}$ Content of Selected Food (μg)

Grain Group		Fruit, Vegetables, and Legumes	
Product 19, Kellogg's, 1 cup	6.0	Apple, 1 raw	0
Total, General Mills, ¾ cup	6.0	Baked beans, 1 cup	0
All-Bran, Kellogg's, ½ cup	1.5	Broccoli, ½ cup	0
French toast, frozen, 1 slice	0.99	Carrots, ½ cup	0
Life cereal, Quaker, ¾ cup	0	Chickpeas, 1 cup	0
Muffin, corn, 2 oz	0.11	Orange, 1 raw	0
White bread, 1 slice	0.01		
Whole wheat bread, 1 slice	0		
Rice, brown or white, 1 cup	0		

Calcium Group

Cottage cheese, 1 cup	1.43
Milk, 1 cup, 1%	0.90
Goat's milk, 1 cup	0.16
Soy milk, 1 cup	0.00
American cheese, 1 oz	0.20
Cheddar cheese, 1 oz	0.23
Edam cheese, 1 oz	0.44
Gruyere cheese, 1 oz	0.45

Protein Group

Liver, beef, 3 oz	71
Beef, 3½ oz	3.8
Fish fillet, 3 oz	1.0
Clams, 3 oz	84.10
Oysters or mussels, 3 oz	20
Lobster or shrimp, 3 oz	1.0–2.0

Miscellaneous

Morningstar breakfast link, 2	3.41
Vegetarian burger, ¼ cup or 2 oz	1.24
Nutritional yeast, 1 tablespoon	4.0[†]

[†]Source: *Journal of the American Dietetic Association,* 97: November 1997, p. 1319.

3-6 Folic Acid

Folic acid is a B vitamin, also known as folacin and folate. Folic acid is needed for proper cell division and protein synthesis. Folic acid, when consumed in adequate amounts, is credited with preventing neural tube defects during pregnancy. It is recommended that all women capable of becoming pregnant consume 400 micrograms (μg) of synthetic folic acid from fortified foods or supplements, in addition to folate from a varied diet. Another study has found that women who get plenty of vitamin B_6 and folic acid from foods or from supplements have about half the risk of heart disease as women who do not. The researchers found 400 μg folic acid and 3 mg of vitamin B_6, amounts higher than the Dietary Reference Intake, were protective against heart disease. Most multivitamin or mineral supplements have 400 μg of folic acid. Processing, canning, and prolonged storage and cooking destroy folic acid. The best sources of folic acid are liver, yeast, leafy vegetables, legumes, and some fruit. As of January 1, 1998, the U.S. FDA requires the addition of folic acid to grain foods (such as bread and cereals) labeled "enriched." The amount added to enriched foods, however, is small and most women will not be able to obtain enough folic acid from their diet alone.

Recommended Daily Dietary Reference Intake for Folic Acid

This table presents Recommended Dietary Allowances (RDA) in **bold type** and Adequate Intakes (AI) in regular type followed by an asterisk (*) (in micrograms [μg]). RDA and AI may both be used as goals for individual intake.

Infants		Males		Females	
Birth to 6 months	65*	9–70+ years	**400**	19–70+ years	**400**
7–2 months	80*			Pregnant	**600**
Children				Lactating	**500**
1–3 years	**150**				
4–8 years	**200**				
9–13 years	**300**				
13–18 years	**400**				

Approximate Folic Acid Content of Selected Foods (μg)

Grain Group		Grain Group	
All-Bran, Kellogg's, ½ cup	100	Puffed rice, 1 cup	3
Basic 4, General Mills, 1 cup	100	Shredded wheat, 1 biscuit	12
Cornflakes, Kellogg's, 1 cup	100	Total, General Mills, 1 cup	400
Frosted Mini-Wheat, Kellogg's, 5 biscuits	100	Corn grits, 1 cup	2
Granola, homemade, ¼ cup	24	Farina, ¾ cup	4
Just Right, Kellogg's, 1 cup	100	Bagel, plain	16
Product 19, Kellogg's, 1 cup	400	Banana bread, homemade, 1 slice, 2 oz	7

Grain Group

Cornbread, from mix, 2 oz	7
French bread, 1 slice	9
Italian bread, 1 slice	9
Pita bread, 6½ inch	14
Raisin bread, 1 slice	9
White bread, 1 slice	9
Whole wheat bread, 1 slice	14
Macaroni, enriched, cooked, 1 cup	10
Brown rice, cooked, 1 cup	8
White rice, enriched, cooked, 1 cup	5
Bulger, cooked, 1 cup	33

Fruit Group

Apple juice, 1 cup	0
Carrot juice, canned, ¾ cup	0
Tomato juice, ¾ cup	36
Apple, 1 raw	4
Banana, 1 medium	22
Orange, 1 medium	44
Pear, 1 medium	12

Vegetable Group

Beets, canned, ½ cup	26
Broccoli, frozen, cooked, ½ cup	52
Brussels sprouts, cooked, ½ cup	47
Carrot, raw 1 medium	10
Chicory greens, raw, ½ cup	99
Green beans, cooked, ½ cup	21
Kale, cooked, ½ cup	9
Lettuce, iceberg, 1 leaf	11
Okra, cooked, ½ cup	116
Peas, frozen, cooked, ½ cup	47
Potato, baked	22
Seaweed, agar, dried, 3½ oz	580
Seaweed, kelp, raw 3½ oz	180
Spinach, cooked, ½ cup	131
Tomato, raw	18
Turnip greens, cooked, ½ cup	85

Protein Group

Beef, 3½ oz	8
Lamb, 3½ oz	19
Pork, 3½ oz	4
Liver (beef), 3½ oz	217
Chicken, 3½ oz	8
Cod, 3 oz	7
Oysters, 3 oz	12
Egg, 1	22
Baked beans, homemade, 1 cup	122
Black beans, cooked, 1 cup	256
Chickpeas, cooked, 1 cup	282
Mung beans, cooked, 1 cup	321

Calcium Group

Milk, 1 cup all types	12
Cheese, american, 1 oz	2
Cheese, cheddar, 1 oz	5

Miscellaneous

Tofu, ½ cup	19
Cashews, 1 oz	20
Peanut butter, 2 tablespoons	29
Sunflower seeds, dry roast, 1 oz	67
Yeast, bakers, 1 package (¼ oz)	164

Sources: *Journal of the American Dietetic Association*, Vol. 98, June 1998, page 701; *Journal of the American Medical Association*, Vol. 279, February 1998, pages 359–364.

Vitamin C, also known as ascorbic acid, is a water-soluble vitamin that can be destroyed by heat and lost in cooking water. It helps keep blood vessels strong, makes scar tissue, helps with the metabolism of protein, boosts the immune system, and assists in the absorption of iron. Vitamin C is abundant in fruits and vegetables. Because the body cannot stockpile vitamin C, a daily supply is needed to maintain optimal health. Good food sources include all citrus fruits and juices, fresh peppers (sweet and hot), tomatoes, and strawberries.

Recommended Daily Dietary Reference Intake for Vitamin C

This table presents Recommended Dietary Allowances (RDA) in **bold type** and Adequate Intakes (AI) in regular type followed by an asterisk (*) (in milligrams [mg]). RDA and AI may both be used as goals for individual intake.

Infants		Males		Pregnant	
Birth to 6 months	40*	14–18 years	**75**	≤18 years	**80**
7–12 months	50*	19–70+ years	**90**	>19 years	**85**

Children		Females		Lactating	
1–3 years	**15**	14–18 years	**65**	≤18 years	**115**
4–8 years	**25**	19–70+ years	**75**	>19 years	**120**
9–13 years	**45**				

Approximate Vitamin C Content of Selected Foods (mg)

Bread Group		Fruit Group	
All-Bran, Kellogg's, ½ cup	15	Peach nectar, 1 cup	13
Cornflakes, Kellogg's, 1 cup	15	Lemonade, frozen concentrate, 1 cup	9
Shredded wheat, 1 oz	0	Capri Sun juice drink, ¾ cup	0
Bagel, 3½ in	0	Grape juice, 1 cup	0
White bread, 1 slice	0		
Whole wheat bread, 1 slice	0	Apple, 1 medium	8
Macaroni, cooked enriched, 1 cup	0	Apricots, raw, 3 medium	11
		Banana, 1 medium	10
Fruit Group		Blueberries, 1 cup	19
Orange juice, fresh, 1 cup	124	Cantaloupe, 1 cup	68
Orange juice, frozen concentrate, 1 cup	97	Cherries, 10	7
Grapefruit juice, frozen concentrate, 1 cup	83	Dates, dried 2	0
Cranberry juice cocktail, 1 cup	67	Fruit cocktail, canned, ½ cup	3
Hawaiian Punch, 1 cup	60	Fruit Roll-up, 1	10
Tomato juice, ¾ cup	33		

Fruit Group

Grapefruit, ½	39
Grapes, 1 cup	4
Honeydew melon, 1 cup	42
Kiwifruit, 1 medium	74
Lemon, 1 medium	31
Mandarin oranges, canned in juice, ½ cup	42
Nectarine, 1 medium	7
Orange, 1 medium	59
Papaya, 1 medium	188
Peach, 1 medium	6
Pear, 1 medium	7
Pineapple, 1 cup	24
Plum, 1 medium	6
Raisins, 2/3 cup	3
Raspberries, 1 cup	31
Strawberries, 1 cup	84
Tangerine, 1 medium	26
Watermelon, 1 cup	15

Vegetable Group

Asparagus, frozen, cooked 4 spears	15
Bamboo shoots, canned, 1 cup	1
Beet greens, cooked, ½ cup	18
Beets, cooked, ½ cup	3
Broccoli,	
raw, ½ cup	41
cooked, ½ cup	58
frozen, cooked, ½ cup	37
Cabbage, green, shredded, cooked, ½ cup	15
Carrots, cooked, ½ cup	2
Cauliflower, cooked, ½ cup	27
Celery, raw, 3½ oz	8
Collards, cooked, 1 cup	15
Corn, cooked, ½ cup	5
Cucumber, raw, ½ cup	3
Eggplant, cooked, ½ cup	1
Garlic, raw, 3 cloves	3
Green beans, cooked, ½ cup	88

Vegetable Group

Kale, cooked, ½ cup	27
Lettuce, 2 leaves	1
Mixed vegetables, canned, ½ cup	4
Mixed vegetables, frozen, ½ cup	3
Mushrooms, cooked, ½ cup	3
Onion, cooked, ½ cup	5
Peas, canned or frozen, ½ cup	2
Pepper, hot chili, ½ cup	45
Pepper, sweet, raw chopped, ½ cup	45
Pepper, large yellow, whole raw, 5 oz	341
Potato, baked, 1 medium	24
Potato, cooked	18
Potato, fried, 10 pieces	3
Potato, mashed, ½ cup	6
Spinach, cooked, ½ cup	9
Squash, summer, cooked, ½ cup	5
Tomato, raw, 1 medium	23
Tomato, stewed, 1 cup	18
Tomato sauce, ½ cup	16

Protein Group

Egg, 1	0
Fish, 3 oz	1
Beef, 3½ oz	0
Poultry, 3½ oz	0
Baked beans, 1 cup	1
Black beans, 1 cup	0
Chick peas, 1 cup	2

Calcium Group

Cheese, 1 oz	0
Milk, 8 oz, 1%	2
Yogurt, 1 cup	0

Miscellaneous

Nuts	0
Margarine	0
Butter	0

Vitamin A is essential for good vision. It prevents night blindness, and it keeps the skin and the lining of the digestive tract healthy. It is a fat-soluble vitamin that can become toxic when consumed in excess. Beta carotene, a precursor of vitamin A, converts to vitamin A in the body. It is found in plants and may help prevent some forms of disease. Good sources of vitamin A include liver, eggs, margarine, fortified milk, pumpkin, winter squash, carrots, sweet red pepper, apricots, mangoes, papaya, and dark green vegetables.

Recommended Daily Dietary Reference Intake for Vitamin A[†]

This table presents Recommended Dietary Allowances (RDA) in **bold type** and Adequate Intakes (AI) in regular type followed by an asterisk (*) (in micrograms [μg]). RDA and AI may both be used as goals for individual intake.

Infants		*Males*		*Pregnant*	
Birth to 6 months	400*	9–13 years	**600**	≤18 years	**750**
7–12 months	500*	14–70+ years	**900**	19–50 years	**770**

Children		*Females*		*Lactating*	
1–3 years	**300**	9–13 years	**600**	≤18 years	**1,200**
4–8 years	**400**	14–70+ years	**700**	19–50 years	**1,300**

Approximate Vitamin A Content of Selected Foods in Retinol Equivalents (RE)[‡] and International Units (IU) where Indicated

Grain Group		*Fruit Group*	
Apple Cinnamon Cheerios, ¾ cup	750 IU	Apple juice, 1 cup	0
Frosted Mini Wheat, 1 cup	0	Grapefruit juice, 1 cup	2
Puffed rice, 1 cup	0	Orange juice, frozen concentrate 1 cup	20
Raisin bran, Ralston Purina, ¾ cup	377 IU	Tomato juice, ¾ cup	102
Shredded wheat, 1 biscuit	0	Apple, 1 raw	7
Bagel, 1, 3½ inch	0	Apricot, 10 dried halves	253
White bread, 1 slice	0	Fruit roll-up Betty Crocker, 1	0
Whole wheat bread, 1 slice	0	Mango, 1 med raw	805
Saltine cracker, 1	0	Peach, 1 raw	47
Whole wheat cracker, 1	0	Pear, 1 raw	3

[†]The vitamin A content of foods is measured as retinol activity equivalents (RAE). One RAE equals the activity of 1 μg of retinol: 1 RAE = 3.33 IU of vitamin A activity on a label. IU is an outdated term still used on labels.

[‡]To calculate RAE from RE of provitamin A carotenoids in foods, divide the RE by 2. For preformed vitamin A in foods or supplements and for provitamin A carotenoids in supplements: 1 RE = 1 RAE.

Vegetable Group

Broccoli, cooked, ½ cup	108
Carrot, medium, raw, 1	2025
Mustard greens, cooked, ½ cup	335
Onion, raw, 1	0
Peas, frozen, cooked, ½ cup	54
Potato, baked	0
Pumpkin, canned, ½ cup	2691
Seaweed, kelp, raw 3-½ oz	12
Spinach, cooked, ½ cup	737
Squash, summer, cooked ½ cup	26
Squash, winter, baked, ½ cup	363
Sweet potato, baked	2,487
Sweet pepper, raw, ½ cup	32
Tomato, raw, 1	76
Turnip greens, cooked, ½ cup	396

Protein Group

Beef, 3½ oz	0
Beef liver, cooked, 3½ oz	10,602
Lamb, 3½ oz	0
Lamb liver, 3½ oz	7,490
Pork, 3½ oz	0
Chicken, 3½ oz	22
Chicken liver, cooked 3½ oz	4,913
Cod, cooked 3 oz	9
Fishstick, 1	9
Egg, 1	84
Egg substitute, frozen, ¼ cup	81

Calcium Group

Milk, 1 %, 1 cup	144
Milk, 2 %, 1 cup	139
Nonfat milk, 1 cup	149
Whole milk, 1 cup	76
Goat milk, 1 cup	137
Soy milk, 1 cup	7
Yogurt, 1 cup	0
American cheese, 1oz	82
Cheddar cheese, 1 oz	86
Cottage cheese, 1 %, 1 cup	25
Cottage cheese, 2 %, 1 cup	45
Goat cheese, soft, 1 oz	80

Miscellaneous

Vegetarian beans, canned, 1 cup	43
Black beans, cooked, 1 cup	2
Chickpeas, cooked, 1 cup	5
Butter, 1 tablespoon	124
Margarine, 1 tablespoon	30

Measuring Vitamin A

Vitamin A refers to three preformed compounds known as retinol, retinal, and retinoic acid. In addition to the preformed vitamin A found in animal products, vitamin A can be metabolized in the body from carotenoids. The most familiar of these is called beta carotene. The amount of vitamin A available from any food depends on how well it is absorbed. Vitamin A can be measured in several ways, depending on the form being measured. The DRI is in micrograms; the content in food is often measured in retinol equivalents (RE) or found on food labels as International Units. To meet the DRI, simply eat vegetables rich in color and select foods with the highest levels listed above. Excessive consumption can be toxic.

3-9 Vitamin D

Vitamin D, also known as cholecalciferol, is essential for proper calcium absorption and healthy bones. Exposure to the sun causes the body to make vitamin D. A severe vitamin D deficiency causes rickets, a deformation of the skeleton. Fortified milk has been successful in eliminating the problem of rickets. People living where sun exposure is reduced may be at greater risk for vitamin D deficiency. Those avoiding the sun and using sunscreen to reduce their cancer risk may not be getting enough vitamin D from sunlight alone. The best food sources of vitamin D include cod liver oil, herring, vitamin D fortified milk, dairy products, and (some) cereal; butter, margarine, eggs, liver, and salmon. Most yogurt and cheese is not made with vitamin D fortified milk.

Recommended Daily Dietary Reference Intake for Vitamin D[†]

This table presents Recommended Dietary Allowances (RDA) in **bold type** and Adequate Intakes (AI) in regular type followed by an asterisk (*) (in micrograms [μg]). RDA and AI may both be used as goals for individual intake.

Infants		Males		Females	
Birth to 12 months	5*	9–50 years	5*	9–50 years	5*
		51–70 years	10*	51–70 years	10*
Children		71+ years	15*	71+ years	15*
				Pregnant	5*
1–8 years	5*			Lactating	5*

[†]Vitamin D is measured in micrograms (μg) and international units (IU). One μg cholecalciferol = 40 IU vitamin D. Vitamin D fortified milk has 10 μg cholecalciferol or 400 IU/qt. Because fortified milk and sun exposure are the best sources of vitamin D and few other foods have significant amounts of vitamin D, a list of vitamin D-rich food is not included here.

Vitamin E, also known as α-tocopherol, helps prevent cell damage and protects tissues of the skin, eye, and liver. Vitamin E deficiency is rare, occurring in premature infants and individuals who do not absorb fat normally. It appears to be a powerful antioxidant and is credited with preventing disease, including cancer and heart disease. Good sources of vitamin E include vegetable oils, peanut butter, and wheat germ.

Recommended Daily Dietary Reference Intake for Vitamin E

This table presents Recommended Dietary Allowances (RDA) in **bold type** and Adequate Intakes (AI) in regular type followed by an asterisk (*) (in milligrams [mg]). RDA and AI may both be used as goals for individual intake.

Infants		Males		Females	
Birth to 6 months	4*	9–13 years	**11**	9–13 years	**11**
7–12 months	5*	14–70+ years	**15**	14–70+ years	**15**
				Pregnant	**15**
Children				Lactating	**15**
1–3 years	**6**				
4–8 years	**7**				

Approximate Vitamin E Content of Selected Foods (mg)

Grain Group		Vegetables	
Granola, Nature Valley, ½ cup	1.97	Broccoli, cooked, ½ cup	1.32
Bagel, plain, 3½ in	0.02	Carrot, raw, 1 medium	0.33
Pita, white	0.02	Corn, frozen, cooked, ½ cup	0.07
Pita, whole wheat	0.6	Peas, frozen, cooked, ½ cup	0.14
Tortilla, flour, 7–8 in	0.44	Tomato, raw, 1	0.47
White bread, 1 slice	0.02		
Whole wheat bread, 1 slice	0.65		

Protein Group	
Beef, cooked, 3½ oz	0.2
Eel, cooked, 3 oz	4.3
Salmon, canned with bones, 3 oz	1.3
Egg, 1	0.53
Egg substitute, frozen, ¼ cup	1.27

Fruit Group	
Apple	.44
Banana	.31
Mango, raw, 10 oz	2.32
Papaya, raw, 10 oz	3.4
Pear, 1 medium	0.83
Orange juice, ½ cup	0.47
Tomato juice, ¾ cup	1.6

Calcium Group

Cheese, 1 oz	0.10
Milk, 1 cup	0.1
Goat's milk, 1 cup	0.22
Soy milk, 1 cup	0.02
Yogurt, plain 1 cup	0.1

Miscellaneous

Corn oil, 1 tablespoon	2.96
Olive oil, 1 tablespoon	1.74
Safflower oil, 1 tablespoon	6.03
Wheat germ oil	26.94
Wheat germ, toasted, ¼ cup	5.26
Almonds, dry roasted, 1 oz	6.72
Peanut butter, 2 tablespoons	3.2
Sunflower seeds, dry roasted, 1 oz	14.25
Chick peas, 1 cup	0.57

3-11 Vitamin K

Vitamin K is consumed in food and made by bacteria in the intestine. It is essential for proper blood clotting. In persons treated with anticoagulant drugs, vitamin K status should be monitored by measuring and maintaining plasma prothrombin concentrations in a normal range. Good sources of vitamin K include green leafy vegetables. Smaller amounts occur in dairy products, meat, eggs, cereal, fruits, and vegetables.

Recommended Daily Dietary Reference Intake for Vitamin K

This table presents Recommended Dietary Allowances (RDA) in **bold type** and Adequate Intakes (AI) in regular type followed by an asterisk (*) (in micrograms [μg]). RDA and AI may both be used as goals for individual intake.

Infants

Birth to 6 months	2.0*
7 months to 1 year	2.5*

Children

1 years	30*
4–8 years	55*

Males

9–13 years	60*
14–18 years	75*
19–70+ years	120*

Females

9–13 years	60*
14–18 years	75*
19–70+ years	90*

Pregnant

≤18 years	75*
19–50 years	90*

Lactating

≤18 years	75*
19–50 years	90*

Approximate Vitamin K Content of Selected Foods (μg)

Grain Group

Oats, dry, 1 oz	18
Whole wheat flour, 1 cup	36
Wheat germ, 1 oz	10

Fruit Group

Apple, raw, 1 medium	4
Orange, raw 1 medium	7
Strawberry, raw, 1 cup	21

Vegetable Group

Asparagus, 4 spears	16
Beets, ½ cup raw	3
Broccoli, frozen, ½ cup	63
Carrot, 1 medium	9
Cauliflower, raw, ½ cup	96
Corn, raw, 1 oz	2
Green beans, frozen, cooked, ½ cup	22
Lettuce, iceberg 1 leaf	22
Potato, baked	6
Seaweed, dulse, dried 3½ oz	1700
Spinach, frozen, ½ cup	131
Turnip greens, raw, ½ cup	182

Protein Group

Egg, 1	25
Beef, 3½ oz	4
Liver, beef, raw, 3½ oz	104

Calcium Group

Milk, 1 cup	10

Legumes

Chick peas, dry, 1 oz	74
Lentils, dry, 1 oz	62

Miscellaneous

Coffee, dry, 1 round teaspoon	96
Tea, green, dry, 1 oz	199
Corn oil, 1 tablespoon	8
Olive oil, 1 tablespoon	0
Soybean oil, 1 tablespoon	76

Pantothenic Acid

Pantothenic acid is part of coenzyme A, which is essential for carbohydrate, protein, and fat metabolism. Good food sources include chicken, beef, potatoes, oats, cereals, tomato products, liver, kidney, yeast, egg yolk, broccoli, and whole grains.

Recommended Daily Dietary Reference Intake for Pantothenic Acid

This table presents Recommended Dietary Allowances (RDA) in **bold type** and Adequate Intakes (AI) in regular type followed by an asterisk (*) (in milligrams [mg]). RDA and AI may both be used as goals for individual intake.

Infants		Males		Females	
0 to 6 months	1.7*	9–13 years	4*	9–13 years	4*
7–12 months	1.8*	14–70+ years	5*	14–70+ years	5*
				Pregnant	6*
Children				Lactating	7*
1–3 years	2*				
4–8 years	3*				

Approximate Pantothenic Acid Content of Selected Foods (mg)

Grain Group

Cream of wheat, instant, cooked, ¾ cup	0.13
Farina, enriched, ¾ cup	0.10
Oatmeal, instant, 1 packet	0.35
All-Bran, Kellogg's, ½ cup	0.49
Cornflakes, General Mills, 1 cup	0
Puffed rice, 1 cup	0.04
Shredded wheat, 1 biscuit	0.2
Bagel, plain, 3½ in	0.26
White bread, 1 slice	0.10
Whole wheat bread, 1 slice	0.15

Fruit Group

Orange juice, 1 cup	0.39
Apple, 1 medium	0.08
Figs, dried 10	0.81
Raisins, ⅔ cup	0.04
Strawberries, 1 cup	0.51

Vegetable Group

Broccoli, ½ cup	0.40
Carrots, 1 raw	0.14
Peas, frozen, cooked, ½ cup	0.11
Potato, baked	0.92

Meat Group

Beef, 3½ oz	0.38
Beef liver, 3½ oz	4.57
Lamb, 3½ oz	0.63
Pork, 3½ oz	0.56
Chicken, 3½ oz	1.1
Cod, 3 oz	0.15
Haddock, 3 oz	0.13
Egg, 1 large	0.7
Egg yolk from 1 egg	0.65
Egg white from 1 egg	0.04

Dairy Group

American cheese, 1 oz	0.14
Cheddar cheese, 1 oz	9.12
Milk, 1%, 1 cup	0.79
Yogurt, plain, 8 oz	0.88

Miscellaneous

Baked beans, homemade, 1 cup	0.39
Black beans, 1 cup	0.42
Chickpeas, cooked, 1 cup	0.47
Peanut butter, 2 tablespoons	0.31
Sunflower seeds, dry roasted, 1 oz	2.0
Peanuts, 1 oz	0.40
Cocoa, 1 oz packet	0.25

Calcium, the predominant mineral in bones and teeth, helps to build and keep them strong. Calcium also helps muscles and nerves work properly. It even plays a role in blood clotting and regulating blood pressure. Calcium deficiency in childhood can show up as stunted bone growth.

In adult women, the condition known as osteoporosis (weak, thin bones) has been linked with inadequate calcium intakes. To get the recommended amount of calcium, eat 2 to 3 servings of calcium-rich foods, such as low-fat dairy foods. Good sources of calcium include all dairy products, fortified soy and rice milk, and calcium-fortified juice. Green leafy vegetables, dried beans, and canned fish with bones are also good calcium sources.

Recommended Daily Dietary Reference Intake for Calcium

This table presents Recommended Dietary Allowances (RDA) in **bold type** and Adequate Intakes (AI) in regular type followed by an asterisk (*) (in milligrams [mg]). RDA and AI may both be used as goals for individual intake.

Infants		Males		Pregnant	
Birth to 6 months	210*	9–18 years	1300*	≤18 years	1300*
7–12 months	270*	19–50 years	1000*	19–50 years	1000*
		51–70+ years	1200*		
Children				Lactating	
1–3 years	500*	Females		≤18 years	1300*
4–8 years	800*	9–18 years	1300*	19–50 years	1000*
		19–50 years	1000*		
		51–70+ years	1200*		

Calcium Content of Foods (mg)

Whole milk, 1 cup	291	Cottage cheese, 1 oz	204
Skim milk, 1 cup	302	Cream cheese, 2 tablespoons	23
Goat's milk, 1 cup	326	Half and half, 1 tablespoon	40
Soy milk, 1 cup	10	Sardines, with bones, 1 oz	90
Soy milk, calcium fortified 1 cup	300	Salmon, canned, with bones, 3 oz	181
Yogurt, vanilla, 8 oz	350	Broccoli, cooked, ½ cup	122
Evaporated milk, 2 tablespoons	80	Turnip greens, cooked, ½ cup	99
Ice cream, vanilla, ½ cup	138	Tofu, ½ cup	130
Frozen yogurt, ½ cup	106	Almonds, 1 oz	73
Cheddar cheese, 1 oz	204	Dried beans, cooked, ½ cup	80

Use food labels to select foods rich in calcium. The calcium content on the Nutrition Facts Panel is listed as a percentage. Foods that have 30% calcium contain approximately 300 mg of calcium. If you are unable to eat the recommended amount of calcium from food, a calcium supplement may be needed.

To get the calcium you need daily:

- Eat three very good sources of calcium
- Look for foods that carry 30% of the daily requirement of calcium on the label
- Consider a supplement if you cannot meet your calcium needs from food

3-14 Copper

Copper helps in the metabolism of iron. Good food sources include organ meats, seafood, nuts, seeds, wheat bran, cereals, whole grain bread and pasta, and foods made with cocoa.

Recommended Daily Dietary Reference Intake for Copper

This table presents Recommended Dietary Allowances (RDA) in **bold type** and Adequate Intakes (AI) in regular type followed by an asterisk (*) (in micrograms [μg]). RDAs and AI may both be used as goals for individual intake.

Infants		Males		Females	
Birth to 6 months	200*	9–13 years	**700**	9–13 years	**700**
7–12 months	220*	14–18 years	**890**	14–18 years	**890**
		19–70+ years	**900**	19–70+ years	**900**
Children				Pregnant	**1000**
				Lactating	**1300**
1–3 years	**340**				
4–8 years	**440**				

Approximate Copper Content of Selected Foods (mg)

Grain Group

Cream of wheat, instant, cooked, ¾ cup	0.069
Farina, enriched, ¾ cup	0.019
Oatmeal, instant, 1 packet	0.097
All-Bran, Kellogg's, ½ cup	0.40
Cornflakes, General Mills, 1 cup	0
Puffed rice, 1 cup	0.024
Shredded wheat, 1 biscuit	0.159
Bagel, plain, 3½ inch	0.116
White bread, 1 slice	0.032
Whole wheat bread, 1 slice	0.08

Fruit Group

Orange juice, 1 cup	0.110
Apple, 1 medium	0.057
Figs, dried, 10	0.585
Raisins, ⅔ cup	0.302
Strawberries, 1 cup	0.073

Vegetable Group

Broccoli, ½ cup	0.034
Carrots, 1 raw	0.034
Peas, frozen, cooked, ½ cup	0.111
Potato, baked	0.675

Meat Group

Beef, 3½ oz	0.164
Beef liver, 3½ oz	4.512
Lamb, 3½ oz	0.123
Pork, 3½ oz	0.113
Chicken, 3½ oz	0.067
Cod, 3 oz	0.031
Haddock, 3 oz	0.028
Egg, 1 large	0.006
Egg yolk from 1 egg	0.004
Egg white from 1 egg	0.002

Dairy Group

American cheese, 1 oz	0.009
Cheddar cheese, 1 oz	0.009
Milk, 1%, 8 oz	0.024
Yogurt, plain, 8 oz	0.020

Miscellaneous

Baked beans, homemade, 1 cup	0.402
Black beans, 1 cup	0.359
Chickpeas, cooked, 1 cup	0.577
Peanut butter, 2 tablespoons	0.165
Sunflower seeds, dry roasted, 1 oz	0.519
Peanuts, 1 oz	0.190
Cocoa, 1 oz packet	0.080

3-15 Iron

Iron is essential in the formation of hemoglobin, the oxygen-carrying factor in blood. The best sources of iron are foods that come from meat and poultry. The form of iron found in animal foods is highly absorbable. Iron from vegetables and grains is not well absorbed, but even consuming a small amount of meat with grains, beans, or vegetables significantly boosts the iron that is absorbed from the meal.

Recommended Daily Dietary Reference Intake for Iron

This table presents Recommended Dietary Allowances (RDA) in **bold type** and Adequate Intakes (AI) in regular type followed by an asterisk (*) (in milligrams [mg]). RDA and AI may both be used as goals for individual intake.

Infants		Males		Females	
Birth to 6 months	0.27*	9–13 years	**8**	9–13 years	**8**
7–12 months	**11**	14–18 years	**11**	14–18 years	**15**
		19–70+ years	**8**	19–30 years	**18**
Children				31–70+ years	**8**
1–3 years	**7**			Pregnant	**27**
4–8 years	**10**			Lactating	
				≤18 years	**10**
				19–50 years	**9**

Approximate Iron Content of Selected Foods (mg)

Grain Group

Cream of wheat, instant, cooked, ¾ cup	9.05
Farina, enriched, dry, ¼ cup	14.39
Oatmeal, instant, 1 packet	6.3
All-Bran, Kellogg's, ½ cup	4.5
Cornflakes, General Mills, 1 cup	8.1
Puffed rice, 1 cup	4.4
Shredded wheat, 1 biscuit	1.0
Rice cereal, Gerber, infant ½ oz	6.8
Bagel, 3½ inch, plain	2.5
White bread, 1 slice	.76
Whole wheat bread, 1 slice	.92

Fruit Group

Orange juice, 1 cup	.25
Apple, 1 medium	.25
Figs, dried, 10	4.17
Raisins, ⅔ cup	1.8
Strawberries, 1 cup	.57

Vegetable Group

Carrots, 1 raw	.36
Peas, frozen, cooked, ½ cup	1.26

Meat Group

Beef, 3½ oz	2.5
Lamb, 3½ oz	2.1
Pork, 3½ oz	1.4
Chicken, 3½ oz	1.3
Cod, 3 oz	0.4
Haddock, 3 oz	1.0
Egg, 1 large	0.6
Egg yolk from 1 egg	0.6
Egg white from 1 egg	0.01

Dairy Group

American cheese, 1 oz	0.11
Cheddar cheese, 1 oz	0.19
Milk, skim, 1%, 2%, – whole fat, 1 cup	0.12
Yogurt, plain, 8 oz	0.1

Miscellaneous

Baked beans, canned, Campbell's, ½ cup	1.4
Black beans, 1 cup	3.6
Chickpeas, 1 cup cooked	4.7
Peanut butter, 2 tablespoons	0.6
Sunflower seeds, dry roasted, 1 oz	1.0

Potassium is a mineral essential to good health. It plays a role in fluid balance, helps the heart beat regularly, and aids in muscle contraction and transmission of nerve impulses. Potassium is abundant in food; however, food processing depletes potassium and increases sodium content. The best sources of potassium can be found in fresh fruit and vegetables and meat.

Dietary Reference Adequate Intake (AI) for Potassium

This table presents Adequate Intakes (AI) in regular type followed by an asterisk (*) (in milligrams [mg]).

Infants		Children		14 years and adults	4,700*
				Pregnant	4,700*
Birth to 6 months	400*	12 months to 3 years	3,000*	Lactating	5,100*
7–12 months	700*	4–8 years	3,800*		
		9–13 years	4,500*		

Approximate Potassium Content of Selected Foods (mg)

Grain Group

Whole wheat bread, 1 slice	71
White bread, 1 slice	30

Fruit Group

Apple, medium	159
Apricot dried, 10 pieces	482
Banana, 1 medium	451
Cantaloupe, cut up, 1 cup	494
Fruit cocktail, canned, ½ cup	115
Fruit roll snack	62
Grapefruit, ½	171
Orange juice, from concentrate, 1 cup	473
Orange drink, canned, ¾ cup	33
Peach, 1 medium	171
Pear, 1 medium	208
Raisins, seedless, ⅔ cup	751
Strawberry, raw, 1 cup	247

Vegetable Group

Tomato sauce, ½ cup	453[†]
Broccoli, cooked, ½ cup	228
Potato, baked	844
Potato, fries, 10 pieces	270[†]

Protein Group

Beef ground, broiled, 3½ oz	292
Beef frank, 2 oz	95[†]
Turkey breast, 2 oz	150
Chicken roasted, 3½ oz	243
Haddock, broiled 3 oz	339
Fish sticks, 3 oz	108[†]
Peanut butter, 2 tablespoons	214[†]

Calcium Group

Milk, 1%, 1 cup	381
Milk, whole, 1 cup	370
Yogurt, 1 cup	351
Morton salt substitute, ¼ tsp	600
Morton Lite salt, ¼ tsp	350[†]

[†]Can be a significant source of sodium.

Iodine, which makes up part of the thyroid hormones, prevents goiter. In 1924, iodized salt was introduced in the United States and the incidence of goiter fell sharply. Good sources of iodine include seafood, iodized salt, eggs, cheese, milk and vegetables grown in iodine-rich soil.

Recommended Daily Dietary Reference Intake for Iodine

This table presents Recommended Dietary Allowances (RDA) in **bold type** and Adequate Intakes (AI) in regular type followed by an asterisk (*) (in micrograms [μg]/100 gram portions). RDA and AI may both be used as goals for individual intake.

Infants		*Males*		*Females*	
Birth to 6 months	110*	9–13 years	**120**	9–13	**120**
7–12 months	130*	14–70+ years	**150**	14–70+ years	**150**
				Pregnant	**220**
Children				Lactating	**290**
1–8 years	**90**				

Approximate Iodine Content of Selected Foods (μg/100 g)[†]

Bread Group		*Vegetable Group*	
Cornflakes, 3½ oz	93	Beets, ½ cup	1
Raisin bran, 3½ oz	19	Corn, canned, ½ cup	8
Shredded wheat, 3½ oz	28	Potato, baked, 1 medium	31
White bread, 1 slice	30	Sweet potato, baked, 1 medium	2
Whole wheat bread, 1 slice	21	Tomato, raw, 1 medium	2
Tortillas, flour, 1, 2 oz	50	Winter squash, ½ cup	1

Fruit Group	
Apple juice, ½ cup	3
Orange juice, ½ cup	1
Apple, raw, 1	1
Fruit cocktail, canned in heavy syrup, ½ cup	33
Prunes, ½ cup	30

Meat Group

Beef, 3½ oz	15
Lamb, 3½ oz	11
Bologna, 3½ oz	21
Chicken, 3½ oz	15
Turkey breast, baked, 3½ oz	40
Egg, 1 (approx)	23
Cod or haddock 3½ oz	116
Fish stick 3½ oz	63
Tuna, canned in oil, 3½ oz	20

Calcium Group

Milk, ½ cup	21
American cheese, 3½ oz	46
Cheese, cheddar, 3½ oz	43

Miscellaneous

Navy beans, cooked, ½ cup	39
Pinto beans, cooked, ½ cup	15
Red beans, cooked, ½ cup	21
Peanut butter, 2 tablespoons	2
Popcorn, popped in oil, 3½ oz	27

[†]100g is approximately 3½ ounces or a ½ cup portion.

Magnesium helps build protein and keep muscles working and teeth strong. All unprocessed food has some magnesium. Good sources include nuts, legumes, whole grain bread, cereal and related products, and green vegetables. Fish, meat, and milk are poor sources.

Recommended Daily Dietary Reference Intake for Magnesium

This table presents Recommended Dietary Allowances (RDA) in **bold type** and Adequate Intakes (AI) in regular type followed by an asterisk (*) (in milligrams [mg]). RDA and AI may both be used as goals for individual intake.

Infants		Males		Pregnant	
Birth to 6 months	30*	14–18 years	**410**	≤18 years	**400**
7 months to 1 year	75*	19–30 years	**400**	19–years	**350**
		31–70+ years	**420**	31–50 years	**360**
Children					
1–3 years	**80**	**Females**		**Lactating**	
4–8 years	**130**	14–18 years	**360**	≤18	**360**
9–13 years	**240**	19–30 years	**310**	19–30 years	**310**
		31–70+ years	**320**	31–50 years	**320**

Approximate Magnesium Content of Selected Foods (mg)

Bread Group

Bran flakes, Post, ¾ cup	60.0
Cornflakes, Kellogg's, ½ cup	1.4
Oatmeal, cooked, 1 cup	56
Shredded wheat, 1 biscuit	32
Rice Crispies, 1¼ cup	16
White bread, 1 slice	6
Bread, whole wheat, 1 slice	24

Fruit Group

Apple juice, ½ cup	3.5
Grapefruit juice, canned, unsweetened, ½ cup	11
Orange juice, canned, ½ cup	12
Apple, 1	7
Banana, 1	33
Pineapple, raw, 1 cup	22

Vegetable Group

Asparagus, canned spears, ½ cup	12
Beans, snap, ½ cup	8.8
Beets, ½ cup	20
Carrots, 1 raw	11
Corn, canned, ½ cup	16.5
Tomato, raw, 1	14
Potato cooked, peeled	30

Protein Group

Pot roast, 1 oz	6.8
Steak, 1 oz	9
Chicken, 1 oz	7
Lamb, 1 oz	6.6
Cod, 1 oz	12
Halibut, 1 oz	30
Egg, 1	5

Calcium Group

Milk, 1 cup	30
American cheese, 1 oz	6
Cheddar cheese, 1 oz	8
Yogurt, plain, 8 oz	26

Miscellaneous

Black beans, 1 cup	120
Chick peas, 1 cup	79
Navy beans, canned, 1 cup	107
Peanut butter, 2 tablespoons	51
Soybean nuts, dry roasted, ½ cup	196
Sunflower seeds, dry roasted, 1 oz	37
Wheat germ, toasted, ¼ cup	93
Quinoa, ½ cup	179
Wheat bran, ½ cup	183

3-19 Manganese

Manganese is involved in bone formation, and is a component of many enzymes. Manganese may be better absorbed from drinking water and supplements than from food. People taking supplements may need to be cautious about consuming large amounts of supplemental manganese. Good sources include nuts, legumes, and whole grain foods.

Recommended Daily Dietary Reference Intake of Manganese

This table presents Recommended Dietary Allowances (RDA) in **bold type** and Adequate Intakes (AI) in regular type followed by an asterisk (*) (in milligrams [mg]). RDA and AI may both be used as goals for individual intake.

Infants		Males		Females	
Birth to 6 months	0.003*				
7–12 months	0.6*	9–13 years	1.9*	9–18 years	1.6*
		14–18 years	2.2*	19–70+ years	1.8*
Children		19–70+ years	2.3*	Pregnant	2.0*
				Lactating	2.6*
1–3 years	1.2*				
4–8 years	1.5*				

Approximate Manganese Content of Selected Foods (mg)

Bread Group

Bran, 100%, ½ cup	2.528
Oatmeal, cooked, 1 cup	1.369
Shredded wheat, 1 biscuit,	0.737
Rice Krispies, frosted, 1 cup	0.210
White bread, 1 slice	0.096
Whole wheat bread, 1 slice	0.651

Vegetable Group

Asparagus, canned spears, ½ cup	0.206
Beets, ½ cup	0.277
Carrots, 1 raw	0.102
Corn, canned, ½ cup	0.142
Tomato, raw, 1	0.129
Potato, baked, no skin	0.265

Fruit Group

Apple juice, 1 cup	.280
Grapefruit juice, canned, 1 cup	0.049
Orange juice, canned, 1 cup	0.035
Apple, 1	0.062
Banana, 1	0.173
Pineapple, raw, 1 cup	2.556

Protein Group

Pot roast, 3 oz	0.017
Ground beef, 3½ oz	0.015
Chicken, 3 oz	0.019
Lamb, 3½ oz	0.025
Cod, 3 oz	0.017
Halibut, 3 oz	0.017
Egg, 1	0.013

Calcium Group

Milk, 1 cup	0.005
American cheese, 1 oz	0.004
Cheddar cheese, 1 oz	0.003
Yogurt, plain, 8 oz	0.009

Miscellaneous

Black beans, 1 cup	0.764
Chick peas, 1 cup	1.689
Navy beans, canned, 1 cup	0.983
Peanut butter, 2 tablespoons	0.597
Soybean nuts, dry roasted, ½ cup	1.878
Sunflower seeds, dry roasted, 1 oz	0.598
Wheat germ, toasted, ¼ cup	5.787
Quinoa, ½ cup	1.921
Wheat bran, ½ cup	3.450

Selenium is a trace mineral, essential to good health. Selenium works with vitamin E to prevent important body compounds from being destroyed. Good sources include seafood, kidney, liver, and meats. Grains and seeds can be good sources, depending on the selenium content of the soils in which they were grown.

Recommended Daily Dietary Reference Intake for Selenium

This table presents Recommended Dietary Allowances (RDA) in **bold type** and Adequate Intakes (AI) in regular type followed by an asterisk (*) (in micrograms [μg]). RDA and AI may both be used as goals for individual intake.

Infants

Birth to 6 months	15*
7–12 months	20*

Children

1–3 years	**20**
4–8 years	**30**

Males

9–13 years	**40**
14–70+ years	**55**

Females

9–13 years	**40**
14–70+ years	**55**
Pregnant	**60**
Lactating	**70**

Approximate Selenium Content of Selected Foods (μg/100g)[†]

Grain Group

All-Bran	9
Bran buds	29
Cheerios	38
Special K	55
Wheaties	5
Bagel	32
Bread, wheat (~3 slice)	31
Bread, white (~ 3 slice)	26
Tortilla, corn	6
Tortilla, flour	22

Fruit Group

Apple juice	0
Orange juice	0
Apple	0
Banana	1
Pineapple	1
Strawberries, sweetened, frozen	1

Vegetable Group

Broccoli, raw	3
Cauliflower, frozen/raw	1
Garlic, raw	14
Peas	0
Spinach, raw	1
Tofu	9

Protein Group

Beef, chuck roast	24
Beef, ground lean	29
Beef liver	58
Bacon, cooked	25
Pork tenderloin	48
Chicken, roasted	26
Chicken liver, broiled	71
Eggs, 2	31
Cod or haddock baked	39
Oysters, cooked	72
Tuna, canned in water	80

Calcium Group

Milk	0
Yogurt	1–2
American cheese	15
Cheddar cheese	14

Miscellaneous

Kidney beans, canned, cooked	1
Cashews, roasted	11
Coconut dried, sweetened	16
Sunflower seed, roasted	78

†100 g is approximately 3½ ounces or a ½ cup portion.

3-21 | Phosphorus

Phosphorus helps keep bones and teeth healthy. It plays a role in many important chemical reactions in the body. Almost all food contains some phosphorus, making deficiencies rare. The best sources of phosphorus include milk, poultry, and fish. Cereal grains can be a good source and additives in convenience foods can have a lot of phosphorus.

Recommended Daily Dietary Reference Intake for Phosphorus

This table presents Recommended Dietary Allowances (RDA) in **bold type** and Adequate Intakes (AI) in regular type followed by an asterisk (*) (in milligrams [mg]). RDA and AI may both be used as goals for individual intake.

Infants		Males		Pregnant	
Birth to 6 months	100*	9–18 years	**1,250**	≤18 years	**1,250**
7 months to 1 year	275*	19–70+ years	**700**	19–50 years	**700**

Children		Females		Lactating	
1–years	**460**	9–18 years	**1,250**	≤18 years	**1,250**
4–8 years	**500**	19–70+ years	**700**	19–50 years	**700**

Approximate Phosphorus Content of Selected Foods (mg)

Grain Group

Bran, 100% ½ cup	340
Cornflakes, Kellogg's, ½ cup	11
Oatmeal, cooked, 1 cup	178
White bread, 1 slice	24
Whole wheat bread, 1 slice	64
Rice, white, ½ cup	12
Noodles, enriched egg, ½ cup	55

Fruit Group

Apple juice, 1 cup	17
Orange juice, 1 cup	40
Prune juice, 1 cup	64
Apple, 1	10
Banana, 1	23
Orange, 1	21

Vegetable Group

Beans, snap, ½ cup	13
Beets, ½ cup	32
Broccoli, ½ cup	46
Carrot, 1	32
Corn, ½ cup	53
Peas, ½ cup	57
Tomato, 1	30
Steak, 1 oz	70
Chicken, 1 oz	60
Cod, 1 oz	40
Egg, 1	89
Tuna, 1 oz	88

Calcium Group

Milk, 1 cup	220
American cheese, 1 oz	211
Cheddar cheese, 1 oz	145
Yogurt, 1 cup	215

Miscellaneous

Black beans, 1 cup	241
Chick peas, 1 cup	276
Navy beans, 1 cup	286
Peanut butter, 2 tablespoons	101
Sunflower seeds, dry roasted, 1 oz	327
Cola, 12 oz	44
Diet cola, 12 oz	32

Zinc is one of the enzymes involved in all major metabolic pathways. It aids in healing wounds, is necessary for a healthy sense of taste, and is an essential element for both plants and animals. Good sources include meat, liver, eggs, and seafood (especially oysters). Whole grain products contain zinc in a less available form.

Recommended Daily Dietary Reference Intake for Zinc

This table presents Recommended Dietary Allowances (RDA) in **bold type** and Adequate Intakes (AI) in regular type followed by an asterisk (*) (in milligrams [mg]). RDA and AI may both be used as goals for individual intake.

Infants		*Males*		*Pregnant*	
Birth to 6 months	2*	9–13 years	**8**	≤18 years	**13**
7–12 months	**3**	14–70+ years	**11**	19–50 years	**11**

Children		*Females*		*Lactating*	
1–3 years	**3**	9–13 years	**8**	≤18 years	**14**
4–8 years	**5**	14–18 years	**9**	19–50 years	**12**
		19–70+ years	**8**		

Approximate Zinc Content of Selected Foods (mg)

Grain Group

Farina, enriched, cooked, ¾ cup	0.12
Oatmeal, 1 packet	0.87
Wheatena, cooked, ¾ cup	1.26
All-bran, Kellogg's, ½ cup	3.75
Corn flakes, General Mills, 1 cup	3.75
Shredded wheat, 1 biscuit	0.79
Wheaties, General Mills, 1 cup	0.60

Vegetable Group

Broccoli, cooked, ½ cup	0.30
Carrot, raw, 1 medium	0.35
Corn, canned, ½ cup	0.32
Mushrooms, raw, ½ cup	0.26
Potato, baked, 1	0.65
Tofu, ½ cup	0.99
Tomato, 1 raw	0.11

Fruit Group

Apple juice, 1 cup	0.07
Orange juice, 1 cup	0.12
Apple, raw, 1 medium	0.06
Banana, 1 medium	0.18
Peach, 1 medium	0.12
Watermelon, 1 cup	0.11

Protein Group

Beef, 3½ oz	6.0
Lamb, 3½ oz	5.5
Pork, 3½ oz	3.0
Liver, beef 3½ oz	6.0
Chicken, dark meat, 3½ oz	2.8
Chicken, light meat, 3½ oz	1.2
Turkey, dark meat, 3½ oz	4.4

Turkey, light meat, 3½ oz	2.0
Egg, 1	0.55
Clams, 3 oz	2.3
Cod, 3 oz	0.49
Haddock, 3 oz	0.41
Mussels, blue, raw, 3 oz	1.36
Oysters, Eastern, canned, 3 oz	77.35
Oyster, Pacific, raw, 3 oz	14.14

Calcium Group

Cheese, 1 oz	0.8
Cow's milk, 8 oz	1.0

Miscellaneous

Baked beans, vegetarian, canned, 1 cup	3.56
Chickpeas, 1 cup	2.51
Wheat germ, toasted, ¼ cup	4.83
Peanut butter, 2 tablespoons	0.89

3-23 Protein

Protein builds and repairs tissues such as skin and muscles. Protein is needed to make antibodies that fight disease and enzymes that aid in digestion. In healthy men and women, it is easy to reach the recommended intake of protein and most Americans exceed their protein requirement. During illness, particularly if weight loss occurs, protein consumption may need to be increased.

Animal foods contain the eight amino acids needed to make new protein. Protein from plant foods, including beans, nuts, and grains, can contribute amino acids that complement each other to make proteins containing all the essential amino acids once they are consumed and digested. Sources of protein include eggs, meat, fish, poultry, milk, yogurt, cheese, beans, soybeans, and peanuts. Grain foods, such as bread, pasta, and cereal, can add up to become significant sources of protein.

Recommended Daily Dietary Reference Intake for Protein

This table presents Recommended Dietary Allowances (RDA) in **bold type** and Adequate Intakes (AI) in regular type followed by an asterisk (*) (in grams [g]). RDAs and AI may both be used as goals for individual intake.

Infants		Males		Females	
Birth to 6 months	9.1*	9–13 years	**34**	9–13 years	**34**
7–12 months	**13.5**	14–18 years	**52**	14–70+ years	**46**
		19–70+ years	**56**	Pregnant	**71**
Children				Lactating	**71**
1–3 years	**13**				
4–8 years	**19**				

Approximate Protein Content of Selected Foods (g)

Grain Group		Grain Group	
Farina, ¾ cup	2.4	White bread, 1 slice	2.0
Oatmeal, instant, 1 packet	4.4	Wheat bread, 1 slice	2.7
All-bran, Kellogg's, ½ cup	3.9	Macaroni, enriched, cooked, 1 cup	6.7
Bran, 100%, ½ cup	3.5	Rice brown, 1 cup	5.0
Granola, homemade, ¼ cup	4.1	Rice white, 1 cup	4.3
Puffed wheat, 1 cup	2.1	Stuffing, ½ cup	3.2
Bagel, 3½ inch	7.5	Tortilla, taco	0.9
Biscuit, 1	2.0	Tortilla, flour	3.0
Cornbread, 2 inch piece	4.4	Pita bread, 6½ inch	5.5
Raisin bread, 1 slice	2.1		

Fruit Group

Apple juice, 1 cup	0.1
Carrot juice, 3-4 cup	1.7
Grapefruit juice, 1 cup	1.4
Orange juice, 1 cup	1.7
Tomato juice, 3-4 cup	1.4
Apple, 1 medium	0.3
Banana, 1 medium	1.2
Peach, 1 medium	0.6
Pear, 1 medium	0.6
Raisins, 2/3 cup	3.0

Vegetable Group

Beets, canned, 1/2 cup	0.8
Carrot, raw, 1	0.7
Corn, frozen, 1/2 cup	2.3
Peas, 1/2 cup	4.0
Potato, baked	4.6
Tofu, 1/2 cup	10
Sweet potato, 3–4 oz	2.0

Protein Group

Beef, pot roast, 3 1/2 oz	33
Beef, lean ground, 3 1/2 oz	24.5
Beef, regular, ground 3 1/2 oz	23
Lamb, 3 1/2 oz	29
Pork 3 1/2 oz	20.4
Bacon, Canadian style, 2 slices	11.4
Bacon, cooked, 3 slices	5.8
Ham, 1 oz	5.4
Veal, 3 1/2 oz	28
Bologna, 1 oz	2.7
Frankfurt, beef, 2 oz	6.8
Salami, ~1 oz	3.5
Chicken, dark meat, 3 1/2 oz	27.4
Chicken, light meat, 3 1/2 oz	30.9
Turkey, dark meat, 3 1/2 oz	28.6

Protein Group

Turkey, light meat, 3 1/2 oz	29.9
Egg, 1 large	6.2
White of 1 egg	3.5
Yolk of 1 egg	2.8
Egg substitute, frozen, 1/4 cup	6.8
Cod, 3 oz	19.4
Fish stick, frozen, 1	4.4

Calcium Group

Milk, 1%, 8 oz	8.0
Milk, whole, 8 oz	8.0
Milk, dry powdered, 1/4 cup	10.8
Soy milk, 8 oz	6.6
Yogurt, 8 oz	8.1
American cheese, 1 oz	6.3
Cheddar cheese, 1 oz	7.1
Cottage cheese, 1 cup	28
Feta cheese, 1 oz	4.0
Mozzarella cheese,1 oz	6.9
Parmesan cheese, 1 oz	10.1

Legumes

Baked beans, 1/2 cup	5.0
Vegetarian beans, canned, 1 cup	12.2
Black beans, 1 cup	15.2
Chickpeas, 1 cup	14.5
Kidney beans, 1 cup	15.3

Miscellaneous

Almonds, dry roasted, 1 oz	4.6
Cashew, dry roasted, 1 oz	4.3
Coconut, dried sweet, 4 oz	3.8
Peanut butter, 2 tablespoons	7.7
Corn oil, 1 tablespoon	0
Olive oil, 1 tablespoon	0
Butter, 1 tablespoon	0
Margarine, 1 tablespoon	0

Eating a variety of plant foods, such as unrefined grains, dried beans, seeds, nuts, and vegetables will provide the amino acids needed to make enough protein for good health.

Try some of these combinations:

- Grain+ nuts (peanut butter sandwich)
- Nuts and vegetables (almonds and green beans)
- Vegetables and legumes (minestrone soup)
- Legumes and beans (beans and rice)
- Grains and vegetable (barley and roasted vegetables)

If appetite is poor, try adding protein to foods in the following way:

- Melt a slice of cheese on toast or crackers
- Serve peanut butter on bread or fruit
- Serve yogurt with fruit or make a fruit and yogurt drink
- Snack on a hard boiled egg
- Fortify liquid milk with 2 tablespoons powdered milk
- Snack on sliced deli meat and cheese roll-ups

Carbohydrates supply calories and spare protein from being used as an energy source, allowing it to be used to build and repair tissue. All carbohydrates have the same calories: 4 calories per gram of weight. It is recommended that most people consume 55% to 60% of calories in the form of carbohydrate. That is approximately 300g for someone eating a 2,000-calorie menu and 375g when eating a 2,500-calorie menu. The RDA is based on carbohydrates' role as the brain's primary energy source.

Recommended Daily Dietary Reference Intake for Carbohydrate

This table presents Recommended Dietary Allowances (RDA) in **bold type** and Adequate Intakes (AI) in regular type followed by an asterisk (*) (in grams [g]). RDA and AI may both be used as goals for individual intake.

Infants		*Children: all ages*	**130**	*Females: all ages*	**130**
Birth to 6 months	60*			Pregnant	**175**
7–12 months	95*	*Males: all ages*	**130**	Lactating	**210**

Approximate Carbohydrate Content of Selected Foods (g)

Grain Group		*Fruit Group*	
Oatmeal, instant, 1 packet	18.1	Apple juice, 1 cup	29
Wheatena, ¾ cup	21.5	Carrot juice, ¾ cup	17.1
All-bran, Kellogg's, ½ cup	23	Grapefruit juice, 1 cup	24
Crackling Oat Bran, Kellogg's, ¾ cup	35.6	Orange juice, 1 cup	26.8
Frosted, mini-wheat, Kellogg's, 1 cup	48	Tomato juice, 3–4 cup	7.7
Oatmeal squares, Quaker, 1 cup	43.3	Apple, medium	21
Puffed wheat, 1 cup	11.1	Cantaloupe, 1 cup	13.4
Shredded wheat, 1 biscuit	19.3	Cherries, 10	8.3
Bagel, 3½ inch	37.9	Fruit roll-up, Betty Crocker, 1	12
Banana bread, 1 slice	32.8	Peach, 1 medium	9.7
Pita bread, 6½ inch	33.4	Pear, 1 medium	25.1
Raisin bread, 1 slice	13.6	Raisins, ⅔ cup	79
White bread, 1 slice	12.9	Watermelon, 1 cup	11.5
Whole wheat bread, 1 slice	12.4		
Macaroni, enriched, cooked, 1 cup	39.7		
Noodles, egg, enriched, cooked, 1 cup	39.7		
Brown rice, 1 cup	44.8		
White rice, 1 cup	44.5		
Tortilla, taco shell, 1 medium	8.1		
Tortilla, flour, 7–8 inch	19.5		

Vegetable Group

Beets, canned, slices, ½ cup	6.1
Broccoli, ½ cup	3.9
Carrot, raw, 1 medium	7.3
Corn, ½ cup	16
Mixed vegetables, canned, ½ cup	7.6
Peas, ½ cup	11
Potato, baked, 6 oz	51
Tomato, 1 raw	5.7

Protein Group

Beef, lamb, pork	0
Frankfurt, 2 oz	1.0
Poultry	0
Egg, 1 large	0.6

Calcium Group

Milk, whole, skim, or 1%	12
Yogurt, plain, 8 oz	19
Yogurt, flavored, 8 oz	48.5
Cheese, hard type, 1 oz	0.5
Cottage cheese, 1 cup	6.1

Miscellaneous

Baked beans, ½ cup	30
Black beans, 1 cup	40
Peanut butter, 2 tablespoons	7
Cooking oils	0

3-25 Fat

Fat is a nutrient as essential to a healthy body as protein and carbohydrate. It plays a critical role in many body functions, including cholesterol metabolism, the transport and absorption of fat-soluble vitamins, and the synthesis of vital hormones and body fluids.

Three fats often included in the discussion of fat and health are saturated, monounsaturated, and polyunsaturated fat. More recently, trans fat or trans fatty acids have been added to the discussion. Saturated fat and trans fat can increase the concentration of harmful fats in our blood, known as LDL or "bad" cholesterol. Saturated fat is found in animal fats, such as meat, butter, cream, coconut oils, and palm kernel oils. Trans fats are in stick margarine and foods that list partially hydrogenated vegetable oil on the ingredient list, including most commercially baked goods, snack foods, and fried foods.

Monounsaturated and polyunsaturated fats are in vegetable oils that remain liquid at room temperature, including corn, safflower and sunflower oil, soft margarine, and salad dressing. Olives, olive oil, peanuts, peanut oil, and canola oil are particularly good sources of monounsaturated fats.

Recommended Daily Dietary Reference Intake for Fat

This table presents Recommended Dietary Allowances (RDA) in **bold type** and Adequate Intakes (AI) in regular type followed by an asterisk (*) (in grams [g]). RDA and AI may both be used as goals for individual intake.

Infants

Birth to 6 months	31*
7–12 months	30*

After the first year of life, no defined fat allowance is set for children or adults, but an Acceptable Macronutrient Range (AMDR) is the range of fat intake in grams associated with a reduced risk of chronic disease while providing intakes of essential nutrients.

Acceptable Macronutrient Distribution Range for Total Fat (g)

Children		Males		Females	
1–3 years	30–40	9–18	25–35	9–18 years	25–35
4–8 years	25–35	19–>70 years	20–35	19–70+ years	20–35
				Pregnant	20–35
				Lactating	20–35

A recommended level of 30% to 35% of calories for total fat and less than 10% for saturated fat is a practical guideline suggested by many nutritionists. For a person eating a 2,000-calorie menu that amounts to 65g of total fat and 20g of saturated fat per day. The Nutrition Facts Panel carries the amount of total and saturated fat contained in each serving of food. Trans fat information will be added to labels in the future.

Sources of fat include butter, margarine, vegetable oils, whole milk dairy products, visible fat on meat and poultry, and invisible fat in fish, shellfish, seeds, nuts, and many baked products.

Polyunsaturated Fatty Acids: Linoleic Acid (Omega-6) and Linolenic Acid (Omega-3)

The major polyunsaturated fats in food are linoleic acid (LA) and linolenic acid (LNA), also called omega-6 and omega-3 fatty acids, respectively. Maintaining a proper ratio of linolenic acid to linoleic acid is thought to be important for disease prevention, including atherosclerosis. Many nutritionists believe omega-3 fatty acid intake is too low and encourage the eating of more foods rich in omega-3 fatty acids. Docosahexaenoic acid (DHA) and eicosapentaenoic acid (EPA) are polyunsaturated fatty acids obtained from food and synthesized from linolenic acid in the body.

Sources of omega-6 fatty acids include nuts, seeds, soybean oil, safflower oil, and corn oil.

Sources of omega-3 fatty acids include soybean oil, canola oil, flaxseed oil, fish oils, and fatty fish, such as salmon and sardines.

Recommended Dietary Reference Intake for Omega-6 and Omega-3 Fatty Acids

This table presents Recommended Dietary Allowances (RDA) in **bold type** and Adequate Intakes (AI) in regular type followed by an asterisk (*) (in grams [g]). RDA and AI may both be used as goals for individual intake.

Infants	Omega-3	Omega-6
Birth to 6 months	0.5*	4.4*
7–12 months	0.5*	4.6*

Males	Omega-3	Omega-6
9–13 years	1.2*	12*
14–18 years	1.6*	16*
19–50 years	1.6*	17*
51–70+ years	1.6*	14*

Females	Omega-3	Omega-6
9–13 years	1.0*	10*
14–18 years	1.1*	11*
19–50 years	1.1*	12*
50–70+ years	1.1*	11*
Pregnant	1.4*	13*
Lactating	1.3*	13*

Children	Omega-3	Omega-6
1–3 years	0.7*	7*
4–6 years	0.9*	10*

Approximate Omega-6 and Omega-3 Fatty Acid Content in Selected Foods (g/100 g)[†]

	Omega-6	Omega-3		
		LNA	EPA	DHA
Protein Group				
Cod, Atlantic	Trace	Trace	0.1	0.2
Haddock	Trace	Trace	0.1	0.1
Halibut, Greenland	0.5	Trace	0.5	0.4
Herring	0.4	0.1	0.7	0.9
Mackerel, Atlantic	1.1	0.1	0.9	1.6
Pollock	Trace	—	0.1	0.4
Salmon, Atlantic	0.7	0.2	0.3	0.9
Snapper, red	0.2	Trace	Trace	0.2
Sole	0.1	Trace	Trace	0.1
Swordfish	—	—	0.1	0.1
Tuna, albacore	—	—	0.4	1.2
Crab, Alaska King	Trace	Trace	0.2	0.1
Lobster, northern	Trace	—	0.1	0.1
Shrimp, Atlantic brown	0.2	Trace	0.2	0.1
Clam, littleneck trace	—	Trace	Trace	
Mussel, blue	0.1	Trace	0.2	0.3
Oyster, pacific	0.3	Trace	0.4	0.2
Scallops	0.1	Trace	0.1	0.1

	Omega-6	Omega-3		
		LNA	EPA	DHA
Fat Group				
Butter	1.8	1.2	—	—
Canola oil	22.2	11.2	—	—
Flaxseed oil	12.7	53.5	—	—
Safflower oil	77.0	1.0	—	—
Soybean oil	51.1	6.8	—	—
Miscellaneous				
Soybean kernels, roasted	11.2	1.5	—	—
Walnuts, black	34.2	3.3	—	—
Walnuts, English	32.3	6.8	—	—

[†]Adapted from Mahan, L. K., and Escott-Stump, S. (2004). *Krause's food, nutrition & diet therapy* (11th ed., 1244–1245). Philadelphia: W. B. Saunders.

Fiber is the part of fruit, vegetables, and grains that is not digested. Two types of fiber—soluble and insoluble—are important to health. Most foods contain some of each; the more processed and refined a food is, the less fiber it is likely to have.

Soluble fiber forms a gel when mixed with water. This is the type of fiber linked with controlling blood sugar and cholesterol levels. It can be found in oat bran, beans, and some fruits, including apricots and blackberries.

Insoluble fiber does not dissolve in water; it acts more like a sponge, absorbing water in the intestine. This type of fiber can help fight constipation by adding bulk to the diet and moving waste through the body more quickly. Foods high in insoluble fiber include wheat bran, whole grains, and many fruits and vegetables.

Recommended Daily Dietary Reference Intake for Total Fiber

This table presents Recommended Dietary Allowances (RDA) in **bold type** and Adequate Intakes (AI) in regular type followed by an asterisk (*) (in grams [g]). RDA and AI may both be used as goals for individual intake.

Infants		Males		Females	
Birth to 6 months	not determined	9–13 years	31*	9–18 years	26*
		14–50 years	38*	19–50 years	25*
7–12 months	not determined	51–70+ years	30*	51–70+ years	21*
				Pregnant	28*
Children				Lactating	29*
1–3 years	19*				
4–6 years	25*				

Approximate Fiber Content of Selected Foods (g)

Grain Group		Grain Group	
Fiber-One, General Mills, ½ cup	13.0	Oatmeal, instant, 1 packet	3.0
All-Bran, Kellogg's, ½ cup	10.0	Life, Quaker, ¾ cup	2.0
Raisin Bran, Kellogg's, ¾ cup	8.2	Cornflakes, Kellogg's, 1 cup	1.1
Cracklin' Oat Bran, Kellogg's, ¾ cup	5.6	Rice Krispies, 1 cup	0.3
Basic 4, General Mills, 1 cup	3.0	Trix, General Mills, 1 cup	0.0
Granola, ⅔ cup	3.0	Whole wheat bread, 1 slice	1.9
Cheerios, 1 cup	3.0	White bread, 1 slice	0.6
Multi Grain Cheerios, 1 cup	3.0	English muffin	1.5
Total, General Mills, ¾ cup	3.0	English muffin, whole wheat	4.4

Grain Group

Bagel	2.0
Saltine crackers, 7	0.7
Triscuit crackers, 7	4.0
Brown rice, 1 cup	3.5
White rice, 1 cup	1.0
Macaroni, cooked, 1 cup	1.8
Macaroni, whole wheat, cooked, 1 cup	3.9

Vegetable Group

Asparagus, ½ cup	1.4
Beets, ½ cup	1.4
Broccoli, ½ cup	2.0
Brussels sprouts, ½ cup	2.0
Cabbage, ½ cup	1.7
Carrots, ½ cup	2.6
Cauliflower, ½ cup	1.7
Corn, ½ cup	2.3
Green beans, ½ cup	2.0
Lettuce, ½ cup	0.5
Mixed vegetables, ½ cup	2.5
Mushrooms, ½ cup	1.7
Okra, ½ cup	2.2
Onions, ½ cup	1.5
Parsnips, ½ cup	3.1
Peas, green, ½ cup	4.0
Peppers, sweet, ½ cup	0.8
Potato without skin	2.5
Potato with skin	4.6
Potato, mashed, ½ cup	2.1
Spinach, ½ cup	2.2
Squash, summer, ½ cup	1.3
Squash, winter, ½ cup	3.5
Sweet potato, mashed, ½ cup	3.0
Tomato, raw, 4 oz	1.4
Turnip, ½ cup	1.6

Protein Group

Fish	0
Egg	0
Beef	0
Poultry	0
Baked beans, 1 cup	12.0
Chili beans, 1 cup	12.0

Protein Group

Bean burrito, frozen, 5 oz	7.0
Chick peas, ½ cup	6.0

Fruit

Apple juice, 1 cup	0.2
Orange juice, 1 cup	0.5
Apple, raw	3.7
Banana	2.7
Cantaloupe, 1 cup	1.3
Cherries, 10	1.1
Fruit salad, canned, ½ cup	1.3
Fruit roll-up	0.0
Grapefruit, ½	1.3
Mandarin oranges, canned, ½ cup	0.9
Orange, 1 medium	3.1
Papaya, 1 medium	5.5
Peach, 1 medium	1.7
Pear, 1 medium	4.0
Pineapple, 1 cup	2.0
Plum, 1 medium	1.0
Prunes, 10	6.0
Raisins, ⅔ cup	4.0
Strawberries, 1 cup	3.4
Watermelon, 1 cup	0.8

Calcium Group

Cheese	0
Milk	0

Miscellaneous

Popcorn, 1 cup	1.0
Potato chips, 1 oz	1.3
Rice cakes, 1	0.3
Peanuts, 1 oz	2.5
Sunflower seeds, 1 oz	3.0

Additional Nutrients for Which Limited Data on Food Sources or Requirements Exists

ARSENIC

Arsenic is needed by animals in very small amounts, but it has no biological function for humans. Dairy products, meat, poultry, fish, grains, and cereals are food sources of arsenic. No Dietary Reference Intake has been established for arsenic.

BIOTIN

Biotin is involved in many reactions related to fat and carbohydrate metabolism. Found primarily in the liver, smaller amounts of it are found in fruits and meats.

Recommended Daily Dietary Reference Intake

This table presents Recommended Dietary Allowances (RDA) in **bold type** and Adequate Intakes (AI) in regular type followed by an asterisk (*) (in micrograms [μg]). RDA and AI may both be used as goals for individual intake.

Infants		Males		Females	
Birth to 6 months	5*	9–13 years	20*	9–13 years	20*
7–12 months	6*	14–18 years	25*	14–18 years	25*
		19–70+ years	30*	19–70+ years	30*
Children				Pregnant	30*
				Lactating	35*
1–3 years	8*				
4–8 years	12*				

BORON

Boron has no clear function in human nutrition, although data indicate it plays a functional role in animals. No Dietary Reference Intake has been established for boron.

CHOLINE

Choline is a simple compound made in the liver and widely distributed in plant and animal food sources. Choline is so abundant in food a deficiency is unlikely to occur. Choline is particularly abundant in milk, liver, eggs, and peanuts.

Recommended Daily Dietary Reference Intake

This table presents Recommended Dietary Allowances (RDA) in **bold type** and Adequate Intakes (AI) in regular type followed by an asterisk (*) (in milligrams [mg]). RDA and AI may both be used as goals for individual intake.

Infants		Males		Females	
Birth to 6 months	125*	9–13 years	375*	9–13 years	375*
7–12 months	150*	14–70+ years	550*	14–18 years	400*
				19–70+ years	425*
Children				Pregnant	450*
				Lactating	550*
1–3 years	200*				
4–8 years	250*				

CHROMIUM

Chromium helps to maintain normal blood sugar levels. It probably does so by entering the cells and increasing the number of insulin receptors or enhancing the movement of sugar across the cell membranes. Although the chromium content of food is limited, the best sources are whole grain cereals, meat, poultry, fish, and beer. The amount of chromium is related to the chromium content of the soil food is grown in.

Recommended Daily Dietary Reference Intake

This table presents Recommended Dietary Allowances (RDAs) in **bold type** and Adequate Intakes (AI) in regular type followed by an asterisk (*) (in micrograms [μg]). RDA and AI may both be used as goals for individual intake.

Infants		Males		Pregnant	
Birth to 6 months	0.2*	9–13 years	25*	≤18 years	29*
7–12 months	5.5*	14–50 years	35*	19–50 years	30*
		50–70+ years	30*		
Children				**Lactating**	
		Females		≤18 years	44*
1–3 years	11*			19–50 years	45*
4–8 years	15*	9–13 years	21*		
		14–18 years	24*		
		19–50 years	25*		
		50–70+ years	20*		

FLUORIDE

Fluoride inhibits the formation of dental cavities and promotes strong bone growth. The most familiar source is in fluoridated water supplies, but it can also be found in tea, salt water fish, and fluoridated dental products.

Recommended Daily Dietary Reference Intake

This table presents Recommended Dietary Allowances (RDAs) in **bold type** and Adequate Intakes (AI) in regular type followed by an asterisk (*) (in milligrams [mg]). RDA and AI may both be used as goals for individual intake.

Infants		*Males*		*Females*	
Birth to 6 months	0.01*	9–13 years	2*	9–13 years	2*
7–12 months	0.5*	14–18 years	3*	14–70+ years	3*
		19–70+ years	4*	Pregnant	3*
Children				Lactating	3*
1–3 years	0.7*				
4–8 years	1*				

MOLYBDENUM

Molybdenum is required by several body enzymes, but no molybdenum deficiency has been observed in people eating a normal diet. Dried beans, grain products, and nuts contain molybdenum.

Recommended Daily Dietary Reference Intake

This table presents Recommended Dietary Allowances (RDAs) in **bold type** and Adequate Intakes (AI) in regular type followed by an asterisk (*) (in micrograms [µg]). RDA and AI may both be used as goals for individual intake.

Infants		*Males*		*Females*	
Birth to 6 months	2*	9–13 years	**34**	9–13 years	**34**
7–12 months	3*	14–18 years	**43**	14–18 years	**43**
		19–70+ years	**45**	19–70+ years	**45**
Children				Pregnant	**50**
1–3 years	**17**			Lactating	**50**
4 to 6 years	**22**				

NICKEL

Plants and animals need nickel, but it serves no clear biological function in humans. It may help with the absorption of iron and the metabolism of microorganisms. Nuts, dried beans, cereal, sweeteners, and chocolate contain nickel. Insufficient data exist to recommend a daily Dietary Reference Intake.

SILICON

Animal studies have found silicon to be involved in bone function. Plant-based foods can contain silicon. Insufficient data exist to establish a recommended daily Dietary Reference Intake.

VANADIUM

Vanadium may play a role in how salt and potassium are transported in the body, but no biological function in humans has been identified. Insufficient data exist to recommend a daily Dietary Reference Intake.

REFERENCES

Arthritis (2004). www.arthritis.org/conditions/DiseaseCenter/oa.asp. Accessed August 18, 2004.

Bent, S., & Ko, R. (2004). Commonly used herbal medicines in the United States: A review. *The American Journal of Medicine, 116,* 478–485.

Blumenthal, M., Goldberg, A., Gruenwald, J., Hall, T., Riggins, C. W., Rister, R. S., Klein, S., & Rister, R.S., trans. (2000). *The Complete Commission E Monographs: Therapeutic Guide to Herbal Medicines* (English Translation). Austin, TX: American Botanical Council; and Boston, MA: Integrative Medicine Communications.

Cholesterol. (2004). Available at: www.cdc.gov/cvh/announcements/cholesterol_education_month.htm. Accessed August 18, 2004.

Covington, M. B. (2004). Omega-3 fatty acids. *American Family Physician, 70,* 133–140.

Center for Science in the Public Interest. (2003). Eight to avoid. *Nutrition Action Health Letter, 30,* 5.

DSHEA. (1994). Dietary Supplement Health Education Act of 1994. Public Law 103-417. October 25, 1994.

U.S. Food and Drug Administration. (1998). FDA determines Cholestin to be an unapproved drug 5/20/98. Available at: www.fda.gov/bbs/topics/ANSWERS/ANS00871.html. Accessed 9/2004

Millen, A. E., Dodd, K. W., & Subar, A. F. (2004). Use of vitamin, mineral, nonvitamin, and nonmineral supplements in the United States: The 1987, 1992, and 2000 National Health Interview Survey results. *Journal of the American Dietetic Association, 104,* 942–950.

Morelli, V., Naquin, C., & Weaver, V. (2003). Alternative therapies for traditional disease states: Osteoarthritis. *American Family Physician,* January 15, 235–241. Available at: www.aafp.org/afp/20030115/339.html. Accessed June 14, 2004.

Morelli, V., & Zoorob, R. J. (2000). Alternative therapies. Part II: Congestive heart failure and hypercholesterolemia. *American Family Physician, 62,* 326.

Sarubin, A. (2000). *The Health Professionals Guide to Popular Dietary Supplements.* American. Chicago, Illinois: American Dietetic Association.

Schardt, D. (2004). The heart of the matter. *Nutrition Action Healthletter, 31,* 8–11.

Sources

Nutrient data

Dietary Reference Intake for Calcium, Phosphorous, Magnesium, Vitamin D, and Fluoride (1997). Food and Nutrition Board, Institute of Medicine, National Academy of Sciences. Washington, DC: National Academy Press. Available on-line at www.nap.edu/books/0309085373/html/.

Dietary Reference Intakes for Calcium, Phosphorous, Magnesium, Vitamin D, and Fluoride (1997). Food and Nutrition Board, Institute of Medicine, National Academy of Sciences. Washington, DC: National Academy Press. Available on-line at http://books.nap.edu/books/0309063507/html/index.html.

Dietary Reference Intakes for Thiamin, Riboflavin, Niacin, Vitamin B_6, Folate, Vitamin B_{12}, Pantothenic Acid, Biotin, and Choline. (1998). Food and Nutrition Board, Institute of Medicine, National Academy of Sciences. Washington, DC: National Academy Press. Available on-line at http://books.nap.edu/books/0309065542/html/index.html.

Dietary Reference Intakes for Vitamins A, Vitamin K, Arsenic, Boron, Chromium, Copper, Iodine, Iron, Manganese, Molybdenum, Nickel, Silicon, Vanadium, and Zinc. (2000). Food and Nutrition Board, Institute of Medicine, National Academy of Sciences. Washington, DC: National Academy Press. Available on-line at http://www.nap.edu/books/0309072794/html/.

Dietary Reference Intakes for Vitamin C, Vitamin E, Selenium, and Carotenoids. (2000). Available on-line at www.nap.edu/books/0309069351/html/.

Dietary Reference Intakes for Energy, Carbohydrate, Fiber, Fat, Fatty Acids, Cholesterol, Protein, and Amino Acids (Macronutrients). (2002). Food and Nutrition Board, Institute of Medicine, National Academy of Sciences. Washington, DC: National Academy Press. Available on-line at www.nap.edu/books/0309085373/html/.

Dietary Reference Intakes for Water, Potassium, Sodium, Chloride, and Sulfate. (2004).

Food and Nutrition Board, Institute of Medicine, National Academy of Sciences. Washington, DC: National Academy Press. Available on-line at http://books.nap.edu/books/0309091691/html/2.html.

Pennington, J. A. T. (1998). *Bowes & Church's Food Values of Portions Commonly Used*, 17th ed. Philadelphia: Lippincott.

Therapeutic Nutrition

Medical nutrition therapy or maintenance of adequate nutrition during acute illness, trauma, or chronic disease is a foundation of good patient care. Poor nutrition can result from decrease in appetite, increase in energy needs, or malabsorption in the digestive tract. The information and the therapeutic diets that follow are intended to offer practical guidance about food choices until an individual can meet with a nutrition professional.

IMPORTANCE OF THERAPEUTIC NUTRITION

Chronic disease, including diabetes, heart disease, and cancer, accounts for 7 of 10 deaths in the United States and affects the quality of life of more than 90 million individuals and their families, according to the National Center for Chronic Disease and Health Promotion (NCCD, 2004). Eating a healthy diet, being active, and avoiding tobacco use can prevent or control the effects of these diseases. Good nutrition plays a role in all areas of healthcare. Use the information in Chapter two to educate patients about what a healthy diet is, in most cases stressing a diet rich in fruits, vegetables, whole grains, and adequate in protein and calcium. Patient education handouts in Section two of this chapter defines whole grains, explains what is a serving of fruit and vegetables, and shows how to reduce sodium and saturated fat. Do not overlook these tools. In many medical conditions, good nutrition alone is not enough. Patients may require advice on altering food choices to relieve symptoms or prevent the progression of a condition. For example when celiac disease is diagnosed, a gluten-free diet is essential. A patient with gout may benefit from a low purine diet during an acute attack. An adjustment in fiber may be advised to aid in a disease of the digestive tract. The patient education handouts are designed to help reinforce the important role diet plays in the comprehensive care of patients

In only a few cases will the dietary recommendations in this section be adequate to answer all questions about nutrition and food choices. Anyone with a chronic disease requiring a modified diet or the elimination of whole food groups should be referred to a registered dietitian for individualized medical nutrition therapy. Several studies support the role of nutrition therapy in the management of disease, including the Diabetes Control and Complications Trial (DCCT) and the Dietary Approach to Stop Hypertension (DASH). The DCCT (DCCT, 1993) proved that intensive diet therapy, including follow-up evaluations and education, could improve diabetic control and reduce complications. The DASH diet (Blackburn, 2001) is one of many studies that supports the role of diet therapy in the control of hypertension. Comprehensive medical nutrition therapy should be an important component in treating any chronic medical conditions, each patient handout contains advice about the importance of finding a registered dietitian.

INSURANCE AND MEDICAL NUTRITION THERAPY

Many healthcare providers incorrectly assume nutrition counseling will not be covered by insurance. Medical Nutrition Therapy (MNT) is the term used to describe nutrition intervention to treat an illness, injury, or condition. As of January 1, 2002, MNT became a distinct Medicare Part B benefit covering MNT when provided by registered dietitians and nutrition professionals to Medicare part B beneficiaries with diabetes or renal disease. Nationwide, health plan and employer coverage of MNT varies. According to the American Dietetic Association, Aetna's national coverage policy and Blue Cross Blue Shield of Massachusetts are examples of third-party payers who provide beneficiaries with access to MNT services provided by a registered dietitian. Individuals should be encouraged to contact their insurance company to ask about coverage.

NUTRITION OVERVIEW OF SELECTED MEDICAL CONDITIONS

Arthritis

According to the National Center for Chronic Disease Prevention and Health Promotion (NCCD, 2004) 1 of 3 Americans have arthritis or chronic joint pain, the leading cause of disability in the United States. Arthritis comprises more than 100 different diseases; the most common include osteoarthritis, rheumatoid arthritis, fibromyalgia, and gout.

OSTEOARTHRITIS

Osteoarthritis, the most frequently diagnosed form of arthritis, involves the destruction of cartilage, causing painful stiff joints. Important nutrition considerations include (Mahan & Escott-Stump, 2004) maintaining a desirable weight and consuming foods rich in B vitamins, calcium, and vitamin D. Glucosamine and chrondroitin sulfate reportedly relieve the pain associated with osteoarthritis. Currently, the National Center for Complementary and Alternative Medicine is conducting a study at 13 research centers across the country to determine the effectiveness of glucosamine and chrondroitin in the treatment of osteoarthritis pain (NIH-NCCAM, 2004). Refer to Box 3-5 to answer questions about supplements used in the treatment of osteoarthritis.

RHEUMATOID ARTHRITIS

Rheumatoid arthritis is a chronic inflammatory autoimmune systemic disease that affects the joints. It is characterized by inflammation of the synovial membranes, which causes atrophy of the joints and osteopenia (too little bone mass). A diet adequate in protein and energy is important. Fasting and vegetarian diets have been useful in the control of joint inflammation; some patients have found benefit in a vegan, gluten-free diet (Muller, de Toledo, & Resch, 2001; Hafstrom, Ringertz, & Spangberg, 2001). Omega-3 fatty acids found in fish, flaxseed, walnuts, and soy and canola oils have been shown to reduce the inflammatory process. Read about omega-3 fatty acids in Section Three.

FIBROMYALGIA

Fibromyalgia is a generalized condition characterized by chronic fatigue and aches that are similar to rheumatoid arthritis. Unlike arthritis, however, the pain is located in the soft tissues around joints and in skin and organs throughout the body. According to the National Fibromyalgia Partnership, (FM Partnership, 2004) 4 to 6 million Americans have the condition and an estimated 80% are women. Gastrointestinal complaints can include irritable bowel syndrome and difficulty swallowing. Treatment aims at managing symptoms. Gentle exercise and proper nutrition can be useful. Sugar, caffeine, and alcohol are thought to irritate muscles and stress the system. One study found a vegan diet to be useful in the treatment of fibromyalgia (Kaartinen, Lammi, & Hypen, 2000). Nutritional programs that dramatically alter a person's traditional diet require the input of a nutritionist familiar with the needs of patients with fibromyalgia. It is appropriate, however, to stress the role of adequate diet, including the use of multivitamin and minerals for those who need them.

GOUT

Gout is a disorder of purine metabolism leading to abnormally high levels of uric acid accumulating in the blood and resulting in acute pain, usually in the big toe. Drugs have replaced the low purine diet as the treatment of choice because 85% of the urate comes from within the body and not from food sources. Nevertheless, many such patients will ask for dietary advice and it is not incorrect to advise a low purine diet during an acute attack. Recently, the role of alcohol, specifically beer, on exacerbating symptoms of gout has been reconfirmed (Choi, Atkinson, & Karlson, 2004). Beer was found to increase the risk of a gout attack, whereas moderate wine consumption did not. A low purine diet is included in Handout 4-17.

RESOURCES

Arthritis Foundation
    www.arthritis.org
National Fibromyalgia Partnership
    www.fmpartnership.org
National Institute of Arthritis, Musculoskeletal and Skin Diseases
    www.nih.gov/niams
Strong Women
    www.strongwomen.com
Nelson, Miriam. (2000). *Strong Women and Men Beat Arthritis*. New York: G. P. Putnam. A scientifically

proven program that allows people with arthritis to take charge of their disease.

CANCER PREVENTION

The American Cancer Society (ACS) issued guidelines for reducing the risk of cancer with healthy food choices and physical activity (Byers, Nestle, & Metieran, 2001). In the United States, about 35% of cancer deaths could be avoided by altering the diet to include more fruit and vegetables, less animal fats and meat, and reduce calories. The American Academy of Family Physicians developed practice guidelines (Ressel, 2002) based on the ACS recommendations, which include the following:

■ Eat a variety of healthy foods: 5 or more fruits and vegetables: limit fried foods; include whole grain foods, such as whole grain rice, bread, pasta, and cereals. Limit red meat and processed meats. Choose fish poultry or beans as an alternative to meat.
■ Adopt a physically active lifestyle: include 30 minutes of moderate activity 5 or more days per week; children and adolescents should aim for 60 minutes of moderate activity.
■ Maintain a healthy weight throughout life.
■ If you drink alcohol, do so in moderation. Men should limit alcohol to two drinks per day; women one drink per day.

Cancer Treatment

Nutrition can play an important role in cancer treatment. Surgery will increase the need for calories and protein; radiation treatment, depending on location, can have an impact on taste, smell, and appetite. Look to patient education Handout 4-24 for advice on increasing calories and protein. Food aversions also can develop during treatment. One study (Menashian, et al., 1992) found a bland, colorless, odorless menu reduced nausea and vomiting associated with cancer treatment. The diet included cottage cheese, unsweetened applesauce, hot cream soup, vanilla ice cream, gelatin, and cola drinks. This is not a balanced diet, but it may be useful in the short term.

Probably the most important nutrition intervention in the treatment of cancer is the routine recording of body weight and preventing weight loss. An unexplained or undesirable weight loss is often the first anthropometric measure of poor nutrition. Monitor the patient's weight weekly and suggest the patient contact a registered dietitian if symptoms that affect eating occur or if an unwanted weight loss develops.

RESOURCES

American Cancer Society
  www.cancer.org
American Institute for Cancer Research
  www.aicr.org
National Cancer Institute
  www.cancer.gov
Oncology Nutrition Practice Group
  www.oncologynutrition.org
Dyer, D. (2002). *A Dietitian's Cancer Story*. 2nd ed. Ann Arbor, Michigan: Swan Press.

CARDIOVASCULAR DISEASE

Cardiovascular disease includes stroke, high blood pressure, and high blood cholesterol.

According to the National Center for Chronic Disease Prevention and Health Promotion (NCCD, 2004) heart disease and stroke—the principal components of cardiovascular disease—are the first and third leading causes of death in the United States, accounting for more than 40% of all deaths. High blood pressure and high blood cholesterol are the most important independent risk factors associated with heart disease. Although perceived as an affliction of older men, cardiovascular disease affects women and people in the prime of their life.

To limit the risk of heart disease:

■ Avoid tobacco
■ Eat healthy
■ Be active

High Blood Pressure

Prevention and control of hypertension would save money and enhance quality of life. Four lifestyle practices can have a significant impact on hypertension (Whelton, et al., 2002). These include weight control, moderate salt intake, moderate alcohol intake, and regular physical activity. The Seventh Report of the Joint National Committee on Prevention Detection, Evaluation and Treatment of High Blood Pressure (The JNC 7 Report) established new guidelines for the management of hypertension. The first three of seven key messages are " (1) in persons older than 50 years, systolic blood pressure (BP) of more than 140 mm Hg is a much more important cardiovascular disease (CVD) risk factor than a diastolic BP; (2) the risk of CVD, beginning at 115/75 mm Hg, double with each increment of 20/10 mm Hg; individuals who are normotensive at 55 years of age have a 90% lifetime risk of developing hypertension; (3) individuals with a systolic BP of 120 to 139 mm Hg or a diastolic BP of 80 to 89 mm Hg should be considered as prehypertensive and

---

BOX 4-1 ■ *Specific Lifestyle Modifications for Primary Prevention of Hypertension*

- Maintain a normal body weight for adults, which is defined as a body mass index (BMI) below 25.
- Reduce sodium intake to 2.4 g of sodium per day
- Limit alcohol consumption to no more than 1 oz of ethanol (24 oz beer, 10 oz wine, or 2 oz 100-proof whisky. Women and lighter weight people should limit daily alcohol consumption to 0.5 oz ethanol or half of the amounts listed above.
- Engage in regular physical exercise, such as a brisk walk, at least 30 minutes most days of the week.
- Maintain an adequate intake of dietary potassium (3,500 mg/day). See Handout 3–16 for a list of foods rich in potassium.
- Consume a diet rich in fruits and vegetables and low-fat dairy products.

---

require health promoting lifestyle modifications to prevent CVD" (Chobanian, 2003). Motivation on the part of the patient is also identified as a key factor in controlling hypertension. Clinicians are encouraged to be both empathetic and positive when treating individuals with hypertension (Box 4-1).

DASH Diet

The DASH Diet (Dietary Approaches to Stop Hypertension) is a diet used to prevent and treat high blood pressure. The DASH diet includes a menu rich in fruits, vegetables, and nonfat dairy foods and low in both saturated and total fat. Adherence to this diet decreased systolic blood pressure and was more effective than just adding fruit and vegetables to the diet. A copy of the DASH diet is found in Section 4 or www.nhlbi.nih.gov/hbp/prevent/h_eating/h_eating.htm

RECOMMENDED READING

Moore, T., Svetkey, L., Pao-Hwa, L., and Karanaja, N. *The DASH Diet for Hypertension Lowers your Blood Pressure in Just 14 Days*. The Free Press, 2003.

American Heart Association. (2001). *American Heart Association Low Salt Cookbook: A Complete Guide to Reducing Sodium and Fat in Your Diet*. 2nd Ed. New York: Crown Publishing.

High Cholesterol

Measurement of total cholesterol has a direct, positive relationship with coronary artery disease. Low-density lipoprotein (LDL) is the primary cholesterol carrier in the blood, making total cholesterol and LDL cholesterol levels highly correlated. The Adult Treatment Panel III (ATP III) (NCEP, 2001) report focuses on LDL cholesterol as a target for lipid-lowering efforts

and measurement and offers the Therapeutic Lifestyle Changes (TLC) Diet to improve lipid levels. Physical activity is an important component of the TLC diet. Refer to Box 3-6 to answer questions about supplements used to lower cholesterol.

Although the TLC diet remains an important part of cholesterol management, the National Cholesterol Education Program released new recommendations that set LDL cholesterol goals for individuals at high risk at <100 mg/dL and individuals at very high risk at <70 mg/dL (Grundy, 2004). These guidelines are likely to increase the use of a LDL-lowering drug, but they do not replace the need for dietary modification in those individuals who can benefit from it (Box 4-2).

Triglycerides

The ATP III report recognizes elevated triglyceride levels as an independent risk factor for coronary artery disease. Triglycerides are the major form of lipid in food and in the body. Obesity, overweight, physical inactivity, smoking, excess alcohol intake, and high carbohydrate diets (>60% of energy intake), particularly from refined grains; several diseases, including diabetes and chronic renal failure; certain drugs; and genetic disorders all can contribute to hypertriglyceridemia, which is often observed in persons with metabolic syndrome (Box 4-3).

Treatment for elevated triglycerides depends on the cause, but weight reduction (including little or no alcohol and reduced sugar intake) and increased activity are the usual cornerstone of treatment. Drug therapy may be part of treatment for those with very high triglyceride levels. The 2000 American Heart Association (AHA) (Kraus, 2000) guidelines report that several studies have shown higher intakes of omega-3 fatty acids (eicosapentenoic [EPA], docosahexenoic [DHA], or fish oils) have been useful in the treatment

---

BOX 4-2 ■ *Nutrition Composition of the Therapeutic Lifestyle Changes (TLC) Diet*

Nutrient	Recommended Intake
Saturated fat*	<7% of calories
Polyunsaturated fat	up to 10% of total calories
Monounsaturated fat	up to 20% of total calories
Total fat	25% to 35% of total calories
Carbohydrate†	50% to 60% of total calories
Fiber	20–30 g/day
Protein	approximately 15% of total calories
Cholesterol	<200 mg/day
Total calories‡	Balance energy intake and expenditure to maintain desirable body weight or prevent weight gain.

*Trans fatty acids are another LDL-raising fat that should be kept at a low intake. (Trans fats are not listed on the Nutrition Facts Panel but partially hydrogenated vegetable oil listed on the ingredient list indicates its presence.)
†Carbohydrates should be derived predominantly from foods rich in complex carbohydrates, including grains, especially whole grains, fruits, and vegetables.
‡Daily energy expenditure should include at least moderate physical activity (contributing approximately 200 kcal/day).
Source: Third Report on Detection, Evaluation and Treatment of High Blood Cholesterol in Adults. www.nhlbi.nih.gov/guidelines/cholesterol/atp3_rpt.htm.

---

of hypertriglyceridemia. For a list of foods rich in these oils see patient education Handout 3–26.

RESOURCES

American Heart Association
www.americanheart.org/
Heart Information Network
www.heartinfo.org/
National Cholesterol Education Program Adult Treatment Panel Guidelines
www.nhlbi.nih.gov/guidelines/cholesterol/atp_iii.htm
American Heart Association. (1998). *American Heart Association Quick and Easy Cookbook*. American Heart Association.
McGowan, M. (2002). *50 Ways to Lower Cholesterol*. New York: McGraw-Hill.

DIABETES MELLITUS

Diabetes affects more than 17 million Americans (NCCD, 2004) and the diagnosis of diabetes increased by 61% since 1991. Diabetes develops when the body does not produce enough insulin or does not respond to the insulin it does make. The three familiar forms of diabetes include type I, type II, and gestational diabetes. Type I diabetes accounts for 5% to 10% of all diagnosis of diabetes. It is often referred to as insulin-dependent diabetes. Type II diabetes, previously called the disease of adults, is now being diagnosed more frequently in children. Type II diabetes mellitus is found in 90% to 95% of people diagnosed with the disease. High blood sugars can increase slowly in type II diabetes, often with weight gain and age. It is estimated that by the year 2050, 29 million Americans will have

---

BOX 4-3 ■ *Metabolic Syndrome (a Cluster of Symptoms Including Three or More Risk Factors)*

Abdominal obesity	(>40 inches for men, >35 inches for women)
High triglyceride levels	(≥150 mg/dL)
Low HDL levels	(<40 mg/dL for men, <50 mg/dL for women)
Blood pressure	(≥130/≤85 mm Hg)
Fasting glucose	(≥110 mg/dL)

Source: *Journal of the American Medical Association* (2001). *16*, 2493.

the condition and 1 of 3 children born in 2000 may develop the disease if they do not adopt a lifestyle that prevents the condition. A healthy diet and regular activity comprise the health prescription of choice. Gestational diabetes is discussed below.

Although proper control is the goal of diabetes management, a recent study found that less the 12% of people diagnosed with diabetes meet the recommended goals for controlling blood glucose, blood pressure, and cholesterol (Saydah, Fradkin, Cowie, 2004).

The goals of medical nutrition therapy for diabetes (ADA, 2004) are to:

1. Attain and maintain optimal metabolic outcomes.
   a. Blood glucose levels in the normal range or as close to normal as is safe to prevent or reduce the risk of complications of diabetes.
   b. Lipid profile that reduces the risk of disease.
   c. Blood pressure that reduces the risk of disease.
2. Prevent and treat the chronic complications of diabetes.
3. Improve health through healthy food choices and physical activity.
4. Address individual needs, taking into account culture, lifestyle, and willingness to change.

Prediabetes or Impaired Fasting Glucose (IFG)

Recently, the Expert Committee on the Diagnosis and Classification of Diabetes Mellitus (Genuth, Alberti, & Bennett, 2003) lowered the criteria for "normal" fasting blood sugar from <110 mg/dL to <100 mg/ dL. Patients with a fasting blood sugar of 100 to 125 mg/dL have impaired fasting glucose (IFG) or prediabetes. Individuals in this group are at high risk for developing diabetes and should start lifestyle changes immediately. In one look at the habits of middle-aged women, those who exercised regularly, ate a healthy diet, drank alcohol in moderation, and most importantly were not overweight, virtually reduced their risk of diabetes to zero (Hu, et al., 2001).

Gestational Diabetes

Gestational diabetes mellitus occurs in about 7% of all pregnancies; it is usually identified in the second or third trimester, probably because the pregnancy affects the ability of insulin to work effectively. This form of diabetes usually disappears after delivery.

Nutrition therapy for gestational diabetes promotes adequate nutrition for both mother and fetus. Adequate energy for appropriate weight gain, maintenance of normoglycemia, and absence of ketones are desired (ADA Pregnancy and Lactation, 2004). Three small-to-moderate sized meals, with an equally divided carbohydrate intake, and 2 to 4 snacks are often advised. The Expert Opinion Recommendations of the American Diabetes Association for nutrition during gestational diabetes include

- The nutrition requirements during pregnancy and lactation are similar for women with and without diabetes.
- MNT for gestational diabetes focuses on food choices for appropriate weight gain, normoglycemia, and absence of ketones.
- For some women with gestational diabetes, modest energy and carbohydrate restriction may be appropriate.

Caloric restriction should be approached with caution because of a reported relationship between elevated maternal serum ketone levels and reduced psychomotor development and IQ at 3 to 9 years of age in children born to mothers with gestational diabetes (Turok, Ratcliffe, & Baxley, 2003).

The patient with newly diagnosed diabetes often wants immediate advise on what to eat. Handout 4–6 *Diabetes: What I Need to Know About Eating and Diabetes* provides patients with sufficient information until they can meet with a diabetes educator or nutrition professional.

RESOURCES

American Diabetes Association
   www.diabetes.org
Children with Diabetes
   www.childrenwithdiabetes.com
International Diabetes Center
   www.idcdiabetes.org
National Institute of Diabetes and Digestive Kidney Diseases
   www.niddk.nih.gov
American Diabetes Association. (2002). *Month of Meals: Classic Cooking Quick & Easy Menus for People with Diabetes*. Alexandria, Virginia.
American Diabetes Association. (2003). *Magic Menus*. 2nd ed. Alexandria, Virginia.
Natow, A., B., Hesling, R. D., and Hesling J. (2003). *The Diabetes Carbohydrate Calorie Counter*. 2nd ed. New York: Pocket Books.
Powers, M. (2003). *American Dietetic Association Guide to Eating Right When You Have Diabetes*. New York: Wiley.
Stanley, K. (2001). *Diabetic Cooking for Seniors*. American Diabetes Association, Alexandria, Virginia.
Warshaw, H. (2002). *The American Diabetes Association Guide to Healthy Restaurant Eating*. American Diabetes Association, Alexandria, Virginia.

Hypoglycemia of Nondiabetic Origin

The word hypoglycemia literally means low (hypo) blood sugar (glycemia). Under normal circumstances, even with wide ranging food and activity patterns, the body can keep blood sugar tightly regulated in the range of 60 to 100mg/dL. Blood glucose regulation is essential for the normal functioning of the brain and central nervous system. When it drops, symptoms related to the function of the brain and central nervous system occur. These include sweating, shaking, weakness, hunger, headache, and irritability.

A glucose fingerstick (taken at the time of symptoms) is often used instead of the Oral Glucose Tolerance Test (OGTT) or a patient can ingest a meal that typically causes symptoms and have a blood glucose reading taken in the office when symptoms occur. To determine a diagnosis of hypoglycemia three features known as Whipple's Triad must be present.

1. A low blood glucose level (usually at 60 mg/dL or below).
2. Symptoms must be present at the time of low blood glucose level.
3. Amelioration of symptoms when hypoglycemia is corrected with food.

Reactive hypoglycemia or postprandial (reactive) hypoglycemia is the term used to describe low glucose levels caused by the body's reaction to a food. Such reactions, which include the above-mentioned symptoms, can develop in response to the over production of insulin, which results in hypoglycemia. Or, an individual may have an increased sensitivity to insulin, which results in low glucose levels and symptoms.

Fasting or (food deprived) hypoglycemia can occur when no food is ingested for a period of time that results in low blood glucose and related symptoms. Symptoms can vary among individuals, but those with nondiabetic hypoglycemia usually report symptoms that are constant to them personally.

The goal of treatment is to adopt eating habits that keep blood glucose levels stable. Individuals may benefit from a referral to a registered dietitian to learn the principle of carbohydrate counting and meal planning. Encourage the following food habits:

1. Eat 5 to 6 small meals and snacks throughout the day.
2. Distribute carbohydrate content. A goal might include 2 to 4 servings of carbohydrate at a meal, for a total of 30 to 60 g and 1 to 2 servings at snacks for a total of 15 to 30 g carbohydrate.
3. Avoid foods with large amounts of carbohydrate, including soft drinks, syrups, candy, and some desserts.
4. Avoid caffeine. Caffeine can make hypoglycemia symptoms worse.

5. Limit alcohol. Alcohol, particularly when consumed on an empty stomach, can lower blood glucose levels by interfering with gluconeogenesis. Individuals who drink should be encouraged to drink with meals.
6. A diet excessive in total fat and high in saturated fat may impair the body's ability to use insulin. Excess body fat can do the same.
7. Refer to Patient Education Handout 4–9.

DIGESTIVE DISORDERS

Patients with a disorder of the digestive tract are probably the ones most likely to ask and expect guidance about food choices. The bland diet once routinely advised has little practical use for the treatment of ulcer disease or even gastritis. Yet the value of thoughtful food selection is not to be ignored. The digestive tract is a complex connection of living tubes, organs, and glands. Within this system, food and liquids must be changed into their smallest parts to allow for absorption into the blood and the nourishing of cells. The sight, smell, and taste of food increase gastrointestinal hormone production and stimulate the digestive tract. Fear, anger, and stress can activate the autonomic nervous system and depress or inhibit peristalsis. Encouraging individual patients to eat a variety of foods and to chew food well and slowly will intuitively make sense to patients and may potentially promote proper digestion.

Dietary treatment for disorders of the digestive tract can include the elimination of food components (e.g., gluten in the case of celiac disease). The prevalence of celiac disease is approximately one case per 250 persons (Nelsen, 2002). Malnutrition, osteoporosis, and anemia can be serious side effects. Antibody tests can identify most patients with a digestive disorder. Antibodies disappear within several months after the institution of a strict gluten-free diet.

Diet therapy can also include the manipulation of macronutrients by increasing or decreasing fat, protein, or fiber to ease symptoms or aid digestion. A person with pancreatitis may feel symptom relief from a low-fat diet; some liver conditions may improve with a high protein diet; a high-fiber diet may be appropriate to control diverticulosis, whereas a low-fiber diet may be needed during a case of diverticulitis. Irritable bowel syndrome (IBS), a disorder that affects one of five Americans, causes extreme distress and discomfort. No cure for IBS currently exists and no one diet prescription suits everyone with IBS. A diet high enough in fiber to prevent constipation, adequate fluid from noncarbonated drinks, and avoiding large meals may be useful. Having patients limit alcohol, caffeine, sorbitol, and fat intake may also be of use (Viera, Hoag, & Shaugnessy, 2002). A lactose-free diet should be implemented only in cases of proven lactase deficiency.

Alteration in fiber, fat, and the volume of meals and the identification of foods that cause an individual problem are important. Discuss diet with anyone experiencing digestive disturbance. Initially, encourage a diet that promotes well-chewed food, small meals, avoids temperature extremes, and eliminates foods known to be problematic. Once a diagnosis is made, a referral to a registered dietitian is advised.

NASH

Nonalcoholic steatohepatitis (NASH) is a common, often symptomless condition once called "fatty liver." It affects 2% to 5% of Americans (NASH-NDDIC 2004) and is becoming more common because of increased obesity. NASH is progressive and can lead to cirrhosis of the liver. Weight loss, when indicated, can provide major improvement as seen postbariatric obesity surgery (Dixon, et al., 2004). Individuals with NASH are advised to lose weight, eat a balanced diet, increase activity, avoid alcohol, and not take any unnecessary medications. Full control of diabetes and hyperlipidemia is critical (Liangpunsakul & Chalasani, 2003).

RESOURCES

Liver Foundation
    www.liverfoundation.org
    www.liver.org
Celiac Disease
    http://digestive.niddk.nih.gov/ddiseases/pubs/celiac/
Crohn's and Colitis Foundation
    www.ccfa.org/
Gastrointestinal Disorders and Treatment (search individual disease)
    www.niddk.nih.gov/health/digest/digest.htm
Nonalcoholic Steatohepatitis
    http://digestive.niddk.nih.gov/ddiseases/pubs/nash/
Bonci, L. (2003). *ADA Guide to Better Digestion*. New York: Wiley.
Magee, E. (2000). *Tell Me What to Eat if I Have Irritable Bowel Syndrome*. Franklin Lakes, New Jersey: Career Press.

KIDNEY DISEASE

The kidneys maintain the homeostatic balance of fluid, electrolytes, and organic solutes. Medical nutrition therapy for the treatment of renal disease may require alterations in protein, sodium, potassium, fluid, energy, and fat. Nutrition care is determined by the portions of the kidney involved in disease and the symptoms associated with it. Managing symptoms and maintaining adequate

nutrition can be extremely complex, requiring the skills of a nutritionist with the appropriate training.

Nephrolithiasis (Kidney Stones)

Kidney stones occur in approximately 10% of all people in the United States at some time in their lives. Stones occur more frequently in men, usually between the ages of 20 and 40 years. Prevention is important in those who have been diagnosed with a kidney stone. Patients should be encouraged to drink enough fluids daily to produce 2 quarts of urine. It is not necessary to avoid foods high in calcium, but calcium supplements may increase the risk of stone formation. Patients susceptible to forming calcium oxalate stones may be asked to limit (not eliminate) foods with a high oxalate content including beets, chocolate, coffee, cola, nuts, rhubarb, spinach, strawberries, tea, and wheat bran.

RESOURCES

The National Kidney Foundation
    www.kidney.org
Oxalosis and Hyperoxaluria Foundation (OHF)
    www.ohf.org
American Foundation for Urologic Disease
    www.afud.org
Lennox Hill Hospital. (1999). *The Gourmet Renal Cookbook*. To order, call 212-434-3266.

OSTEOPOROSIS

Osteoporosis is the loss of bone tissue, resulting in an increase risk of bone fracture. It occurs more often in women than in men, but screening is advised for both. The U.S. Preventive Services Task Force (USPSTF) recommends screening for women over age 65 and older and at age 60 for those at increased risk (USPSTF, 2004). Three factors influence bone health: diet, exercise, and estrogen. Diet and lifestyle can be significant; good nutrition, including adequate calcium and vitamin D, not smoking, and avoidance of alcohol all affect bone health. The Dietary Reference Intake (DRI) for calcium for adults is 1,000 to 1,300 mg/day. See Handout 3–13 for calcium sources and amounts by age. The need for vitamin D is 5 to 15 μg/day. See Handout 3–9 for more information about vitamin D. Vitamin D deficiency is of particular concern for Americans living in northern latitudes where sun exposure is less. Exposure to the sun causes the body to make vitamin D and it is one of our best sources of vitamin D. Vitamin D is often measured in international units in vitamin supplements (10 μg cholecalciferol = 400 IU vitamin D). Cholecalciferol is the form of vitamin D produced when the skin is exposed to sunlight.

RESOURCES

National Osteoporosis Foundation
   www.nof.org
Nelson, M. E. (2000). *Strong Women, Strong Bones.*
   New York: Berkley Publishing Group.

PATIENT EDUCATION HANDOUTS

Use the patient education handouts that follow to effectively answer your patient's questions. If your patient has in-depth questions about nutrition, a referral to a registered dietitian is to be encouraged.

The handouts are as follows:

4-1	The DASH Diet
4-2	Low Cholesterol, Low Saturated Fat Diet
4-3	Ten Steps to Lower Your Cholesterol
4-4	What Do the Numbers Mean?
4-5	Triglycerides: What Are They and What Can I Do About Them?
4-6	Diabetes: What I Need to Know About Eating and Diabetes
4-7	Warning Signs of a Diabetic Low Blood Sugar
4-8	Do You Have Prediabetes?
4-9	Hypoglycemia for People Who Do Not Have Diabetes
4-10	Low-sodium Diet
4-11	High-potassium Diet
4-12	Low-potassium Diet
4-13	High-fiber Diet
4-14	Low-fiber Diet
4-15	Low-fat Diet
4-16	Liquid Diet
4-17	Low-purine Diet for Gout
4-18	Gluten-free Diet for Celiac Disease
4-19	Lactose-restricted Diet
4-20	Diet for Heartburn and Gastroesophageal Reflux Disease
4-21	Diet and Gas
4-22	Diet and Constipation
4-23	Diet and Diverticular Disease
4-24	High Protein, High Calorie Diet

Sources (unless stated otherwise on the patient education handout):

American Dietetic Association. (2000). *Manual of Clinical Dietetics* (6th ed.).

Mahan, K., & Escott-Stump, S. (2004). *Krause's Food, Nutrition & Diet Therapy* (11th ed.). Philadelphia: W.B. Saunders.

Shils, M. E., Shike, M., & Olson, J. A. (1999). *Modern Nutrition in Health and Disease* (9th ed.). Philadelphia: Lippincott Williams & Wilkins.

The DASH diet is rich in fruits, vegetables, and low-fat dairy foods, and low in saturated and total fat. It is also low in cholesterol; high in dietary fiber, potassium, calcium, and magnesium; and moderately high in protein. The DASH eating plan shown below is based on a 2,000-calories-a-day eating plan. Depending on your caloric needs, your number of daily servings in a food group may vary from those listed.

GRAIN AND GRAIN PRODUCTS: MAJOR SOURCES OF ENERGY AND FIBER

7–8 daily servings of grains and grain products, including whole wheat bread, English muffin, pita bread, bagel, cereals, grits, and oatmeal.

Serving size: 1 slice bread, 1 oz dry cereal, ½ cup cooked rice, pasta, or cereal.

VEGETABLE GROUP: RICH SOURCE OF POTASSIUM, MAGNESIUM, AND FIBER

4–5 daily servings, including tomatoes, potatoes, carrots, peas, squash, broccoli, turnip greens, collard greens, kale, spinach, artichokes, beans, and sweet potatoes.

Serving size: 1 cup raw leafy vegetable, ½ cup cooked vegetable, or 6 oz vegetable juice.

FRUIT GROUP: IMPORTANT SOURCE OF POTASSIUM, MAGNESIUM, AND FIBER

4–5 daily servings, including apricots, bananas, dates, grapes, oranges, orange juice, grapefruit, grapefruit juice, mangoes, melons, peaches, pineapples, prunes, raisins, strawberries, and tangerines.

Serving size: 6 oz fruit juice, 1 medium fruit, ¼ cup dried fruit, or ½ cup fresh, frozen, or canned fruit.

DAIRY FOODS: MAJOR SOURCE OF CALCIUM AND PROTEIN

2–3 daily servings, including skim or 1% milk, skim or low-fat buttermilk, nonfat or low-fat yogurt, part skim milk mozzarella cheese, and nonfat cheese.

Serving size: 8 oz milk, 1 cup yogurt, or 1.5 oz cheese.

MEAT, FISH, AND POULTRY GROUP: RICH SOURCE OF PROTEIN AND MAGNESIUM

2 or fewer daily servings. Select only lean portions; trim away visible fats; broil, roast, or boil instead of frying; remove skin from poultry.

Serving size: 3 oz cooked meats, poultry, or fish.

NUTS, SEEDS, AND DRIED BEANS: RICH SOURCES OF ENERGY, MAGNESIUM, POTASSIUM, PROTEIN, AND FIBER

4–5 servings per week, including almonds, filberts, mixed nuts, peanuts, walnuts, sunflower seeds, kidney beans, and lentils.

Serving size: 1.5 oz or ⅓ cup nuts, ½ oz or 2 tablespoons seeds, or ½ cup cooked legumes.

FATS AND OILS

DASH has 27 percent of calories as fat, including fat in or added to foods.

2–3 servings daily, including soft margarine, low-fat mayonnaise, light salad dressing, and vegetable oils (olive, corn, canola, or safflower).

SWEETS

Sweets should be low in fat.

5 per week, including maple syrup, sugar, jelly, jam, fruit-flavored gelatin, jelly beans, hard candy, fruit punch, and sorbet.

Serving size: 1 tablespoon sugar, 1 tablespoon jelly or jam, ½ oz jelly beans, or 1 cup lemonade.

A DASH DIET SAMPLE MENU: APPROXIMATELY 2,000 CALORIES PER DAY

Breakfast

Orange juice	6 oz (¾ cup)
1% low fat milk	8 oz (1 cup)
Corn flakes (with 1 teaspoon sugar)	1 cup
Banana	1 medium
Whole wheat bread (with 1 tablespoon jelly)	1 slice
Soft margarine	1 teaspoon

Lunch

Chicken salad	¾ cup
Pita bread	½, large

Raw vegetable medley:
   3–4 sticks each carrots and celery
   2 sliced radishes
   2 leaves loose-leaf lettuce
Part skim mozzarella cheese   1.5 oz
1% low fat milk   8 oz
Fruit cocktail in light syrup   ½ cup

Dinner

Herbed baked cod   3 oz
Scallion rice   1 cup
Steamed broccoli   ½ cup
Stewed tomatoes   ½ cup
Spinach salad:
   ½ cup raw spinach
   2 cherry tomatoes
   2 slices cucumber
Light Italian dressing   1 tablespoon
Whole wheat dinner roll   1 small
Soft margarine   1 teaspoon
Melon balls   ½ cup

Snacks

Dried apricots   ¾ cup
Mini-pretzels   ¾ cup
Mixed nuts   ⅓ cup
Diet ginger ale   12 oz

Total number of servings in 2,000 calories/day menu

Grains   8
Vegetables   4
Fruits   5
Dairy foods   3
Meat, poultry, and fish   2
Nuts, seeds, and legumes   1
Fats and oils   2.5

Reprinted from the The DASH (Dietary Approaches to Stop Hypertension) Eating Plan. Available at: www.nhlbi.nih.gov/health/public/heart/hbp/dash/.

TIPS ON EATING THE DASH WAY

- Start small. Make gradual changes in your eating habits.
- Center your meal around carbohydrates (pasta, rice, beans), or vegetables.
- Treat meat as one part of the whole meal, instead of the focus.
- Use fruits or low-fat, low-calorie food (sugar-free gelatin) for desserts and snacks.

Remember! If you use the DASH Diet to help prevent or control high blood pressure, make it part of a lifestyle that includes choosing foods lower in salt and sodium, keeping a healthy weight, being physically active, and, if you drink alcohol, doing so in moderation.

Where Can I Get More Information?

To learn more about high blood pressure, call 1-800-575-WELL or visit the National Heart, Lung, and Blood Institute (NHLBI) available at: www.nhlbi.nih.gov/health/public/heart/hbp/dash/.

To find a registered dietitian in your area, go to www.eatright.org and click: Find a Nutrition Professional or call the American Dietetic Association at 1-800-366-1655.

Low Cholesterol, Low Saturated Fat Diet

Cholesterol is a soft, waxy substance the body needs for proper health and brain function, but too much cholesterol in the blood increases the risk for heart disease. Blood cholesterol levels are affected by saturated fat, trans fat, and cholesterol in food and by cholesterol made in the liver. Saturated fat is found in meat, whole-fat dairy products, hard cheese, and some snack foods. It is the saturated fat in food that raises blood cholesterol levels more than anything else we eat. Trans fats are produced when oils are hydrogenated and used in prepared foods, including commercially made baked and fried foods. Lowering blood cholesterol levels can reduce the risk of heart disease and a heart attack. Eating foods rich in fiber, controlling weight, and getting regular exercise are important to heart health too.

BEVERAGES

Fruit-flavored drinks, lemonade, fruit punch, soda, and cola can be included. They do not contain cholesterol or saturated fat, but they can be a significant source of calories and can increase another type of fat called "triglyceride." (Read about triglycerides below.) Limit liquid calories if you are overweight. Avoid beverages made with cream or whole milk.

CEREALS

Include cereal with whole oats, whole wheat, corn, or multigrain. Read labels to look for those high in fiber (>3 g per serving) and no or low in saturated fat.

BREADS

Include whole grain breads, English muffins, bagels, rolls, and corn or flour tortilla. Read labels to avoid bread with saturated fat, which may include bread made with cheese, butter, or egg as a major ingredient.

DESSERTS AND SWEETS

Sugar, syrup, honey, jam, jelly, and candy made without fat and fruit-flavored gelatin contain no cholesterol. Frozen desserts including nonfat and low-fat yogurt, and ice cream; sherbet and sorbet; fruit and Italian ice, and popsicles contain little or no fat. Ginger snaps, fig bars, fruit bar cookies, and angel food cake are good low-cholesterol choices. Cookies, cake, pie, and pudding made with egg whites, egg substitutes, skim and 1% milk, liquid vegetable oil, or soft margarine can be included.

Limit candy made with milk chocolate, chocolate, coconut oil, palm kernel oil, or palm oil. Also limit regular and premium ice cream, which can be a rich source of cholesterol and saturated fat, commercially made pies, cakes, and doughnuts, high-fat cookies, and cream pies.

FATS

Include canola, olive, safflower, sunflower, corn, soybean, cottonseed, and peanut oil. Margarine made from those oils and light or diet margarine, especially soft or liquid forms, are good choices, as is spray margarine or oil. Include salad dressings made from the oils listed above and include (these can be high in calories) avocado, olives, seeds, nuts, and peanut butter in your diet.

Limit salad dressing made with egg yolk, cheese, sour cream, or whole milk.

FRUIT

Include all fruit—fresh, frozen, or canned, including fruit juice. Avoid coconut. Avocado and olives are included in the fat list.

MEAT AND OTHER PROTEIN FOODS

Choose lean cuts of beef, pork, or lamb; poultry without skin, fish and shellfish, lean processed meats, dry beans, tofu, tempeh, and low-fat or nonfat soy burgers or meatless vegetarian burgers.

Avoid fried fish and chicken, poultry with skin, regular ground beef, fatty cuts of meat, including spare ribs, organ meats, and regular luncheon meats.

Choose egg whites (two egg whites can be substituted for one egg in most recipes) or egg substitute. A suggested egg limit for those with high blood cholesterol is two to four per week, including eggs in cooking and baking. Avoid bacon and sausage when eating eggs.

DAIRY FOODS AND CALCIUM

Include skim, ½%, or 1% fat milk; buttermilk, nonfat or low-fat yogurt, 1% or nonfat soy or rice beverages, and low-fat cheese. Avoid whole milk, whole milk yogurt, and regular cheeses.

POTATO, RICE, AND PASTA

Include potatoes, pasta, and rice in your diet. Try whole grain versions as often as possible, including whole wheat pasta and brown rice. Avoid dishes made with egg, cream, or butter, as well as fried potatoes.

SOUP

Include broth-based soups with low-fat ingredients, such as chicken, vegetable, and bean soups. Avoid soup made with whole milk, cream, fatty meats, and poultry fat or skin.

VEGETABLES

Include all fresh, frozen, or canned vegetables* without added fat or sauce. Avoid fried vegetables.

MISCELLANEOUS

Salt, pepper, and most seasonings contain no saturated fat or cholesterol.

Where Can I Get More Information?

American Heart Association available at: www.americanheart.org/.

Heart Information Network available at: www.heartinfo.org/.

To find a registered dietitian in your area go to www.eatright.org and click: Find a Nutrition Professional or call the American Dietetic Association at 1-800-366-1655.

---

*Canned vegetables can be high in sodium.

4-3 Ten Steps to Lower Your Cholesterol Level

Read this list. Chose two steps to practice and add a new one every week until you have included all ten into a new healthy lifestyle.

1. Read and follow the Low Cholesterol, Low Saturated Fat Food Guidelines in Patient Education Handout 4-2.
2. Eat at least five or more fruits and vegetables daily.
3. Include 3 servings (or more) of whole grain food every day.
4. Keep your intake of meat, poultry, and fish to approximately 6 oz per day.
5. Enjoy 2 or more servings of fish each week.
6. Maintain a level of physical activity that keeps you fit and matches the number of calories you eat. Walk or do other activities for 30 minutes on most days.
7. Achieve and maintain a healthy body weight.
8. Read labels. Keep total cholesterol and saturated fat low. On a 2,000-calorie diet, healthy people should eat less than 300 mg cholesterol per day and less than 20 g of saturated fat. On a 2000-calorie, low-cholesterol diet, eat less than 200 mg cholesterol and 14 g of saturated fat.
9. To raise your high-density lipoprotein (HDL) (good) cholesterol, increase your activity, stop smoking, and lose weight (if you are overweight).
10. To lower your low-density lipoprotein (LDL) (bad) cholesterol:
    - Substitute polyunsaturated and monounsaturated fats (soft margarine, olive oil, canola oil) for saturated fats (butter, cream). Margarines fortified with plant stanol may be beneficial. These are available in most grocery stores.
    - Eat a menu rich in soluble fiber (oats, bananas, oranges, carrots, barley, and kidney beans). Soluble fiber can lower LDL cholesterol.
    - Include soy proteins to replace animal meats (recent studies have shown that including 20–50 g of soy protein in the diet significantly reduces LDL cholesterol).
    - Avoid food containing trans fat. Trans fats are found in prepared foods containing partially hydrogenated vegetable oils (e.g., cookies, crackers, commercially prepared fried foods, and some margarine).

TRIGLYCERIDES

Triglycerides, the major form of fat in foods, is also the major form of energy storage in the body. Individuals with elevated triglycerides should try to reduce weight (if needed), increase physical activity, and reduce carbohydrate intake. Carbohydrate sources should come from whole grains, fruits, and vegetables instead of sugar and refined white flour products. High intakes of fatty fish could result in an intake of omega-3 fatty acids or "fish oils" that might be beneficial in the treatment of hypertriglyceridemia. In addition, increased alcohol can aggravate hypertri-glyceridemia. Limit or avoid alcohol altogether.

Where Can I Get More Information?

American Heart Association available at: www.americanheart.org.

National Heart, Lung, and Blood Institute available at: www.nhlbi.nih.gov/.

To find a registered dietitian in your area, go to www.eatright.org and click: Find a Nutrition Professional or call the American Dietetic Association at 1-800-366-1655.

Sources: American Heart Association Dietary Guidelines. (2000). *Circulation, 102*, 2284–2299.
National Cholesterol Education Program. (2001). Expert Summary of the Third Report of the National Cholesterol Education Program (NCEP) Expert Panel on Detection, Evaluation, and Treatment of High Blood Cholesterol in Adults (Adult Treatment Panel III). *Journal of the American Medical Association, 285*, 2486–2497.

4-4 What Do the Numbers Mean?

Cholesterol levels are interpreted based on your health and the heart disease risk factors you might have. The risk factors include:

Smoking	Diabetes
A low HDL (good cholesterol)	A high LDL (bad cholesterol)
Elevated triglycerides	High blood pressure

A family history of early onset heart disease, obesity, inactivity, and stress can also play a role.

The more risk factors you have, the more important it becomes to lower your cholesterol. Those with few risk factors may not require treatment. LDL cholesterol is usually considered more important than total cholesterol when evaluating risk for disease.

What Causes High Cholesterol?

Cholesterol levels are determined by a person's genetic makeup and partly by lifestyle, including diet and exercise. Sometimes a person can be thin, active, eat a low-fat diet and still have a high cholesterol level. In this case, high cholesterol is caused by genetic factors.

Why Is Blood Sugar Important?

People with impaired glucose metabolism, a state between "normal" and "diabetes," are at risk of developing diabetes and diabetes is a risk factor for heart disease and stroke.

What Can I Do?

■ Be active every day for 30 minutes. Walk, bike, do active work around the house, or a combination of these.

■ Eat at least 5 or more servings of fruits and vegetables.

■ Select a diet that is low in saturated fat and total cholesterol.

■ Eat most of your bread, cereal, and pasta in the whole grain form.

■ Lose weight, if you are overweight.

■ If you smoke, quit!

Where Can I Get More Information?

American Heart Association available at: www.americanheart.org.

National Heart, Lung, and Blood Institute available at: www.nhlbi.nih.gov/.

To find a registered dietitian in your area, go to www.eatright.org. and click: Find a Nutrition Professional or call the American Dietetic Association at 1-800-366-1655.

4 Triglycerides: What Are They and What Can I Do About Them?

Triglyceride is a type of fat found in food as well as in the body and blood. It is normal to have triglycerides in the blood, but levels that are too high can increase the risk for coronary artery disease. Elevated triglycerides occur most often in people who are overweight or have diabetes.

Triglycerides are made from the extra calories we eat that are not needed right away and get stored as fat (triglyceride). Between meals, the body can release triglycerides from fat tissue. Alcohol and foods high in sugar tend to raise triglyceride levels.

The National Cholesterol Education Program Guidelines for Fasting Triglycerides are

Normal	Less than 150 mg/dL
Borderline-high	150 to 199 mg/dL
High	200 to 499 mg/dL
Very high	500 mg/dL or higher

To lower triglyceride levels, look at your diet and lifestyle.

- Eat the right amount of calories for your activity level; about 15 calories for each pound you weigh, if you are moderately active. Less-active people need to drop that number to 13 calories per pound. This is the calorie intake you need to maintain weight. Eat 250 calories less every day to lose ½ pound per week
- Reduce your intake of alcohol.
- Limit foods high in sugar: desserts, sweetened drinks (including juice) and high sugar snacks.
- Choose more carbohydrate sources from fruits, vegetables, and whole grains.
- Do not cut out all fat. Eliminating good fats may lower HDL "good" cholesterol. Choose fat sources that are rich in monounsaturated fat and polyunsaturated fat. These healthy fats can be found in canola oil, olive oil, and liquid margarine.
- High triglyceride levels can increase the risk of heart disease. Limit foods high in cholesterol and saturated fats (butter, cream, whole milk cheese, and fatty meats) to reduce your risk.
- Omega-3 fatty acids can improve triglyceride levels. Fish is a rich source of omega-3 fatty acids; try to eat fish twice per week. Mackerel, lake trout, herring, sardines, canned light tuna, and salmon are good sources.
- Other sources of omega-3 fatty acids include green leafy vegetables, soybeans, nuts, and flaxseed and canola oil.
- Try to get 30 minutes of exercise on most days.

- When planning meals, choose lean meat, poultry without skin, fish, and fat-free milk and cheese. Try to eat more whole grains and choose snacks low in sugar.

- Keep your blood pressure under control and do not smoke.

Where Can I Get More Information?

American Heart Association available at www.americanheart.org.

To find a registered dietitian in your area, go to www.eatright.org and click: Find a Nutrition Professional or call the American Dietetic Association at 1-800-366-1655.

Diabetes: What I Need To Know About Eating and Diabetes

HOW FOOD AFFECTS YOUR BLOOD GLUCOSE

Whether you have type 1 or type 2 diabetes, what, when, and how much you eat all affect your blood glucose. Blood glucose is the main sugar found in the blood and the body's main source of energy.

If you have diabetes (or impaired glucose tolerance), your blood glucose can go too high if you eat too much. If your blood glucose goes too high, you can get sick.

Your blood glucose can also go too high or drop too low if you don't take the right amount of diabetes medicine.

How Can I Keep My Blood Glucose at a Healthy Level?

1. Eat about the same amount of food each day. (Your blood glucose goes up after eating. If you eat a big lunch one day and a small lunch the next day, your blood glucose levels will change too much).

2. Eat your meals and snacks at about the same time each day.

   (Keep your blood glucose at a healthy level by eating about the same amount of carbohydrate foods at the same times each day. Carbohydrate foods also called carbs, provide glucose for energy. Starches, fruits, milk, starchy vegetables such as corn and sweets are all carbohydrate foods).

3. Do not skip meals or snacks (talk with your doctor or diabetes teacher about how many meals and snacks to eat each day).

4. Take your medicine at the same time each day. What you eat and when affects how your diabetes medicines work. Talk with your doctor or diabetes teacher about the best time to take your medicines based on your meal plan.

5. Exercise at about the same time each day. Exercise should be safe and enjoyable—talk to your doctor about what types of exercises are right for you.

HYPOGLYCEMIA

You should know the signs of hypoglycemia (low blood sugar), such as feeling weak, dizzy, sweating more, noticing sudden changes in your heartbeat, or feeling hungry. If you experience these feelings, stop exercising and test blood glucose. If it is 70 or less, eat one of the following right away:

   2 or 3 glucose tablets

   ½ cup any juice

   ½ cup of a regular (not diet) soft drink

1 cup milk

5 or 6 pieces hard candy

1 to 2 teaspoons of sugar or honey.

After 15 minutes, test your blood glucose again. Once blood glucose is stable, if it will be at least an hour before your next meal, it's a good idea to eat a snack.

How Much Should I Eat Each Day?

Have about 1,200 to 1,600 calories a day if you are a small woman who exercises, a small or medium woman who wants to lose weight, or a medium woman who does not exercise much. Choose this many servings from these food groups to have 1,200 to 1,600 calories a day*:

6 starches	2 milk and yogurt
3 vegetables	2 meat or meat substitute
2 fruit	up to 3 fats

Have about 1,600 to 2,000 calories a day if you are a large woman who wants to lose weight, a small man at a healthy weight, a medium man who does not exercise much, or a medium to large man who wants to lose weight. Choose this many servings from these food groups to have 1,600 to 2,000 calories a day*:

8 starches	2 milk and yogurt
4 vegetables	2 meat or meat substitute
3 fruit	up to 4 fats

How Can I Satisfy My Sweet Tooth?

It's okay to have sweets once in a while. Try having sugar-free popsicles, diet soda, fat free ice cream or frozen yogurt, or sugar-free hot cocoa mix.

ALCOHOL

Alcohol has calories but no nutrients. If you drink alcohol on an empty stomach, it can make your blood glucose level too low. Alcohol also can raise your blood fats. If you want to drink alcohol, talk with your doctor or diabetes teacher about how it fits into your plan.

WHEN YOU ARE SICK

If you can't eat your usual food, try drinking juice or eating crackers, popsicles, or soup. Make sure you check your blood glucose. Your blood glucose may be high even if you're not eating.

---

*Talk with your diabetes teacher to make a meal plan that fits the way you usually eat, your daily routine, and your diabetes medicines. Then make your own plan.

Call your doctor right away if you throw up more than once or have diarrhea for more than 6 hours.

Where Can I Get More Information?

The National Diabetes Information Clearinghouse (NDIC) provides information about diabetes to people with diabetes; contact them at ndic@info.niddk.nih.gov or go to their web page: http://diabetes.niddk.nih.gov/dm/pubs/hypoglycemia/index.htm.

To find a diabetes teacher near you, call the American Association of Diabetes Educators at 1-800-832-6874 or go to www.diabeteseducator.org and click: Find a Diabetes Educator.

To find a dietitian near you, call the American Dietetic Association at 1-800-366-1655 or go to www.eatright.org and click: Find a Nutrition Professional.

This information was reprinted from the National Diabetes Clearinghouse publication *What I Need To Know About Eating and Diabetes*. The full document can be read at http://diabetes.niddk.nih.gov/dm/pubs/eating_ez/index.htm (page 1–27).

Hypoglycemia, also called low blood sugar, occurs when your blood glucose (blood sugar) levels drops too low to provide enough energy for your body's activities.

Symptoms can include the following:

- Hunger
- Nervousness and shakiness
- Perspiration
- Dizziness or light-headedness
- Sleepiness
- Confusion
- Difficulty speaking
- Feeling anxious

Hypoglycemia might also happen at night while sleeping. You might

- Cry out or have nightmares
- Find that your pajamas or sheets are damp from perspiration
- Feel tired, irritable, or confused when you wake up

CAUSES OF HYPOGLYCEMIA

In people taking certain blood-glucose lowering medications, blood glucose can fall too low for a number of the following reasons:

- Meals or snacks that are too small, delayed, or skipped
- Excessive doses of insulin, or some diabetes medications, including sulfonylureas and meglitinides (although alpha-glucosidase inhibitors, biquanides, and thiazolidinediones alone should not cause hypoglycemia, they can when used with other diabetes medicines).
- Increased activity or exercise
- Excessive drinking of alcohol

PREVENTION

- Ask your healthcare provider if your diabetes medication can cause hypoglycemia.
- Meet with a registered dietitian and develop a meal plan that fits your life. Eat a regular meal, have enough food at each meal, and try not to skip meals or snacks.
- Ask your healthcare provider about having a snack before being active, particularly if you will be doing something that is not part of your normal routine (e.g., shoveling snow).

- Drinking an alcoholic beverage on an empty stomach can cause low blood sugar. Always have a snack or meal when you drink an alcoholic beverage.
- Know what is a normal blood sugar range for you and learn how to treat hypoglycemia.

TREATMENT

If you think your blood glucose is too low, use a blood glucose meter to check your level. If it is 70 mg/dL or below, have one of these "quick fix" foods right away to raise your blood glucose level:

- 2 or 3 glucose tablets
- ½ cup (4 oz) of any fruit juice
- ½ cup (4 oz) of a regular (not diet) soft drink
- 1 cup (8 oz) of milk
- 5 or 6 pieces of hard candy
- 1 or 2 teaspoons of sugar or honey

After 15 minutes, check your blood glucose level again to make sure that it is no longer too low. If it is still too low, have another serving. Repeat these steps until your blood glucose is at least 70 mg/dL. Then, if it will be an hour or more before your next meal, have a snack.

It is especially important to prevent hypoglycemia while driving a vehicle. Checking blood glucose level frequently and snacking (as needed) to keep your blood glucose above 70 mg/dl will help prevent accidents.

Where Can I Get More Information?

The National Diabetes Information Clearinghouse (NDIC) provides information about diabetes to people with diabetes; contact them at ndic@info.niddk.nih.gov or go to their web page at: http://diabetes.niddk.nih.gov/dm/pubs/hypoglycemia/index.htm

To find a diabetes teacher near you, call the American Association of Diabetes Educators at 1-800-832-6874 or go to www.diabeteseducator.org and click Find a Diabetes Educator.

To find a registered dietitian in your area go to www.eatright.org and click: Find a Nutrition Professional or call the American Dietetic Association at 1-800-366-165.

This information is reprinted from the National Diabetes Information Clearinghouse publication *Hypoglycemia*. The full article can be obtained at http://diabetes.niddk.nih.gov/dm/pubs/hypoglycemia/index.htm (page 1–12)

4-8 Do You Have Prediabetes?

Prediabetes is the term used to describe people who have blood sugar levels that are higher than normal, but not yet high enough to be considered diabetes. People with prediabetes are more likely to develop diabetes within 10 years and also are more likely to have a heart attack or stroke. At least 16 million Americans have prediabetes. Although 17 million Americans have diabetes, one third of those do not know it.

Your risk for diabetes develops as you get older. It also rises if you have the following risk factors:

1. You are overweight. Most individuals are overweight if their body mass index (BMI) is ≥25. If you are Asian American, a BMI ≥23 puts you at risk. If you are a Pacific Islander, a BMI ≥26 puts you at risk. Ask your healthcare provider to calculate your BMI.

2. You have a parent, brother, or sister with diabetes.

3. Your family background is African American, American Indian, Asian American, Hispanic/Latino, or Pacific Islander.

4. You had gestational diabetes or gave birth to one baby weighing 9 pounds or more.

5. You have high blood pressure.

6. Your cholesterol levels are not normal. Your HDL (good) cholesterol is less than 40 (for men) or less than 50 (for women), or your triglyceride level is 250 or higher.

7. You exercise fewer than three times a week.

What Can I Do About My Risk?

You can do a lot to lower your chances of getting diabetes. Exercising regularly, reducing fat and calorie intake, and losing weight can all help you reduce your risk of developing type 2 diabetes. Try these steps and talk to your healthcare provider about blood tests and a referral to a dietitian for an individualized diet plan.

- Reduce serving sizes of main courses (such as meat), desserts, and foods high in fat. Increase the amounts of fruits and vegetables you eat.

- You may need to reduce the number of calories you eat each day. Research shows that overweight people reducing their daily calorie intake by 450 calories, significantly reduced the risk of developing diabetes.

- Be active every day. Exercise will help you lose weight, lower your cholesterol, lower blood pressure, and help your body use insulin better. Walking 5 days a week for 30 minutes can be very effective. If you are not active now, start slowly and aim for 30 minutes in the future.

Reprinted from *Your Game Plan for Preventing Type 2 Diabetes: Information for Patients* (NIH Publication No. 01-4155) and *Am I at Risk for Type 2 Diabetes?* (NIH Publication No. o4-4805) Publications developed by the National Diabetes Education Program a joint program of the National Institutes of Health and the Centers for Disease Control. Learn more about the Small Steps Big Rewards program (Prevent type 2 Diabetes) available at: www.ndep.nih.gov.

Where Can I Get More Information?

Contact the National Diabetes Education Program at 1-800-438-5383 or http://ndep.nih.gov/ or the National Diabetes Information Clearinghouse 1-800-860-8747 or www.niddk.nih.gov.

To find a nutrition professional in your area, go to www.eatright.org and click: Find a Nutrition Professional.

4-9 Hypoglycemia for People Who Do Not Have Diabetes

Two types of hypoglycemia (low blood sugar) can occur in people who do not have diabetes: reactive (postprandial, or after meals) and fasting (postabsorptive). Reactive hypoglycemia is not usually related to any underlying disease; fasting hypoglycemia often is.

SYMPTOMS

Symptoms of both types of hypoglycemia resemble the symptoms that people with diabetes and hypoglycemia experience: hunger, nervousness, perspiration, shakiness, dizziness, light-headedness, sleepiness, confusion, difficulty speaking, and feeling anxious or weak.

If you are diagnosed with hypoglycemia, your doctor will try to find the cause by using laboratory tests to measure blood glucose, insulin, and other chemicals that play a part in the body's use of energy.

REACTIVE HYPOGLYCEMIA

In reactive hypoglycemia, symptoms appear within 4 hours after you eat a meal.

Diagnosis

To diagnose reactive hypoglycemia, your doctor may:

- Ask about signs and symptoms
- Test your blood glucose while you are having symptoms
- Check to see whether your symptoms ease after your blood glucose level returns to 70 mg/dL or above (after eating or drinking)

A blood glucose level of less than 70 mg/dL at the time of symptoms and relief after eating will confirm the diagnosis.

The oral glucose tolerance test is no longer used to diagnose hypoglycemia; experts now know that the test can actually trigger hypoglycemic symptoms.

To relieve reactive hypoglycemia, some health professionals recommend taking the following steps:

- Eat small meals and snacks about every 3 hours
- Exercise regularly
- Eat a variety of foods, including meat, poultry, fish, or non meat sources of protein; starchy foods such as whole-grain bread, rice, and potatoes; fruits; vegetables; and dairy products
- Choose high fiber foods
- Avoid or limit foods high in sugar, especially on an empty stomach

FASTING HYPOGLYCEMIA

Diagnosis

Fasting hypoglycemia is diagnosed from a blood sample that shows a blood glucose level of less than 50 mg/dL after an overnight fast, between meals or after exercise.

It can be caused by certain medications, alcohol, illness, and hormonal deficiencies.

Points to Remember

- In reactive hypoglycemia, symptoms occur within 4 hours of eating. People with this condition are usually advised to follow a healthy eating plan recommended by a registered dietitian.
- Fasting hypoglycemia can be caused by certain medications, illness, inherited conditions and needs to be treated by identifying and treating the underlying cause.

Where Can I Get More Information?

American Diabetes Association 1-800-232-3472 or www.diabetes.org.

To find a registered dietitian in your area, go to www.eatright.org and click: Find a Nutrition Professional.

This report was reprinted from the National Institute of Diabetes and Digestive and Kidney Disease publication: *Hypoglycemia* (page 6– 9). The full publication can be accessed at http://diabetes.niddk.nih.gov/dm/pubs/hypoglycemia/index.htm.

Low-sodium Diet

Sodium is a natural and essential mineral found in food and water. Table salt is made of sodium plus chloride. The words sodium and salt are often used interchangeably. Many people get far more sodium than they need. A low-sodium diet can be useful when the body retains fluid. Conditions such as high blood pressure, congestive heart failure, and some forms of kidney disease may require a low-sodium diet. The following diet provides about 2000 mg or 2 g of sodium.

BEVERAGES

Include all fruit juice and salt-free vegetable juices, and low-sodium carbonated beverages.

Limit buttermilk and milk-based drinks (shakes and chocolate milk). Commercially softened water can be high in sodium.

DESSERTS AND SWEETS

Include most desserts, but milk-based pudding should be consumed within milk allowance.

CEREALS

Most dry cereals are allowed, but read labels for sodium content and choose the one with lower sodium.

BREADS

Include most sliced breads and rolls, but avoid those with salted tops. Choose snacks or crackers low in sodium.

Many commercial crackers are high in sodium; for example, Nabisco Cheese Tidbits contain 420 mg sodium in 32 pieces; one 1 oz matzo cracker has 1 mg sodium and can be a good low-sodium alternative. Self-rising flours can be high in sodium and commercial muffins, biscuits, and stuffing mixes can have more sodium than the homemade version.

FAT AND OIL

Include butter and margarine, all cooking oils, and sour, light, and heavy cream.

Limit salted salad dressing to one serving per meal. Limit butter and cream if your doctor has told you your cholesterol is elevated.

FRUIT

Include all fruit—fresh, canned, or frozen.

Avoid dried fruit with salt added.

MEAT AND OTHER PROTEIN SOURCES

Include fresh or frozen beef, lamb, pork, poultry, and fish and rinsed canned fish. Choose low-sodium cheese (1 oz regular American cheese contains 406 mg sodium, 1 cup regular cottage cheese has 918 mg sodium). Choose low-salt peanut butter and unsalted nuts. Eggs and egg substitute are allowed.

Avoid high-sodium meats, including bacon, cold cuts, ham, hot dogs, sausage, sardines, and marinated herring. Avoid pickled eggs and pickled meats. Choose frozen dinners or meals with <500 mg sodium per serving.

DAIRY FOODS AND CALCIUM

Include milk in moderation; each 8 oz cup of milk contains 122 mg sodium; a limit of 16 oz per day is suggested.

POTATO, RICE, AND PASTA

Include white rice, brown rice, and all whole grains packaged without salt: noodles, spaghetti, and pasta cooked without salt; white or sweet potatoes and winter squash, fresh or frozen without salt.

All commercially packaged rice, macaroni, potatoes, and packaged stuffing are to be avoided unless labeled low in salt.

SOUP

Include specially labeled low-sodium soups or homemade soup made with allowed ingredients.

Canned chicken soup (½ cup) contains 980 mg sodium. Dehydrated soups and ready-to-heat soups are likely to be very high in sodium.

VEGETABLES

Include fresh and frozen vegetables (without high-sodium sauces) and low-salt canned vegetables.

Regular canned vegetables, sauerkraut, pickled vegetables, or vegetables seasoned with cheese; bacon and ham are to be avoided. Spaghetti and tomato sauce can contain 738 mg sodium in ½ cup and must be limited.

MISCELLANEOUS

Most herbs and spices are allowed, with the exception of garlic salt or onion salt. Lemon, lime, and vinegar can be useful low-sodium seasonings.

Sea salt, meat tenderizers, soy sauce, barbecue sauce, steak sauce, Worcestershire sauce, and canned gravy are high in sodium. Ask you doctor about the use of salt substitutes; some individuals should avoid the extra potassium a salt substitute may contain.

Where Can I Get More Information?

American Heart Association available at: www.americanheart.org.

National Heart, Lung, and Blood Institute available at: www.nhlbi.nih.gov/hbp/prevent/sodium/tips.htm.

To find a registered dietitian in your area, go to www.eatright.org and click: Find a Nutrition Professional or call the American Dietetic Association at 1-800-366-1655.

Potassium is abundant in many foods. Milk, fruit, vegetables, beef, poultry, and fish are rich sources of potassium. The elderly or seriously ill individual may need to eat a high-potassium diet because of poor diet, diarrhea, over use of laxatives, and vomiting. Some blood pressure medications can lower blood potassium levels, requiring a high potassium intake. A patient with kidney disease should not eat a high-potassium diet or take potassium supplements unless told to do so by a healthcare provider.

FOOD PREPARATION HINTS

Potassium can leach out of food during cooking. To retain potassium, stew, bake, or steam food instead of boiling and use as much of the cooking water to make soup, sauces or gravies as is practical. To get an adequate amount of potassium from food, eat at least 2 to 3 servings of fruit or juice daily and at least 2 to 3 servings of a vegetable daily.

The Dietary Reference Intake of potassium for adults is set at 4,700 mg. Refer to Handout 3–16 for a list of approximate potassium content in select foods.

BEVERAGES

Include skim, low-fat, and whole milk; and 100% fruit drinks such as orange, pineapple, and grapefruit.

Coffee, tea, and water contain little potassium. Fruit drinks made with small amounts of real fruit juice are usually low in potassium.

BREADS

Include all bread, rolls, and crackers.

This food group is not usually a rich source of potassium, but do not avoid it either.

CEREAL

Include all cereal, hot and cold.

Cereals are not usually a rich source of potassium unless served with milk or fruit.

DESSERTS AND SWEETS

Include pudding and custard made with milk or fruit and most fruit-based desserts.

Honey and jelly contain small, but potentially significant, amounts of potassium, if used liberally.

FATS AND OIL

Include all fats and oils and avocado, which is a true fruit, but is listed here because of its fat content.

Butter and margarine are very poor sources of potassium.

FRUIT

Fruits are your best source of potassium. Apricots, bananas, dates, melons, papayas, plantains, pomegranates, prunes, and raisins are very rich sources of potassium.

Try to eat at least 3 servings of fruit daily. A serving should be ½ cup or more.

MEAT AND OTHER PROTEIN FOODS

Include all meat, fish, and poultry; beans, peanut butter, eggs, tofu, cottage cheese, yogurt, and cheese.

One cup of beans can supply 500 to 1,000 mg potassium. One cup cottage cheese contains 1,000 mg potassium.

DAIRY FOODS AND CALCIUM

Include milk and yogurt.

One cup of yogurt contains over 400 mg of potassium.

POTATO, RICE, AND PASTA

Include all foods in this group.

Rice, pasta, and boiled potatoes do not provide much potassium unless topped or combined with vegetables, fruit, or cheese.

SOUP

Include soup made with vegetables or milk.

VEGETABLES

Include all vegetables and vegetable juices.

One half cup of most vegetables has about 200 mg potassium.

MISCELLANEOUS

Herbs and seasoning, including spices, mustard, or catsup, contribute little potassium.

Where Can I Get More Information?

Recipes for fruits and vegetables can be found at www.5aday.gov.

To find a registered dietitian in your area go to www.eatright.org and click: Find a Nutrition Professional or call the American Dietetic Association at 1-800-366-1655.

A low-potassium diet may be indicated to prevent high blood levels of potassium—a condition called hyperkalemia. Hyperkalemia can result from kidney disease or the use of some medications. Potassium is abundant in fresh fruits, vegetables, and meats. It is difficult to eat a low-potassium diet and still maintain adequate nutrition. The absence of a food on the following list does not mean it is low in potassium. The following guidelines will alert you to very high and low potassium sources, but the diet should only be used under the guidance of a dietitian. The amount of potassium an individual may need varies and often depends on blood potassium levels. See Handout 3–16 for more information about potassium and ask your local hospital dietitian for guidance.

POTASSIUM CONTENT OF SELECTED FOOD GROUPS

Milk and dairy foods have approximately 185 mg potassium per ½ cup.

Meat (poultry and beef) contains approximately 100 mg potassium per 1 ounce.

Starches (bread, crackers, and cereal) contain approximately 35 mg potassium per serving.

Fats and oils (margarine, oils salad dressing) contain approximately 10 mg potassium per serving.

VEGETABLES LOW IN POTASSIUM

Alfalfa sprouts

Bamboo shoots, canned

Green and wax beans

Bean sprouts

Cabbage

Chard

Cucumber peeled

Endive

Escarole

Lettuce

Green and sweet pepper

Water chestnuts, canned

Watercress

FRUITS LOW IN POTASSIUM

Applesauce

Blueberries

Cranberries

Cranberry juice cocktail

Grape juice

Lemon (½)

Papaya nectar

Peach nectar

Pears, canned

Pear nectar

BEVERAGES LOW IN POTASSIUM

Carbonated soda, except Moxie, colas, and pepper-type

Lemonade

Limeade

Mineral water

VEGETABLES HIGH IN POTASSIUM

Asparagus

Avocado

Beets

Brussels sprouts

Celery, cooked

Kohlrabi

Mushrooms

Okra

Parsnips

Pepper, chili

Potato

Pumpkin

Rutabaga

Tomato

Tomato juice

Tomato paste, puree and sauce

Vegetable juice cocktail

Bamboo shoots fresh

Beet greens

Chard, cooked

Spinach, cooked

Sweet potato

Winter squash

FRUITS HIGH IN POTASSIUM

Apricots

Banana

Cantaloupe

Dates

Figs

Honeydew melon

Kiwi

Nectarine

Orange juice

Orange

Pear, fresh

Prune juice

Prunes

MISCELLANEOUS

All types of broth, bouillon, and consommé are very high in potassium.

Where Can I Get More Information?

National Digestive Diseases Information Clearinghouse http://digestive.niddk.nih.gov.

Go to www.eatright.org and click: Find a Nutrition Professional to locate a professional dietitian in your area.

Fiber is the indigestible part of food; it is especially abundant in fruit, vegetables, and whole or minimally processed foods. Some fiber, called insoluble fiber, acts like a sponge; it absorbs water in the intestine and is best known for its effect on preventing constipation and normalizing bowel movements. It is found in bran cereal, whole wheat bread, fruit, and vegetables. Another type of fiber called soluble fiber is abundant in oatmeal, barley, kidney beans, lima beans, and fruit (e.g., bananas and blackberries), and vegetables (e.g., carrots). Soluble fiber forms a gel when mixed with water and can help improve blood sugar and cholesterol levels when consumed as part of a regular diet.

The best sources of fiber are found in fruit, vegetable, and whole-grain food, such as cereal, bread, whole wheat pasta, and brown rice. To consume enough fiber, start the day with a whole grain cereal and eat at least two fruits and three vegetables along with other whole grain food during the day.

The Recommended Dietary Allowance or Adequate Intakes varies with age. Adult men over age 19 are advised to ingest 38 g per day, women 26 g. See Handout 3-27 for fiber recommendations by age.

FOOD PREPARATION HINTS

Fiber will not be destroyed in cooking, but removing skin from fruit and vegetables reduces intake. The fiber content of food is listed on labels; use it to compare foods before buying. It is recommended that fluid intake be increased when starting a high-fiber diet. Fluid works with fiber to aid digestion.

BEVERAGES

Include fruit smoothies (if made with whole fruit) and unstrained vegetable juice.

Liquids, such as coffee, tea, or sodas, do not contain any fiber. Milk and milk-based drinks contain no fiber, unless pureed with fruit.

CEREALS

Include brands such as Fiber One and All-Bran, bran, and oatmeal.

Cereal made with corn, rice, or white flour are low in fiber. Choose a cereal that provides at least 3 g of fiber per serving.

BREADS

Include whole wheat, rye, and pumpernickel bread, and crackers made with whole grains.

Choose bread that has at least 2 g of fiber per slice.

DESSERTS AND SWEETS

Include dessert made with whole fruit (apple crisp, pumpkin pie, fruited gelatin), whole grains (oatmeal cookies), nuts (pecan pie), and dried fruit (raisin cookies).

Discourage plain cookies and cake.

FATS AND OILS

Include nuts of any type.

Butter, margarine, and cooking oil contain no fiber.

FRUIT

Include all fruit, especially fresh and dried fruits.

Try to consume 3 or more servings per day (½ cup = serving). Edible skin should not be removed.

MEAT AND OTHER PROTEIN FOODS

Include all meat, fish, poultry, legumes, and nuts.

Try to consume at least 2 serving of beans, lentils, or dried peas daily.

DAIRY FOODS AND CALCIUM

Cheese and milk contain no fiber, unless combined with fiber-containing foods.

POTATO, RICE, AND PASTA

Include whole grain pasta, popcorn, brown rice, wild rice, sweet potato, and unpeeled potatoes.

SOUP

Include soup made with beans or vegetable.

VEGETABLES

Include all vegetables, especially asparagus, celery, green beans, broccoli, cabbage, carrots, cauliflower, leafy vegetables, onion, squash, and canned tomato.

Try to eat 3 servings daily either raw or cooked.

MISCELLANEOUS

All condiments are allowed.

Include plenty of fluids from water, soup and beverages.

Where Can I Get More Information?

Food and Nutrition Information Center available at: www.nal.usda.gov/fnic.

Wheat Foods Council available at: www.wheatfoods.org.

To find a registered dietitian in your area, go to www.eatright.org and click: Find a Nutrition Professional or call the American Dietetic Association at 1-800-366-1655.

A low-fiber diet limits the nondigestible carbohydrate (fiber) that is not broken down in the digestive tract. The diet restricts vegetables, fruits, and whole grains. It can be used for a limited time, for instance, when the digestive tract is irritated or inflamed, to minimize fecal volume before or after surgery, and during the acute phase of a digestive disorder, including ulcerative colitis, Crohn's disease, and diverticulitis. Once symptoms are relieved, a diet rich in fiber may be advised to prevent a recurrence of symptoms. Use the recommendations below as a guide. For more advice, read about fiber in patient education Handout 3-27. Use the nutrition label to select foods with the lowest fiber content within a food group. A low-fiber diet will contain approximately 16 g of dietary fiber. Ask your doctor if this is an amount appropriate for you.

BEVERAGES

Include coffee, tea, soft drinks, strained fruit juice, and fruit drinks.

Limit juices that contain pulp. Prune juice, although not high in fiber, may not be well tolerated in those with digestive disorders.

CEREALS

Include refined, cooked cereals, including grits and farina, and cold cereals made with refined grains, including puffed rice and puffed wheat.

Avoid whole grain cereals, including oatmeal, bran, shredded wheat, granola type cereal, and cereals containing seeds, nuts, coconut, and dried fruit. Read labels looking for a cereal with a low fiber content. One cup of Rice Krispies contains <1 g of fiber.

BREADS

Include refined white bread (<1 g fiber per slice), rolls, biscuits, muffins, crackers, and pancakes made with refined white flour.

Avoid any products made with whole grain flour, including whole wheat (~2 g fiber per slice), bran, bread with seeds, nuts, dried fruit, and coconut, or graham crackers.

DESSERTS AND SWEETS

Include plain cake and cookies, pie made with allowed fruits, plain sherbet, fruit ice, Italian ice, sorbet, frozen pops, gelatin, jelly, plain hard candy, marshmallows, and plain ice cream.

Avoid desserts made with whole grain flour, bran, seeds, nuts, coconut, or dried fruit.

FATS AND OIL

Include margarine, butter, salad oils, strained salad dressings, mayonnaise, bacon, and plain gravy.

Avoid any oil and butters with herbs, nuts, seeds, or dried fruit.

FRUIT

Include most canned or cooked fruits, including applesauce and canned fruit cocktail.

Avoid fresh fruit or fruit with skins.

MEAT AND OTHER PROTEIN FOODS

Include beef, lamb, ham, veal, pork, poultry, fish, organ meat, and eggs. Tough, fibrous meats may not be higher in fiber, but may not be easy to chew or digest well.

Avoid any foods prepared with whole grain ingredients, seeds, nuts, dried beans, peas, lentils, legumes, and peanut butter.

DAIRY FOODS AND CALCIUM

Include milk, yogurt, custard, and cheese.

Avoid yogurt or milk shakes made with whole fruit or any foods with seeds, nuts, or dried fruit. Although not high in fiber, these foods may be restricted for individuals following a low-residue diet.

POTATO, RICE, AND PASTA

Include cooked, white and sweet potato without the skin, white rice, refined pasta, and noodles.

Avoid brown rice, whole wheat pasta, barley, or other whole grains.

SOUP

Include clear broth and bouillon and cream soup made with allowed ingredients.

Avoid soups made with vegetables or beans.

VEGETABLES

Include well-cooked and canned vegetables without seeds, peel, or skin. Strain vegetable juice.

MISCELLANEOUS

Salt, pepper, sugar, spices, herbs in small amounts, vinegar, ketchup, and mustard without seeds are allowed.

Avoid nuts, coconut, foods with seeds, and popcorn.

Where Can I Get More Information?

Food and Nutrition Information Center available at: www.nal.usda.gov/fnic.

National Digestive Diseases Information Clearinghouse at: http://digestive.niddk.nih.gov.

To find a registered dietitian in your area, go to www.eatright.org and click: Find a Nutrition Professional or call the American Dietetic Association at 1-800-366-1655.

A lowfat diet may be useful in controlling diarrhea, heartburn, flatulence, and abdominal pain caused by diseases of the liver, gall bladder, and pancreas, or conditions that cause malabsorption of dietary fat. Fat is most prevalent in meat, whole milk dairy products, butter, margarine, and cooking oils. Individuals on very lowfat diets should seek the help of a registered dietitian in planning their diet.

LOWFAT DIET (50 g)

To keep in a 50 g fat range, limit meat to 6 oz per day, choose low or no-fat dairy foods, and limit the servings of fat or oil (butter, margarine or oil) to the equivalent of 20 g of fat or 4 teaspoons of butter (each serving has 5 g of fat). Read fat serving sizes below.

VERY LOWFAT DIET (25 g)

On a very lowfat (25 g) diet, choose only 4 oz of lean meat and fat-free dairy products and only 1 teaspoon of butter, margarine, or oil per day. Read fat serving sizes below.

BEVERAGES

Include coffee, tea, Postum, fruit juice, soft drinks, cocoa made with cocoa powder and skim milk, and fat-free powdered drinks.

Avoid beverages made with whole milk or cream.

CEREALS

Include plain, nonfat cereals, cooked cereals, and cereals without nuts or fat.

Avoid granola type cereal.

BREADS

Include whole-grain breads, enriched breads, saltines, soda crackers, bagels, English muffins, and plain or low fat tortillas.

Avoid biscuits, breads containing egg or cheese, most pastry, pancakes, waffles, French toast, doughnuts, fritters, popovers, snack chips, stuffing, fried tortillas, and popcorn prepared with fat.

DESSERTS AND SWEETS

Include nonfat sherbet, fruit ice, gelatin, and fruit popsicles; angel food cake, lowfat cookies, including vanilla wafers, graham crackers, meringues, fat-free baked goods, jelly, jam, marmalade, honey, syrup, molasses, sugar, hard candy, fondant, gumdrops, jelly beans, marshmallows, cocoa powder, fat-free chocolate sauce, and red and black licorice.

Avoid regular cakes, cookies, pie, and pastry. Avoid candy made with chocolate, nuts, butter, and cream or fat of any kind.

FATS AND OIL

The following foods contain approximately 5 g of fat in the portion listed; read individual product labels for specific fat content.

Unsaturated Fats

Margarine (1 teaspoon), diet margarine (1 tablespoon), mayonnaise (1 teaspoon), reduced calorie mayonnaise (1 tablespoon), creamy salad dressing (2 teaspoons), reduced calorie (1 tablespoon), and all vegetable oils (1 teaspoon). Nuts: cashews (1 tablespoon or 2 nuts), whole almonds (6), peanuts (20 small or 10 large), peanut butter (2 teaspoons), cashew butter (2 teaspoons), walnuts (2 whole), pistachios (18 whole), and other nuts (1 tablespoon).

Saturated Fats

Bacon (1 slice), butter (1 teaspoon), whipped butter (2 teaspoons), chitterlings (½ oz), shredded coconut (1 tablespoon), cream; half & half (2 tablespoons), heavy cream (1 tablespoon), sour cream (2 tablespoons), cream cheese (1 tablespoon), light cream cheese (2 tablespoons), shortening (1 teaspoon), and salt pork (¼ oz).

FRUIT

Include fresh, frozen, canned, or dried fruit and fruit juices. Limit avocado.

MEAT AND OTHER PROTEIN FOODS

Include fish, poultry without skin, lean veal, beef, pork, and lamb. One ounce contains 3–5 g of fat; 4 oz water-packed tuna contains ~5 g fat and 3 oz tofu or tempeh carries ~5 g of fat. Eggs contain 5 g of fat per egg; egg whites are fat free.

Avoid fried meat, fish, or poultry, sausage, spareribs, poultry with skin, duck and goose, luncheon meats (unless low fat), gravy (unless fat free), fish packed in oil, and peanut butter.

DAIRY FOODS AND CALCIUM

Include skim milk or buttermilk made with skim milk, powdered and evaporated skim milk; tofu in allowed amounts, nonfat soymilk, and nonfat yogurt. Also, low-fat cheese containing <5 g of fat (use sparingly), nonfat cottage cheese, and ricotta cheese. Avoid whole milk products, including ice cream, puddings, and custards made with whole milk; whole milk yogurt, whole milk-based drinks, and all regular cheese.

POTATO, RICE, AND PASTA

Include potatoes, rice, barley, noodles, and pasta made without egg yolks. Avoid fried potatoes, fried rice, potato chips, crisp chow mein noodles, ramen noodles, and dishes prepared with extra fat.

SOUP

Include fat-free broth, fat-free vegetable soups, and no-fat cream soups made with skim milk.

Avoid chowders and cream soup made with cream or whole milk and ramen noodle soup.

VEGETABLES

Include all fresh, frozen, or canned vegetables prepared without added fat. Avoid buttered, au gratin, creamed, or fried vegetables unless made with allowed fat.

MISCELLANEOUS

Include condiments such as ketchup, chili sauce, vinegar, pickles, vanilla flavoring, unbuttered popcorn, mustard, herbs, and seasonings. Avoid cream sauces, regular gravy, and buttered popcorn.

Where Can I Get More Information?

National Digestive Diseases Information Clearinghouse at: http://digestive.niddk.nih.gov.

To find a registered dietitian in your area, go to www.eatright.org and click: Find a Nutrition Professional or call the American Dietetic Association at 1-800-366-1655.

Clear or full liquid diets may be prescribed before or after surgery, before tests, or as a temporary meal choice when food is not appealing.

CLEAR LIQUID DIET (ANY LIQUID YOU CAN SEE THROUGH)

Include clear broth, bouillon, clear juices (e.g., apple, cranberry, or grape), strained grapefruit, orange juice, or lemonade; plain or flavored gelatin; frozen pops or fruit ices made from clear fruit juice; plain tea, black coffee, clear carbonated beverages (e.g., ginger ale, 7-up, Sprite), sugar, honey if dissolved in a beverage, and hard candy.

FULL LIQUID DIET (ANY FOOD LIQUID AT ROOM TEMPERATURE)

Include all foods listed in the clear liquid diet above, all forms of milk, strained cream soups, plain or flavored yogurt without seeds or pieces of fruit, pudding, custard, milk shakes, eggnog, ice cream, vegetable juice, fruit juice, refined strained cooked cereal (e.g., farina), butter, margarine, oils, cream, sugar, honey, syrup, and any type of tea or coffee.

Liquid Meal Replacements

Available in the supermarket for use on a full liquid diet are Carnation Instant Breakfast (Nestle) and Ultra Slim Fast (Slim Fast Food Co.), which can be mixed with milk and consumed while on a full liquid diet. An 8-oz beverage prepared with milk will provide approximately 280 calories and most essential nutrients.

Lactose-free Ready-to-drink Formulas

Pharmaceutical companies make ready-to-drink fortified milkshakes, which are available in pharmacies and many supermarkets. These products have the advantage of being a good source of calories and nutrition without containing any lactose. Lactose is the naturally occurring milk sugar that some individuals can have difficulty digesting, particularly during illness that affects the digestive tract.

Where Can I Get More Information?

For additional information about these products and those listed below, go to the company web page or ask your local pharmacist for helping you choose the right product.

Boost made by Mead Johnson available at: www.meadjohnson.com.

Complete and Fibersource made by Novartis available at: www.novartis.com.

Ensure and Jevity made by Ross available at: www.ross.com.

To find a registered dietitian in your area, go to www.eatright.org and click: Find a Nutrition Professional or call the American Dietetic Association at 1-800-366-1655.

Low-purine Diet for Gout

Gout is one of the oldest ailments to affect mankind. High levels of uric acid accumulate in the blood and form crystals that accumulate in joints and cause pain. Drug treatment is the most effective way to manage gout, but a low-purine diet may be useful during an acute attack. Uric acid is metabolized from purines. Purines from within the body are a far greater source than dietary sources.

A low-fat, moderate protein intake is advised, along with drinking plenty of fluids. Drinking alcohol is discouraged. A purine-free diet is impossible, but a restriction of 100 to 150 mg/day has been suggested in severe cases of gout. Tofu (bean curd) may be a preferable protein source over beef and poultry.

FOODS HIGHEST IN PURINE (150–825 mg/100 g)

Anchovies

Bouillon, broth, consommé

Brains

Kidney, heart

Game meats

Gravies

Herring

Liver, kidney

Mackerel, herring

Meat extracts

Mincemeat

Sardines

Scallops, mussels

Sweetbreads

Yeast (taken as a supplement)

FOODS HIGH IN PURINE (50–150 mg/100 g)

Asparagus

Breads, cereals, and whole grains

Cauliflower

Eel

Fish, fresh and saltwater

Legumes, such as beans, lentils, and peas

Meat (beef, lamb, pork, veal)

Meat soups and broths

Mushrooms

Oatmeal

Peas, green

Poultry (chicken, duck, turkey

Shellfish (crab, lobster, oysters)

Spinach

Wheat germ and bran

FOODS LOWEST IN PURINE (10–50 mg/100 g)

Coffee, tea, sodas, postum

Breads and cereals, except whole grains, crackers

Cheese

Eggs, custard

Fats

Fish roe

Fruit and fruit juices

Gelatin

Milk, ice cream

Nuts

Sugars (syrups and sweets)

Vegetables, except those listed above

Vegetable and cream soups

Where Can I Get More Information?

Arthritis Foundation available at: www.arthritis.org.

To find a registered dietitian in your area, go to www.eatright.org. and click: Find a Nutrition Professional or call the American Dietetic Association at 1-800-366-1655.

This information is from Mahan, S., and Escott-Stump, K. (2004). *Krause's Food, Nutrition, & Diet Therapy* (11th ed., p. 1135). Philadelphia: W.B. Saunders; and Pennington, J. (1999). *Bowes and Church's Food Values of Portions Commonly Used* (17th ed., p. 391). Philadelphia: J.B. Lippincott.

Celiac disease (also called celiac sprue and gluten-sensitive enteropathy) is an autoimmune inflammatory disease of the digestive tract that occurs in people who cannot tolerate gluten in food; it is often genetic. Gluten is a protein found in wheat, rye, barley, and possibly oats. When individuals with celiac disease consume food containing gluten, the immune system responds by provoking an immune response, damaging the small intestine. Symptoms vary widely and can be mild to severe, including, abdominal bloating and pain, chronic diarrhea, weight loss, gas, bone pain, muscle cramps, delayed growth, and pain in the joints. Exclusion of gluten results in healing and resolves malabsorption.

GLUTEN-FREE DIET

A gluten-free diet means avoiding all foods that contain wheat (including spelt, triticale, and kamut), rye, barley, and possibly oats— most grain, pasta, cereal, and many processed foods. Instead of wheat flour, use potato, rice, soy, or bean flour. Or, buy gluten-free bread, pasta, and other products from special food companies. Following is a list of foods allowed and those to be avoided. It is not a complete list. Because a gluten-free diet is complicated, contact a dietitian or healthcare professional who specializes in food and nutrition for help. Contact the organizations listed below for more in-depth information.

BREADS, CEREAL, RICE, AND PASTA

Recommended Foods

Breads or bread products made from corn, rice, soy, arrowroot, corn or potato starch, pea, potato, or whole-bean flour; tapioca, sago, rice, bran, cornmeal, buckwheat, millet, flax, teff, sorghum, amaranth, or quinoa.

Hot cereals made from soy, hominy, hominy grits, brown and white rice, buckwheat groats, millet, cornmeal, and quinoa flakes.

Puffed corn, rice, or millet, and other rice and corn made with allowed ingredients.

Rice, rice noodles, and pasta made from allowed ingredients.

Some rice crackers and cakes, and popped corn cakes made from allowed ingredients.

Foods to Omit

Breads and baked products containing wheat, rye, triticale, barley, oats, wheat, germ or bran, graham, gluten or durum flour, wheat starch, oat bran, bulgur, farina, wheat-based semolina, spelt, and kamut.

Cereals made from wheat, rye, triticale, barley, and oats; and cereals with added malt extract and malt flavorings.

Pastas made from the ingredients listed above.

Most crackers.

Tips

Use corn, rice, soy, arrowroot, tapioca, and potato flours (or a mixture) instead of wheat flours in recipes. Experiment with gluten-free products. Some may be purchased from your supermarket, health food store, or directly from the manufacturer.

VEGETABLES

Recommended are all plain, fresh, frozen, or canned vegetables made with allowed ingredients.

Omit any creamed or breaded vegetables (unless allowed ingredients are used), canned baked beans, and some French fries.

Tips

Buy plain, frozen, or canned vegetables and season with herbs, spices, or sauces made with allowed ingredients.

FRUITS

Recommended are all fruits and fruit juices.

Omit some commercial fruit pie fillings and dried fruit.

MILK, YOGURT, AND CHEESE

Recommended are all milk and milk products, except those made with gluten additives and aged cheese.

Omit malted milk, some milk drinks, and flavored or frozen yogurt.

Tips

Contact the food manufacturer for product information if the ingredients are not listed on the label.

MEATS, POULTRY, FISH, DRY BEANS AND PEAS, EGGS, AND NUTS

Recommended are all meat, poultry, fish, and shellfish, and eggs; dry beans, peas, nuts, peanut butter, and soybeans; cold cuts, frankfurters, or sausage made without fillers.

Omit any food prepared with wheat, rye, oats, barley, gluten stabilizers, or fillers, including some frankfurters, cold cuts, sandwich spreads, sausages, and canned meats; self-basting turkey, and some egg substitutes.

Tips

When dining out, select meat, poultry, or fish made without breading, gravies, or sauces.

FATS, SNACKS, SWEETS, CONDIMENTS, AND BEVERAGES

Recommended are butter, margarine, salad dressings, sauces, soups, and desserts made with allowed ingredients; sugar, honey, jelly, jam, hard candy, plain chocolate, coconut, molasses, marshmallows, and meringues; pure instant or ground coffee, tea, carbonated drinks, wine (made in United States), rum; and most seasonings and flavorings.

Omit commercial salad dressings, prepared soups, condiments, sauces, and seasonings prepared with ingredients to be omitted. Also, hot cocoa mixes, nondairy cream substitutes, flavored instant coffee, herbal tea, alcohol distilled from cereals (e.g., gin, vodka, whisky, and beer); ale, cereal, malted beverages, and licorice.

Tips

Store all gluten-free products in your refrigerator or freezer because they do not contain preservatives. Remember to avoid sauces, gravies, canned fish, and other products with hydrolyzed vegetable protein or hydrolyzed plant protein (HVP/HPP) made from wheat protein.

Where Can I Get More Information?

Glucose Intolerance Group of North America available at: www.gluten.net.

To find a registered dietitian in your area, go to www.eatright.org and click: Find a Nutrition Professional or call the American Dietetic Association at 1-800-366-1655.

This report was reprinted from *Celiac Disease* (p. 4–8) by the National Digestive Diseases Information Clearinghouse (NDDIC). The full publication can be obtained at: http://digestive.niddk.nih.gov/ddiseases/pubs/celiac/index.htm.

Lactose is the name of the naturally occurring sugar found in milk and foods made with milk. Individuals who cannot digest lactose need to follow a lactose-restricted diet to avoid symptoms, which can include nausea, cramps, bloating, gas, and diarrhea. Symptoms begin 30 minutes to 2 hours after ingesting lactose. Many individuals can tolerate small amounts of lactose and recent research shows the lactose contained in yogurt is well tolerated and can be a good source of calcium. It is important to establish an individual tolerance level and to ensure calcium intake is adequate. Calcium can be obtained from supplements, calcium-fortified juice, and lactose-free dairy products.

BEVERAGES

Include soybean milks, coffee, tea, and carbonated beverages.

Avoid milk-based beverages, including powdered milk breakfast drinks and meal replacement drinks.

CEREALS

Include any cereal that does not contain lactose.

BREADS

Include French, Italian, and Syrian bread made with water; matzoh, soda crackers; whole grain and enriched flour breads that do not contain milk or milk products.

Avoid quickbreads, muffins, biscuits, pancakes, and rolls made with milk. Fruit juice and soymilk are good milk replacements when making muffins or quick breads.

DESSERTS AND SWEETS

Include water and fruit ices, gelatin desserts, angel food cake, pie, cake, and cookies made from allowed ingredients.

Avoid commercially made desserts made with milk or milk products.

FATS AND OIL

Include butter or margarine, salad dressings, nondairy creamer, and all cooking oils.

Avoid any foods prepared with lactose-containing ingredients.

FRUIT

Include all fruits and juices.

MEAT AND OTHER PROTEIN FOODS

Include all meats, poultry, fish, eggs, peanut butter, dried peas and beans, and hard aged processed cheese, if tolerated.

DAIRY FOODS AND CALCIUM

Include Lact-Aid milk, yogurt and hard cheese (if tolerated), soymilk fortified with calcium, and calcium-fortified orange juice.

Avoid milk and milk products or acidophilus milk.

POTATO, RICE, AND PASTA

Include potatoes, rice, barley, noodles, spaghetti, macaroni, and other pastas.

Avoid potatoes or substitutes made with milk or mixes made with lactose-containing ingredients.

SOUP

Include broth-based soups, bouillon, and soups or chowder made with allowed ingredients.

Avoid soup or chowder made with milk or milk products.

VEGETABLES

Include all vegetables.

Avoid vegetables prepared with milk or milk products.

MISCELLANEOUS

Include all seasonings, spices and flavorings that are allowed.

Avoid any with milk or milk products added.

CALCIUM AND LACTOSE CONTENT IN COMMON FOODS

Food	Calcium (mg)	Lactose (g)
1 cup calcium-fortified orange juice	320	0
1 cup soymilk	200	0
1 cup raw broccoli	90	0

Food	Calcium (mg)	Lactose (g)
½ cup pinto beans	40	0
Salmon, canned 3 oz with bones	205	0
Lettuce greens, ½ cup	10	0
Yogurt, 1 cup	415	5
Milk, 1 cup	295	11
Swiss cheese, 1 oz	270	1
Ice cream, ½ cup	85	6
Cottage cheese, ½ cup	75	2–3

Where Can I Get More Information?

Gastrointestinal Disorders and Treatment available at: www.niddk.nih.gov/health/digest/digest.htm.

To find a registered dietitian in your area, go to www.eatright.org and click: Find a Nutrition Professional or call the American Dietetic Association at 1-800-366-1655.

Diet for Heartburn and Gastroesophageal Reflux Disease

Gastroesophageal reflux disease (GERD) occurs when the ring of muscle (lower esophageal sphincter [LES]) that separates the stomach from the throat (esophagus) does not close or tighten properly. This allows stomach acid to regurgitate back into the throat, causing a burning sensation known as heartburn. Presence of a hiatal hernia can contribute to reflux disease by making it easier for stomach acid to wash back up into the esophagus. Diet can have an impact on symptoms. Individuals with GERD are advised to avoid reclining after meals, alcohol, overeating, and certain foods that cause symptoms. Foods commonly identified as being problematic include citrus juices, chocolate, and coffee (with or without caffeine), mint flavorings, carbonated beverages, and tomato-based foods. Weight loss is advised for those who are overweight and foods high in fat are thought to make symptoms worse.

Eating three small meals, with appropriate snacks, and not lying down after meals can improve symptoms. Recommended food guidelines follow.

BEVERAGES

Include skim milk, 1%, 2%, low-fat milk, buttermilk, noncitrus juices, and decaffeinated non-mint tea.

Avoid whole milk, chocolate milk, chocolate, and coffee, including decaffeinated and regular. Limit consumption of carbonated beverages.

CEREALS

Include all types, with or without whole grain ingredients. Look for cereals with a low fat content.

BREADS

Include bread, rolls, bagels, corn tortillas, and muffins made with low-fat ingredients.

Avoid foods with higher fat content, such as croissants, doughnuts, sweet rolls, regular muffins, and waffles or pancakes, if not well tolerated.

DESSERTS AND SWEETS

Include angel food cake, sponge cake, low-fat cookies, gelatin, frozen desserts, sherbet, fruit ice, low-fat yogurt, low-fat ice cream and milk-based desserts made with skim, 1%, or 2% low-fat milk.

Avoid pies, cookies, cakes, regular ice cream, and chocolate desserts.

FATS AND OIL

Include nonfat and low-fat dressings and mayonnaise; nonfat liquid or powdered cream substitutes, and nonfat sour cream.

Avoid full-fat cream and sour cream, and limit gravies, bacon, butter and margarine, and vegetable oils, which are rich in fat.

FRUITS

Include fruit of all types, including fresh, frozen, or canned.

Avoid orange, lemon, tangerine, pineapple, or grapefruit juice.

MEAT AND OTHER PROTEIN FOODS

Include lean meat, poultry (without skin), lean pork, fish, tofu, dried beans (including fat free refried beans) and peas, and eggs.

Avoid fried meat, poultry, fish, and eggs; regular deli meats, including hot dogs and sausages, and canned beans with fat added.

DAIRY FOODS AND CALCIUM

Include nonfat and low-fat yogurt, milk, or cheese.

Avoid whole milk, yogurt, and cheese.

POTATO, RICE, AND PASTA

Include baked, boiled, and mashed potatoes: prepared rice with little fat added, and cooked pasta, including noodles, spaghetti, and macaroni served with allowed ingredients.

Avoid fried potatoes and chips, and pasta served with cream or cheese sauces.

SOUP

Include fat-free or homemade soups made with allowed ingredients.

Avoid regular cream soup and chowders and tomato-based soups.

VEGETABLES

Include all plain fresh, frozen, and canned vegetables prepared with little added fat or cheese.

Avoid fried or creamed vegetables and tomatoes and tomato-based products.

MISCELLANEOUS

Include salt, garlic, oregano, sage, pepper, and other spices and herbs.

Avoid spices and herbs in tomato-based sauces, spearmint, peppermint, chili and jalapeno peppers, and vinegar.

Where Can I Get More Information?

National Digestive Diseases Information Clearinghouse available at: http://digestive.niddk.nih.gov.

To find a registered dietitian in your area, go to www.eatright.org and click: Find a Nutrition Professional or call the American Dietetic Association at 1-800-366-1655.

WHY DO I HAVE GAS?

Everyone has gas. How much gas the body makes and how sensitive a person is to gas in the large intestine determine how uncomfortable having gas is.

WHAT CAN I DO ABOUT GAS?

Changing what you eat and drink can help prevent or relieve gas.

1. Cut down on foods that cause gas including:

   - Beans
   - Vegetables such as broccoli, cabbage, brussel sprouts, onions, artichokes, and asparagus
   - Fruits such as pears, apples, and peaches
   - Whole grains such as whole wheat and bran
   - Soft drinks and fruit drinks
   - Milk and milk products, such as cheese and ice cream
   - Packaged foods that have lactose in them, such as bread, cereal, and salad dressing
   - Dietetic foods and sugar-free candies and gums

2. Drink plenty of water, non-"fizzy" liquids, and clear soup.

   Try not to drink liquids that cause gas, like soda and beer. If you do drink these liquids, pour them into a glass first to let some of the "fizz" out.

3. Reduce the amount of air you swallow. Here are some ways to avoid swallowing air:

   - Eat slower and chew more to cut down on the amount of air you swallow when you eat.
   - Avoid chewing gum and eating hard candy.
   - If you smoke, try to cut down or quit.
   - If you have false teeth, see your dentist to make sure they fit right.

4. Keep a diary.

   Write down the foods (and the amounts) that seem to cause you the most problems. Also keep track of the number of times you pass gas. Take the diary with you to the doctor to answer questions about eating habits and symptoms.

Where Can I Get More Information?

National Digestive Diseases Information Clearinghouse available at: http://digestive.niddk.nih. gov.

To find a registered dietitian in your area, go to www.eatright.org and click: Find a Nutrition Professional or call the American Dietetic Association at 1-800-366-1655.

Reprinted from the National Digestive Diseases Information Clearinghouse (NDDIC). *What I Need to Know About Gas* NIH No. 04-415. January 2004 (p.1–3). The full report can be obtained at http://digestive.niddk.nih.gov/ddiseases/pubs/gas_ez

Constipation is the most common gastrointestinal complaint in the United States. To understand constipation, it helps to know how the colon (large intestine) works. As food moves through it, the colon absorbs water while forming waste products (stool). Muscle contractions in the colon push stool toward the rectum. By the time stool reaches the rectum, it is solid because most of the water has been absorbed. The hard and dry stool of constipation occurs when the colon absorbs too much water. This happens because the colon's muscle contractions are slow or sluggish in moving the stool through the colon.

COMMON CAUSES OF CONSTIPATION

- Not enough fiber in diet
- Not enough liquids
- Lack of exercise
- Medications
- Irritable bowel syndrome
- Changes in life or routine such as pregnancy, older age, and travel
- Abuse of laxatives
- Ignoring the urge to have a bowel movement
- Specific disease such as multiple sclerosis and lupus
- Problems with the colon and rectum
- Problems with intestinal function (chronic idiopathic constipation)

Diet

The most common cause of constipation is a diet low in fiber found in vegetables, fruits, and whole grains and high in fats found in cheese, eggs, and meats. People who eat plenty of high-fiber foods are less likely to become constipated.

Fiber, soluble and insoluble, is the part of fruits, vegetables, and grains that the body cannot digest. Soluble fiber dissolves easily in water and takes on a soft, gel-like texture in the intestines. Insoluble fiber passes almost unchanged through the intestines. The bulk and soft texture of fiber help prevent hard, dry stools that are difficult to pass.

On average, Americans eat about 5 to 20 g of fiber daily, short of the 20 to 35 g recommended by the American Dietetic Association.

High-fiber foods include beans, whole grains and bran cereals, fresh fruits, and vegetables such as asparagus, brussel sprouts, cabbage, and carrots.

Not Enough Liquids

Liquids such as water and juice add fluid to the colon and bulk to stools, making bowel movements softer and easier to pass. People who have problems with constipation should drink eight 8-oz glasses of liquid daily.

Lack of Exercise

Lack of exercise can lead to constipation, although doctors do not know precisely why. For example, constipation often occurs after an accident or during an illness when one must stay in bed.

POINTS TO REMEMBER

1. Constipation affects almost everyone at one time or another.
2. Many people think they are constipated when, in fact, their bowel movements are regular.
3. The most common causes of constipation are poor diet and lack of exercise.
4. Additional causes of constipation include medications, irritable bowel syndrome, abuse of laxatives, and specific diseases.
5. A medical history and physical examination may be the only diagnostic tests needed before the doctor suggests treatment.
6. Most people with mild constipation do not need laxatives. Doctors may recommend laxatives for a limited time for people with chronic constipation.
7. In most cases, following these simple tips will help relieve symptoms and prevent recurrence of constipation.
   - Eat a well-balanced, high-fiber diet that includes beans, bran, whole grains, fresh fruits, and vegetables.
   - Drink plenty of liquids.
   - Exercise regularly.
   - Set aside time after breakfast or dinner for undisturbed visits to the toilet.
   - Do not ignore the urge to have a bowel movement.
   - Understand that normal bowel habits vary.
   - Whenever a significant or prolonged change in bowel habits occurs, check with a doctor.

A SAMPLE HIGH-FIBER MENU

Food	Fiber (g)	Food	Fiber (g)
Breakfast		*Lunch*	
Orange juice, ¾ cup	0.2	Turkey sandwich made with	
Fiber One cereal, ½ cup	13	2 slices whole wheat bread	6
Whole wheat bread, 1 slice	3	Lettuce and tomato	0.5
Margarine, 1 teaspoon	0	Coleslaw, ½ cup	2.5
Milk, 1 cup	0	Apple, 1 medium with peel	3
Coffee or tea	0		

Food	Fiber (g)	Food	Fiber (g)
Dinner		*Snack*	
Baked fish, 4 oz	0	Orange, 1	<u>3</u>
Baked potato with skin	5	Total fiber content	41.7
Mashed winter squash, ½ cup	2.5		
Spinach, cooked, ½ cup	2		
Butter or margarine, 2 teaspoons	0		
Cantaloupe, cubed, 1 cup	1		

Where Can I Get More Information?

National Digestive Diseases Clearinghouse. The clearinghouse provides information about diseases to people with digestive disorders and to their families, healthcare professionals, and the public.
E-mail: nddic@info.niddk.gov.
http://digestive.niddk.nih.gov.

To find a registered dietitian in your area, go to www.eatright.org and click: Find a Nutrition Professional or call the American Dietetic Association at 1-800-366-1655.

This report was reprinted from a National Digestive Diseases Information Clearinghouse article "Constipation" (p. 1–13). The complete publication is available at: http://digestive.niddk.nih.gov/ddiseases/pubs/constipation/.

Diverticulosis occurs when small pouches (diverticula) form in the colon (large intestine). About 30% of people over the age of 50 have diverticulosis and by age 80 almost everyone has the condition. A low-fiber diet is believed to be the main cause of diverticular disease. The disease is rare in countries where people eat a fiber-rich diet. A high-fiber diet is recommended to prevent constipation, which can increase pressure in the colon causing diverticula.

TREATMENT FOR DIVERTICULOSIS

A high-fiber diet is the usual treatment for diverticulosis. A high-fiber diet keeps stools soft, prevents constipation, and lowers pressure in the large intestine. The recommended adequate intake (AI) of fiber is 21 to 38 g per day for adults. It may take several months before the benefits of a high-fiber diet take affect.

Usually, no symptoms are associated with diverticulosis, but if the pouches become infected or inflamed the condition is called diverticulitis. Abdominal pain and tenderness on the left side is a common symptom of diverticulitis. A high-fiber diet is not recommended during an acute diverticulitis attack.

FIBER CONTENT OF SELECTED FOOD (g)

Fiber One, ½ cup	13
All-Bran, ½ cup	10
Raisin Bran, 1 cup	8.2
Cheerios, 1 cup	3
Cornflakes, 1 cup	1.1
Trix, 1 cup	0
Whole wheat bread, 1 slice	1.9
White bread, 1 slice	0.6
Brown rice, 1 cup	3.5
White rice, 1 cup	1.0
Apple juice, 1 cup	0.2
Apple, raw	3.7
Banana	2.7
Prunes, 10	6.0

Raspberries, 1 cup*	8.4
Strawberries, 1 cup*	3.4
Asparagus, ½ cup	1.4
Broccoli, ½ cup	2.0
Carrots, ½ cup	2.6
Sweet potato, ½ cup	3.0
Cheese	0
Baked beans, 1 cup	12.0
Peanuts, 1oz	2.5

Increase the fiber intake in the diet by eating at least 2 servings of fruit and three servings of vegetables daily. Choose high-fiber and whole grain cereals, breads, and rice whenever possible. Drink plenty of fluids to aid with digestion.

For information on a low-fiber diet see Patient Education Handout 4–14.

Where Can I Find More Information?

National Digestive Diseases Information Clearinghouse available at: http://digestive.niddk.nih.gov.

To find a registered dietitian in your area, go to www.eatright.org and click: Find a Nutrition Professional or call the American Dietetic Association at 1-800-366-1655.

---

*Until recently, many doctors suggested avoiding all foods with small seeds (e.g., tomatoes or strawberries) because they believed that particles could lodge in the diverticula and cause inflammation. This is now a controversial point. The seeds in tomatoes, zucchuni, cucumbers, strawberries, rasberries and poppy seeds are generally considered harmless but nuts, popcorn hulls, sunflower seeds, pumkin seeds, caraway seeds and sesame seeds should be avoided. Source: Diverticulosis and Diverticulitis NIH Publication No. 04-1163, August 2004. http://digestive.niddk.nih.gov/ddiseases/pubs/diverticulosis/index.htm, accessed 5/21/05.

A high-protein, high-calorie diet is indicated when unwanted weight loss occurs from loss of appetite, the increased calorie needs of surgery, or as a side effect of medical treatment. Protein is needed to build and repair tissue, making it essential for healing. Calories are required for energy and to ensure the protein in food is spared from being used for fuel so it can be used to heal and repair tissue.

HIGH-PROTEIN FOODS

Include eggs, meat, fish, poultry, milk, cheese, eggnog, custard, yogurt, peanut butter, almond butter, dried beans, and peas. On a high-protein diet, include 2 to 3 servings of protein-rich food daily.

Tips to boost calories and protein:

- In most cases, use whole milk dairy foods for the extra calories, not low-fat versions.
- Most grains and starch have only 2 to 3 g of protein per serving, but they accumulate to be a good protein source and can be combined with other foods to add protein. For example, toast topped with melted cheese and rice pudding made with milk, rice, and egg.
- Vegetables and fruit are not rich in protein or calories, but they can be combined with other foods to add flavor and nutrition. For example, vegetable with butter and fruit with cream.
- Fats and oils are also not rich in protein, but they have a significant amount of calories; butter, margarine, and cooking oils contain 45 calories per teaspoon and mayonnaise or salad dressing contains 45 calories per tablespoon. Spread butter on bread generously, melt on vegetables, and melt into cooked dishes.
- Fortify milk: Mix 2 to 4 tablespoons nonfat dry milk with 1 cup whole milk, which boosts protein by 6 to 12 g per cup.
- Evaporated milk is twice as rich in protein and calories as fluid milk; use it in casseroles, baked goods, and cooked cereals.
- Eggs: Each egg has 7 g protein; scramble eggs into soup, pasta dishes, and mashed potatoes.
- Cheese has 100 calories per ounce; melt cheese on vegetables, in casseroles, and eat as a snack.
- Sour cream has 26 calories per tablespoon; add sour cream to vegetables, soup, and mix in sauces.
- Peanut butter has 100 calories per tablespoon; serve peanut butter on fruit, toast, and waffles.
- Carnation Instant Breakfast has 130 calories per packet; mix with whole (not skim milk) for a 250-calorie beverage.
- Use cream instead of milk to make milk shakes.

■ Yogurt smoothie: Blend 8 oz yogurt, 1 cup fruit, ½ cup half and half cream for 300+ calories.

Where Can I Get More Information?

Food and Nutrition Information Center available at: www.nal.usda.gov/fnic.

To find a registered dietitian in your area, go to www.eatright.org and click: Find a Nutrition Professional or call the American Dietetic Association at 1-800-366-1655.

REFERENCES

American Diabetes Association. (2004). American Diabetes Association Nutrition Principles and Recommendations in Diabetes. *Diabetes Care, 276,* (Suppl 1), S36–S46.

American Diabetes Association (2004). Pregnancy and lactation 2004. American Diabetes Association Nutrition Principles and Recommendations in Diabetes. *Diabetes Care,* 27 (Suppl 1), s42–s43.

Blackburn. G. L. (2001). The Public Health Implications of the Dietary Approaches to Stop Hypertension Trial. *American Journal of Clinical Nutrition, 74,* 1–2.

Byers, T., Nestle, M., Mctiernan, A., Doyle, C., Currie-Williams, A., & Gansler, T. M. (2001). American Cancer Society guidelines on nutrition and physical activity for cancer prevention: Reducing the risk of cancer with healthy food choices and physical activity. *CA: A Cancer Journal for Clinicians, 52,* 92–119. Full text article online at: caonline.amcancersoc.org

Chobanian, A. V. (2003). The Seventh Report of the Joint National Committee on Prevention, Detection, Evaluation, and Treatment of High Blood Pressure. *Journal of the American Medical Association, 289,* 2560–2572.

Choi, H. K., Atkinson, K., Karlson, E. W., Willett, W., & Curhan, G. (2004). Alcohol intake and risk of incident gout in men: a prospective study. *Lancet, 363,* 1277–1281.

Diabetes Control and Complications Trial Research Group. (1993). The effect of intensive treatment of diabetes on the development and progression of long-term complications in insulin-dependent diabetes mellitus. *New England Journal of Medicine, 329,* 977–986.

Dixon, J. B., Bhathal, P. S., Hughes, N. R., & O'Brien, P.E (2004). Nonalcoholic fatty liver disease: Improvement in liver histological analysis with weight loss. *Hepatology, 39,* 1647–1654.

FM Partnership (2004). Available at: www.fmpartnership.org.

Grundy, S. (2004). NCEP Report: Implications of Recent Clinical Trials for The National Cholesterol Education Program Adult Treatment Panel III Guidelines. *Circulation, 110,* 227–239. Available at: http://circ.ahajournals.org/cgi/content/abstract/110/2/227. Accessed September 4, 2004.

Genuth, S., Alberti, K. G., Bennett, P., Buse, J., Defronzo, R., Kahn, R., et al. (2003). Expert Committee on the Diagnosis and Classification of Diabetes Mellitus. *Diabetes Care, 26,* 3160–3167.

Hu, F. B., Manson, J. E., Stampfer, M. J., Colditz, G., Liu, S., Solomon, C. G., et al. (2001). Diet, lifestyle, and the risk of type 2 diabetes mellitus in women. *New England Journal of Medicine, 345,* 790–797.

Hafstrom, I., Ringertz, B., Spangberg, A., von Zweibergk, L., Brannemark, S., Nylander, I., et al. (2001). A vegan diet free of gluten improves signs and symptoms of rheumatoid arthritis: The effects on arthritis correlate with a reduction in antibodies to food antigens. *Rheumatology, 40,* 1175–1179.

Kaartinen, K., Lammi, K., Hypen, M., Nenonen, M., Hanninen, O., & Rauma, A. I. (2000). Vegan diet alleviates fibromyalgia symptoms. *Scandinavian Journal of Rheumatology, 29,* 308–313.

Kraus, R. M. (2000). AHA Dietary Guidelines Revision 2000: A statement for healthcare professionals from the Nutrition Committee of the American Heart Association. *Circulation, 102,* 2284–2299.

Liangpunsakul, S., & Chalasani, N. (2003). Treatment of nonalcoholic fatty liver disease. *Current Treatment Options in Gastroenterology, 6,* 455–463.

Mahan, S., & Escott-Stump, K. (2004). *Krause's food, nutrition & diet therapy* (11th ed., p. 1126). Philadelphia: WB Saunders.

Menashian, L., Flam, M., Douglas-Paxton, D., & Raymond, J. (1992). Improved food intake and reduced nausea and vomiting in patients given a restricted diet while receiving cisplatin chemotherapy. *Journal of the American Dietetic Association, 92,* 58–61.

Muller, H., de Toledo, F. W., & Resch, K. L (2001). Fasting followed by vegetarian diet in patients with rheumatoid arthritis: A systematic review. *Scandinavian Journal of Rheumatology, 30,* 1–10.

National Cholesterol Education Program. (2001). Expert Summary of the Third Report of the National Cholesterol Education Program (NCEP) Expert Panel on Detection, Evaluation, and Treatment of High Blood Cholesterol in Adults (Adult Treatment Panel III). *Journal of the American Medical Association, 285,* 2486–2497.

National Institutes of Health National Center for Complementary and Alternative Medicine. (2004). Available at: http://nccam.nih.gov.

National Center for Chronic Disease and Health Promotion. (2004). Available at: www.cdc.gov/nccdphp.

Nelsen, D. A. (2002). Gluten-sensitive enteropathy (celiac disease): More common than you think. *Journal American Family Practice, 66,* 2259–2266.

Nonalcoholic Steatohepatitis. National Digestive Diseases Information Clearinghouse (NDDIC) (2004). Available at: http://digestive.niddk.nih.gov/ddiseases/pubs/nash/index.htm.

Pennington, J. (1999). *Bowes and Church's food values of portions commonly used.* (17th ed., p. 39): Philadelphia: JB Lippincott.

Ressel, G. W. (2002). Practice Guidelines. American Cancer Society releases guidelines on nutrition and physical activity for cancer prevention. *American Family Physician, 66,* 1555,1559, 1560,1562.

Saydah, S. H., Fradkin, J., & Cowie, C. C. (2004). Poor control of risk factors for vascular disease among adults with previously diagnosed diabetes. *Journal of the American Medical Association, 291,* 335–342.

Turok, D. K., Ratcliffe, S. D., & Baxley, E. G. (2003). Management of gestational diabetes mellitus. *American Family Physician, 68,* 1767–1772.

United States Preventive Services Task Force. (2004). Available at: www.ahrq.gov/clinic/uspstfab.htm. Accessed September 2, 2004.

Viera, A. I., Hoag, S., & Shaughnessy, J. (2002). Management of irritable bowel syndrome. *American Family Physician, 66,* 1867–1874.

Whelton, P. K., He, J., Appel, L. J., Cutler, J. A., Havas, S., & Kotchen, T. A. (2002). Primary prevention of hypertension: Clinical and public health advisory from the National High Blood Pressure Education Program. *Journal of the American Medical Association, 288,* 1882–1888.

Family Nutrition

Pregnancy, birth, and well-child visits provide the ideal opportunity for healthcare providers to discuss diet, food choices, and eating habits with their patients. The "Nutrition Talking Points at Well-Child Visits" discussed in Section One can provide a foundation for integrating nutrition into healthcare. The "Healthy People 2010" objectives related to nutrition are also goals that can guide healthcare providers. "Healthy People 2010" is built on initiatives that began over two decades ago with the 1979 Surgeon General's Report *Healthy People* followed by *Healthy People 2000*. The most recent objectives *Healthy People 2010* have set are specific goals for maternal, infant, and child health that address infant mortality, prenatal and obstetrical care, prevention of disabilities, reducing prenatal substance exposure, and promoting breastfeeding. Objectives related to nutrition and diet include adequate growth and reducing iron deficiency in the number of children with dental carries in primary teeth. (The full outline of objectives can be read at www.health.gov/healthypeople.) Adequate nutrition and proper diet are essential to maternal and child health to meet these goals. The patient education handouts that follow at the end of this section will assist providers in answering their patients' questions about diet and nutrition and it can provide them with resources for additional information.

NUTRITION DURING PREGNANCY

The role of diet and nutrition during pregnancy and infancy is critical. Yet, everyone does not obtain optimal nutrition and the results of poor diet can have a major impact on health. Preventable birth defects, including spina bifida and other neural tube defects, could be reduced by half if women consumed adequate folic acid while pregnant (Czeizel 1992). Poor fetal nutrition, as measured by low birth weight, can force the fetus to adapt to being undernourished, which permanently increases the risk for chronic disease including heart disease, high blood pressure, type 2 diabetes, metabolic syndrome, and obesity in adulthood (Barker 1999).

No specific diet is recommended for pregnant women. Cultures around the world meet their nutrient needs from a wide variety of foods. It is the nutrients that are important, not the source. Consumption of calcium, protein, folic acid, and iron are especially important during pregnancy. A wide variety of foods rich in these nutrients can be found listed in Section Three. A balanced diet that meets the dietary guidelines and supplies enough calories to meet but not exceed the recommended weight guidelines is the goal. Being a pregnant teenager with poor weight gain increases the risk for poor pregnancy outcome. Folate is recommended for all pregnant women and many physicians will prescribe a prenatal vitamin with folic acid and iron as part of routine care. A suggested diet during pregnancy is given in Boxes 5-1 through 5-3.

GESTATIONAL DIABETES

Gestational diabetes is the form of diabetes that occurs during pregnancy. Patients diagnosed with gestational diabetes will need to monitor their blood glucose levels, exercise consistently, and learn food and menu choices to maintain normoglycemia. Treatment goals include maintaining fasting capillary blood glucose <95 to 105 mg/dL. A postprandial treatment goal of 140 mg/dL at 1 hour and 120 mg/dL at 2 hours is an expected goal. Women not meeting these goals need to start insulin therapy (Turok 2003). Refer patients to

BOX 5-1 ■ *Nutritional Needs During Pregnancy*

Nutrient (unit)	Amount needed daily
Protein (g)	71
Calcium (mg)	1,300 ≤18 years
	1,000 >19 years
Magnesium (mg)	400 ≤18 years
	350 19 to 30 years
	360 31 to 50 years
Iron (mg)	27
Zinc (mg)	13 ≤18 years
	11 >19 years
Iodine (μg)	220
Selenium (μg)	60
Vitamin A (μg)	≤750
	770 >9 years
Vitamin D (μg)	5
Vitamin E (mg)	15
Vitamin C (mg)	80 ≤18 years
	85 >19 years
Thiamin (mg)	1.4
Riboflavin (mg)	1.4
Niacin (mg)	18
Vitamin B_6 (mg)	1.9
Folate (μg)	600
Vitamin B_{12} (μg)	2.6

Source: Dietary Reference Intakes for Calcium, Phosphorous, Magnesium, Vitamin D, and Fluoride (1997). Dietary Reference Intakes for Thiamin, Riboflavin, Niacin, Vitamin B_{12}, Pantothenic Acid, Biotin and Choline (1978). Dietary Reference Intakes for Vitamin C, Vitamin E, Selenium, and Carotenoids (2000) and Dietary Reference Intakes for Vitamin A, Vitamin K, Arsenic, Boron, Chromium, Copper, Iodine, Iron, Manganese, Molybdenum, Nickel, Silicon, Vanadium, and Zinc (2001): National Academy of Sciences.

BOX 5-2 ■ *Recommended Weight Gains During Pregnancy*

	Total weight gain	First trimester	Weekly weight gain Second and third trimesters
Underweight (BMI <19.8)	28–40 pounds	5.0 pounds	1.07
Normal Weight (BMI 19.8–26)	25–35 pounds	3.5 pounds	0.97
Overweight (BMI >26–29)	15–25 pounds	2.0 pounds	0.67
Obese (BMI >29)	At least 15 pounds		

Young adolescents and Black women should strive for gains at the upper end of the recommended level. Short women (<62 inches) should strive for gains at the lower recommended range. The weight range for women carrying twins is 35 to 45 pounds.

BMI, Body Mass Index.
Source: Subcommittee of Nutritional Status and Weight Gain during Pregnancy and Subcommittee on Dietary Intakes and Nutrient Supplements during Pregnancy, Food, and Nutrition Board, National Academy of Sciences. (1990). *Nutrition During Pregnancy* (Parts I and II). Washington, DC: National Academy Press.

BOX 5-3 ■ *Weight Distribution During Pregnancy*

Fetus	7.5–8.5 pounds
Stored fat and protein	7.5 pounds
Blood	4.0
Tissue fluids	2.7
Uterus	2.0
Amniotic fluids	1.8
Placenta and umbilical cord	1.5
Breasts	1.0
Total	28–29 pounds

Source: Mahan, S., & Escott-Stump, K. (1992). *Krause's Food, Nutrition, and Diet Therapy* (11th ed., p. 183). Philadelphia: WB Saunders.

Handout 4-6, *Diabetes: What I Need To Know About Eating and Diabetes* for general guidelines and Handout 5-6, *Gestational Diabetes: What It Means for Me and My Baby*.

POSTPARTUM WEIGHT LOSS

Postpartum weight loss concerns many new mothers and retention of unwanted weight contributes to long-term obesity (Keppel 1993). Gestational weight gain is the greatest factor influencing postpartum weight retention (Somvanshi 2002), exceeding age, parity, employment status, and race. Adolescents and Black women are at the greatest risk for retaining postpartum weight, potentially increasing the prevalence of obesity-related illnesses in these patient populations. Women should be cautioned during pregnancy about weight gain that exceeds the Institute of Medicine's pregnancy weight gain recommendations. After delivery, realistic weight goals, emphasizing slow, steady weight loss, should be encouraged. Lactation does not guarantee weight loss for all women, particularly if calorie intake is high and exercise is not part of a daily routine (read about breastfeeding below). Women can expect to lose the greatest amount of weight in the first 3 months postpartum, followed by a slower weight loss that can continue until 6 months.

BREASTFEEDING

In 1931, breastfeeding was the norm for American women for the first four months of an infant's life. After World War II, with more women in the work force and the promotion of commercial formula, breastfeeding declined. The American Academy of Pediatrics (AAP) strongly recommends breastfeeding for all infants, in-cluding premature infants. Breastfeeding imparts immunologic, allergenic, economic, and psychological advantages not found in commercial feeding. The Healthy People 2010 objective (objective 16-191-c) is to increase the rate of breastfeeding to 75% at birth and 50% at 6 months and 25% at 1 year of age (Polhamus 2001). In the 2001 Pediatric Nutrition Surveillance Report (PedNSS), 50.9% of infants were never ever breastfed, 20.8% were breastfed for at least 6 months, and 13.6% were breastfed for at least 12 months.

According to the AAP, the women least likely to breastfeed are Black and Hispanic women; those with less education, and those who are single, young, and already have children. Employment is also linked to lower rates of breastfeeding.

Despite long-held concerns that a mother's food choices will effect milk composition, breast milk remains remarkably consistent in nutrition quality despite a mother's diet. Protein, calcium, and fluid are important as are adequate calories to meet the demand of breast milk production and a mother's energy needs. Fatigue is often cited as a reason for poor milk production and stopping breastfeeding. A complete list of nutrients needed during lactation is found under individual nutrients listed in Section Three. Vegetarian mothers who eat no animal foods, dairy, or eggs will need a vitamin B_{12} supplement to meet nutrient needs.

Weight loss while breastfeeding can be unpredictable. The tenth edition of the *Recommended Dietary Allowances* set the energy requirement for lactation at 2,700 calories daily, an amount many nutritionists believe is too high for today's sedentary mother. Recent research found that a caloric restriction of 500 calories per day plus 45 minutes of exercise 4 days per week produced a weight loss of approximately 1 pound per week and did not affect the growth of the nursing infant (Lovelady 2000). The Institute of Medicine encourages an energy intake of at least 1,800 calories for all lactating women. Intakes below 1,500 calories per day are not recommended at any time during lactation, although fasting less than 1 day has not been shown to decrease milk production. Liquid diets or weight loss medications are not recommended (IOM 1991).

The AAP recommends the following guidelines while breastfeeding. (A suggested patient education eating guide during lactation can be found in Handout 5-5.)

- Avoid alcohol; it can pass through breast milk. Women who choose to drink should do so after nursing.
- Do not smoke. It is dangerous to newborns and increases the risk of sudden infant death syndrome (SIDS).
- Avoid excessive caffeine. Caffeine can accumulate in the body and be passed to the infant through breast milk, potentially causing irritability and sleeplessness.

Discuss medications with your pharmacist or healthcare provider. Take medications after nursing rather than before (Box 5-4).

RESOURCES

Maternal and Child Health Resource Center
    www.mchirc.net
National Women's Health Information Center
    www.4woman.gov
La Leche League International
    www.lalecheleague.org

CHILDHOOD NUTRITION

Iron deficiency anemia is the most common known nutrient deficiency in the world. In the 2001 PedNSS, the highest rate of iron deficiency anemia occurs in children

---

BOX 5-4 ■ *Nutritional Needs During Lactation*

Nutrient (unit)	Amount needed daily
Protein (g)	71
Calcium (mg)	1,300 ≤18 years
	1,000 >19 years
Magnesium (mg)	360 ≤18 years
	310 19–30 years
	320 31–50 years
Iron (mg)	10 ≤18 years
	9 >19 years
Zinc (mg)	14 ≤18 years
	12 >9 years
Iodine (μg)	290
Selenium (μg)	70
Vitamin A (μg)	1200 ≤18 years
	1300 >19 years
Vitamin D (μg)	5
Vitamin E (mg)	19
Vitamin C (mg)	115 ≤18 years
	120 >19 years
Thiamin (mg)	1.4
Riboflavin (mg)	1.4
Niacin (mg)	17
Vitamin B$_6$ (mg)	2.0
Folate (μg)	500
Vitamin B$_{12}$ (μg)	2.8

Source: Dietary Reference Intakes for Calcium, Phosphorous, Magnesium, Vitamin D, and Fluoride (1997). Dietary Reference Intakes for Thiamin, Riboflavin, Niacin, Vitamin B$_{12}$, Pantothenic Acid, Biotin, and Choline (1978). Dietary Reference Intakes for Vitamin C, Vitamin E, Selenium, and Carotenoids (2000), and Dietary Reference Intakes for Vitamin A, Vitamin K, Arsenic, Boron, Chromium, Copper, Iodine, Iron, Manganese, Molybdenum, Nickel, Silicon, Vanadium, and Zinc (2001): National Academy of sciences.

under age 2 (between ages 6 and 11 months). The rate of anemia declines with age. The highest rate of anemia was among Black children. According to the PedNSS, the children under age 2 are considered anemic if their hemoglobin (Hb) concentration is <11.0 g/dL or hematocrit (Hct) level is <33.0%. Besides iron, calcium, zinc, vitamin B_6, and vitamin A are important nutrients for children and can be easily obtained from eating a diet of fruits, vegetables, fortified or whole grains, lean protein, and those containing good calcium.

True malnutrition in the United States is rare, but the complaint of "picky eaters" is extremely common and feeding habits in the first years of life can lay the groundwork for a lifetime of eating habits. Food surveys find that only 30% of children age 2 to 11 actually consumes the recommended servings of the essential food groups (Munoz 1997). Overconsumption of high-calorie snack foods and the accompanying rise in childhood obesity is a serious nutrition issue among children. The well-child visit provides an opportunity to discuss nutrition issues and food practices before problems can develop. Refer to Section One to find a list of "Talking Points" intended to help practitioners guide parents and children toward eating habits that will reduce the risk of obesity and optimize food choices and family meal time.

RESOURCES

Bright Futures
    www.brightfutures.org/
National Center for Education in Maternal and Child
    Health
    www.ncemch.org

Dental Caries

Early childhood caries or "baby bottle tooth decay" is a common chronic disease for some children. It is caused by the continuous consuming of fruit juice and sweetened beverages (including milk) in a bottle or "sippy" cup through the day and night. Dipping a pacifier in a sweetened substance also increases the risk of early childhood caries. To prevent caries, parents should be encouraged to limit their child's juice to 4 to 6 oz per day, served in a cup, not in a bottle. Putting the child to bed with a bottle of juice, formula, or milk is also to be discouraged.

RESOURCES

National Oral Health Information Clearinghouse
    www.nohic.nidcr.nih.gov

FOOD ALLERGY

Allergic disease affects 50 million Americans each year and accounts for more than 16.7 million doctor's office visits. Food allergy is the cause of 100 deaths (mostly children) each year.

It is estimated that 8% of children under age 6 will experience a food allergy as will approximately 1% to 2% of adults (NIAID, NIH 2002). Food allergy refers to an adverse immunologic response to food. IgE antibodies are directed to specific food proteins affecting the skin, gastrointestinal tract, and the respiratory system (Sicherer, 1999). Virtually any food can cause a reaction, but only a small number of foods account for 90% of all cases of food allergy and most patients are sensitive to fewer than three foods. Egg, milk, peanuts, soy, wheat, tree nut, and fish are the foods to which children are most likely to react. Adults react to peanuts, tree nuts (walnuts, cashews), fish, and shellfish most often. Children often lose their sensitivity to egg, milk, wheat, or soy with age, but those allergic to peanuts, tree nuts, fish, and shellfish may find it persists into adulthood. Children requiring the elimination of entire food groups will benefit from a referral to a registered dietitian to plan a menu that provides all nutrients.

The first step in food allergy treatment is to confirm the suspected diagnosis through careful testing, which can include skin prick tests, radioallergosorbent test (s), and possibly oral food challenges. Food challenges should be done only under the care and supervision of a board-certified allergist prepared to respond to a potentially life-threatening response. Once a potentially anaphylactic food allergy is identified, parents must eliminate the offending food (in all forms), and they must be instructed in the use of epinephrine. The prompt use of epinephrine in response to a serious reaction is extremely important.

Parents of young children need to educate all those in contact with the child regarding the allergy, with the goal of being prepared in the event the child inadvertently consumes a causal food and to respond to an anaphylaxis crisis. Recognizing the importance of being prepared for an emergency, an Emergency Healthcare Plan for Food Allergy is included in Handout 5-11 (Sicherer 1999). Any parent with a child having a food allergy should have such a plan in place at facilities where the child is likely to spend time.

Refer parents to Handout 5-10 for information about food allergy. General food guidelines for allergy to wheat, soy, peanut, milk, and egg can be found in Handout 5-12 to 5-16. Food intolerances (e.g., gluten and lactose) are not to be identified with food allergies that can trigger a life-threatening anaphylaxis response. Information about a gluten-restricted diet is included in Section Four Handout 4-16 and a lactose restricted diet is found in patient education Handout 4-5. For more information, refer patients to The Food Allergy and Anaphylaxis Network, an organization created to provide educational materials and resources to parents, educators, and healthcare providers. It has a 12-member medical advisory board comprised of leaders in food allergy research.

RESOURCES

The Food Allergy and Anaphylaxis Network
   www.foodallergy.org.
American Academy of Allergy, Asthma, and Immunology
   www.aaaai.org
American Celiac Society
   973-325-8837
Gluten Intolerance Group of North America
   www.gluten.net

VEGETARIAN NUTRITION

Eight to ten million Americans consider themselves to be vegetarian. One's personal definition of vegetarianism can be the exclusion of all animal-based foods, including milk and eggs, or it may mean avoiding only red meat (Box 5-5).

Nutritional Adequacy of a Vegetarian Diet

A well-planned vegetarian diet can meet the needs of infants, children, pregnant women, lactating women, and even professional athletes. A vegetarian food pyramid can be found in Section Two Handout 2-4. Protein is the nutrient of most concern, but this is often an unnecessary worry because protein is abundant in many nonmeat foods. Protein can be obtained in dairy foods, egg, soymilk, soy products, beans, and grains. If energy and total calories are adequate and a wide variety of foods are consumed, all age groups can meet their nutrition needs on a vegetarian diet. Infants need to consume energy-dense food to meet their calorie needs. Good sources of nutrition and energy for infants (after 7 to 8 months of age) can include, tofu, well-cooked beans, tempeh, cheese, and egg yolks (egg white after 1 year of age). Despite the avoidance of iron-rich red meats, iron deficiency anemia is not common among vegetarians. Vitamin C intake is high in a vegetarian diet and vitamin C enhances iron absorption, which reduces the risk of iron deficiency anemia.

SUPPLEMENTS FOR VEGAN DIETS

For those individuals on a vegan diet, consider the following nutrient supplement guidelines: (ADA 6th edition).

Vitamin B_{12}

Vitamin B_{12} is found in animal-based foods (including dairy products and eggs) or fortified cereals and grains. Adults need 2.4 µg/day, and 2.6 µg during pregnancy and lactation (see Handout 3-5 for vitamin B_{12} needs by age.) A daily supplement of 5 µg B_{12} or a weekly supplement of 2,000 µg is recommended for those on a vegan diet (Messina 2003). The Institute of Medicine recommends that all individuals over age 50, regardless of diet, take a multivitamin containing B_{12} to optimize health (FAB, IOM, DRI 1998).

BOX 5-5 ■ *Names Used To Describe Vegetarian Diets*

Name	Foods included	Foods excluded
Lacto-ovovegetarian	Fruits, grains, legumes, nuts Seeds, vegetables, milk, Milk products, eggs	Meat, poultry, seafood
Lacto-vegetarian	Fruits, grains, legumes, nuts, seeds, vegetables, milk, milk Products	Meat, poultry, seafood, eggs
Ovo-vegetarian	Fruits, grains, legumes, nuts seeds, vegetables, eggs	Meat, poultry, seafood, milk and Milk products
Vegan	Fruits, grains, legumes, nuts, Seeds, vegetables	Meat, poultry, seafood eggs, milk products, Honey
Fruitarians	Raw fruits, nuts, seeds, and berries	All other foods

Vitamin D

Vitamin D is found in dairy products, fish, and fortified milk. Individuals need food sources or a supplement supplying 5 μg daily (10 μg for ages 50 to 70; 15 μg for those over age 70) or mid morning to afternoon sunlight exposure on forearms and face. For light skinned people, 10 to 15 minutes of sunlight; for dark skinned people, 30 minutes or more sunlight exposure is recommended.

Omega-3 Fatty Acids

Omega-3 fatty acids are found in marine animals, seeds, nuts and some oils. Individuals will need to include 1 to 2 servings daily (pregnant and lactating women 2 servings) of foods rich in omega-3 fatty acids. A serving includes 1 teaspoon flaxseed oil, 3 tablespoons walnuts, 4 teaspoons canola or soybean oil, or 6 oz tofu.

RESOURCES

Vegetarian Resource Group
    www.vrg.org
North American Vegetarian Society
    www.navs-online.org

ROUTINE CHILDHOOD ILLNESS

Many routine childhood illnesses, including colic, colds, stomachache, headache, and sore throat, have no medical cures. Time and rest are the treatment of choice. Food offers a way for parents to provide comfort, symptom relief, and to participate in care. Refer parents to the patient education tools that follow, which address colic, constipation, diarrhea, and stomachache and use the infant and toddler feeding guide to promote a healthy diet to prevent illness as often as is possible.

RESOURCES

Academy of Family Physicians
    www.familydoctor.org (Family Health Information resource) or www.aafp.org
American Academy of Pediatrics
    www.aap.org

Eating Disorders

Most children need to eat less and exercise more. When a normal weight or underweight child becomes committed to weight loss and excessive exercise or develops unwarranted concerns about weight, parents and healthcare providers should take notice.

Five warning signs have been suggested as indicators of a childhood and early adolescent eating disorder (Woodside 1995). These include dieting with:

1. A decreasing weight goal
2. Increasing criticism of body
3. Increasing social isolation
4. Disruption of menses
5. Purging

Ideally, a multidisciplinary treatment team will be available to the family with a child suspected of an eating disorder; realistically, this may not be the case. A *Wall Street Journal* article (March 30, 2004 D1) "The Informed Patient: Amid Focus on Obesity and Diet, Anorexia, Bulimia Are on the Rise" by Laura Landro, reveals that only 500 inpatient beds in the country are devoted to the problem of eating disorders and the cost is very expensive. The National Eating Disorders Screening Program www.mentalhealthscreening.org has outreach programs across the country, including anonymous online screening programs that reached >14,000 individuals in 2003 identified as being "at risk." Such a program may be useful. A patient education Frequently Asked Questions About Eating Disorders can be found in Handout 5-22. This includes additional resources for parents and patients.

RESOURCES

National Association of Anorexia Nervosa and Associated Disorders
    847-831-3438
National Eating Disorders Organization
    www.kidsource.com/nedo
The National Women's Health Information Center
    www.4women.gov
Additional Resources for Family Health
American Academy of Pediatrics
    www.aap.org/
University of Washington (pediatric nutrition in the community)
    http://depts.washington.edu/nutrpeds
National Center for Education in Maternal and Child Health
Bright Futures: Nutrition in Practice
    www.brightfutures.org/nutrition/index.html
National Center for Health Statistics
Healthy People 2010: Objectives for Improving Health
    www.health.gov/healthypeople/

PATIENT EDUCATION HANDOUTS

Infant Feeding Guide: Tips to Keep First Meals Safe and Healthy

Introduce only one new food at a time; wait 1 week before adding another.

Remember, formula or breast milk will be your infant's most important source of nutrition. Do not worry about how much your little one "eats" at those first feedings.

Always use a spoon, do not mix and feed solids from a bottle.

Infant food does not need salt or sugar.

When serving juice, try it in a cup and not a bottle (this may help prevent cavities).

Do not serve from the jar; take what you need for one feeding and keep the rest refrigerated (this will prevent spoilage).

Be careful when cooking or reheating in the microwave. Check food temperature before serving it to your baby.

Smile when you feed your baby, let the baby know mealtime is a pleasurable experience right from the start.

Never leave your infant alone in a high chair and use the high chair's safety straps.

A SUGGESTED FEEDING SCHEDULE FOR INFANTS

Check with your own health care provider for guidance.

0–4 Months*

Breast milk or formula. No cow's milk.

4–6 Months

Breast milk or formula. Infant cereal can be introduced. Mix cereal with water, formula, or breast milk.

6-8 Months

Breast milk or formula

Strained or mashed foods:

All varieties of infant cereal can be offered (none with honey, nuts, or dried fruit), including an infant teething biscuit. Try serving infant juice with vitamin C in a cup. Offer a dark green or dark orange vegetable every other day. Offer fresh or cooked fruit (mash or puree; no skin, peels, or seeds).

---

*The American Academy of Pediatrics supports exclusive breastfeeding for the first 6 months, but does recognize that infants are often interested and developmentally ready to accept solid food at 4 to 6 months of age. When formula is introduced, iron-fortified formula is the type of formula recommended for most infants.

8–10 Months

Breast milk or formula (still no cow's milk)

Mashed or finely minced foods:

Offer 2 to 3 small servings of grain type food such as infant cereal, cream of wheat, toast, bagel, rice, or noodles. Offer 1 to 2 servings of fresh or cooked chopped fruit (try soft ripe bananas, peaches, or pears). Offer 4 oz of 100% fruit juice in a cup, not a bottle. Most cooked or mashed vegetables can be served, offer 1 to 2 tablespoons twice a day. Include lean protein foods: lean beef, chicken, egg yolk, plain yogurt, dried beans, peanut butter, and cottage cheese.

10–12 Months

Breast milk or formula (cow's milk can be offered after the first birthday).

Minced, chopped foods: All unsweetened cereal, rice, noodles, crackers, and spaghetti. Two servings daily of peeled, canned (no sugar-added), ripe, or cooked fruit and most vegetables. Offer protein foods, including lamb, beef, poultry, eggs, cheese, yogurt, beans, and tofu.

12–36 Months

Breast milk, cow's milk, or other calcium-rich foods such as yogurt.

Chopped table foods: Most cereal (low sugar), enriched pasta, rice, or bread. Offer at least one whole grain food every day. Limit juice to 4 oz per day; satisfy thirst with water. Offer at least two servings of fresh, canned (no sugar), or cooked fruit every day. Offer vegetables prepared to match chewing ability. Offer protein-rich foods, including meat, fish, poultry, eggs, nuts, peanut butter, beans, or tofu.

What not to feed an infant

- Honey and corn syrup
- Very salty and very sweet foods
- Hard, round foods that tend to cause choking (carrots, hot dogs, grapes, round candy, and lollipops)
- Cow's milk, especially low-fat or nonfat

BASIC BABY FOOD RECIPE

½ cup peeled, seeded, vegetable or fruit cut into ½ inch cubes

2–4 tablespoons unsweetened fruit juice, water, or formula

In a small saucepan, combine the fruit or vegetables with liquid, cover and cook until tender. Cool slightly; puree in a food mill, blender, or food processor; add additional liquid if needed. Strain for first time eaters.

Where Can I Get More Information?

American Academy of Pediatrics available at: www.aap.org.

WebMDHealth, which provides information on a wide range of health issues, is available at: www.webmd.com.

Food and Nutrition Information Center, a directory to credible, accurate resources about food and nutrition, is available at: www.nal.usda.gov/fnic.

To find a nutrition professional in your area, contact www.eatright.org and click Find a Nutrition Professional or call the American Dietetic Association at 1-800-366-1655.

RECOMMENDED READING

- *American Academy of Pediatrics Guide to Your Child's Nutrition* by William H. Dietz and Loraine Stern. American Academy of Pediatrics, 1999.
- *Child of Mine: Feeding with Love and Good Sense* by Ellyn Satter. Bull Publishing, 2000.
- *Feeding Your Child for Lifelong Health: Birth Through Age Six* by Susan Roberts. Bantam Publishers, 1999.
- *Fit Kids: Raising Physically and Emotionally Strong Kids with Real Food* by E. Behan. Pocket Books, 2002.

Toddler and Child Feeding Guide

Use this information as a guide to balance your child's diet. If you serve the recommended food groups in the suggested amounts on most days, your child will be eating a "balanced" diet. Most children will have room for more food, including dessert or snacks.

Encourage children to eat sitting down, so they can concentrate on chewing. An adult should always be supervising. Try to eliminate distractions, including loud music, toys, or games, at the table. Most children learn healthy eating habits and table manners if the TV is not on. Avoid eating in the car because it will be impossible to help a child who starts to choke. Eating at times not associated with meals can promote overeating. Do not use food as an activity to ease boredom; use toys, games, or music while driving and at home.

AGE 2 TO 3 YEARS

Milk and Dairy: ½ cup milk or yogurt 4 to 5 times a day for a total of 16 to 20 oz.

Meat, Fish, Poultry, or Equivalent: 1 to 2 oz, twice a day for a total of 2 to 4 oz.

Vegetable and Fruit: 4 to 5 servings per day. A serving is 2 to 3 tablespoons of cooked vegetables, or ½ or 1 small piece of fruit, 2 to 4 tablespoons canned fruit, or 3 to 4 oz juice.

Grain Products: 3 to 4 servings each day. A serving is ½ to1 slice bread or ¼ to ½ cup cooked cereal, rice, or noodles, or ½ to 1 cup dry cereal.

AGE 4 TO 6 YEARS

Milk and Dairy: ½ to ¾ cup 3 to 4 times per day for a total of 24 to 32 oz.

Meat, Fish, Poultry, or Equivalent: 1 to 2 oz, twice a day for a total of 2 to 4 oz.

Vegetable and Fruit: 4 to 5 servings per day. A serving is 3 to 4 tablespoons vegetables, ½ to 1 small piece of fruit, 4 to 6 tablespoons canned fruit, or 4 oz juice.

Grain Products: 3 to 4 servings every day. A serving equals 1 slice of bread, ½ cup cooked cereal, rice, or pasta, or 1 cup dry cereal.

AGE 7 TO 12 YEARS

Milk and Dairy: ½ to 1 cup 3 to 4 times a day for a total of 24 to 32 oz.

Meat, Fish, Poultry, or Equivalent: 2 oz 3 to 4 times per day for a total of 6 to 8 oz.

Vegetable and Fruit: 4 to 5 servings per day. A serving is ¼ to ½ cup vegetables, 1 medium piece of fruit, ¼ to ½ cup canned fruit, or 4 oz juice.

Grain Products: 4 to 5 servings per day. A serving is 1 slice of bread, ½ to 1 cup cooked rice, cereal, or noodles or 1 cup dry cereal.

COMMENTS

Milk substitutions: ½ cup milk can be replaced with ½ to ¾ oz cheese, ½ cup yogurt, or 2½ tablespoons nonfat dry milk.

Protein substitutions: 1 egg, 2 tablespoons peanut butter, 2 to 4 oz tofu, or 4 to 5 tablespoons cooked beans can be substituted for 1 oz meat, fish, or chicken.

Fruit and vegetable choices: Include one green leafy vegetable or yellow vegetable every day for vitamin A. Good choices include carrots, spinach, broccoli, winter squash, or greens. Include one serving most day of a vitamin C-rich food (orange, grapefruit, strawberries, melon, tomato, or broccoli).

Grain substitutions: For 1 slice of bread, substitute ⅓ cup spaghetti, macaroni, noodles, or rice; 5 saltines, ½ English muffin, ¼ bagel, or 1 tortilla. Offer your child at least one serving of whole grain bread, pasta, cereal, or brown rice each day.

Fats and oils: Include some fat in your child's diet everyday (e.g., soft margarine, cooking oil, such as canola or olive oil, nuts, or salad dressing). Fat is needed for vitamins, calories, and proper growth.

This feeding guide is adapted from the American Academy of Pediatrics. (2004). *Pediatric Nutrition Handbook* (5th ed., p. 129).

Where Can I Get More Information?

American Academy of Pediatrics available at: www.aap.org.

WebMDHealth, provides information on a wide range of health issues, is available at: www.webmd.com.

Food and Nutrition Information Center, a directory to credible, accurate resources about food and nutrition, is available at: www.nal.usda.gov/fnic.

To find a nutrition professional in your area, contact www.eatright.org and click Find a Nutrition Professional or call the American Dietetic Association at 1-800-366-1655.

RECOMMENDED READING

- *American Academy of Pediatrics Guide to Your Child's Nutrition* by William H. Dietz and Loraine Stern
- *Child of Mine: Feeding with Love and Good Sense* by Ellyn Satter
- *Feeding Your Child for Lifelong Health: Birth Through Age Six* by Susan Roberts
- *Fit Kids: Raising Physically and Emotionally Strong Kids with Real Food* by Eileen Behan

HEALTHY EATING TIPS FOR PREGNANCY

- Talk to your healthcare provider about how much weight you should gain
- Eat food rich in folic acid, iron, calcium, and protein, or take a supplement with these nutrients.
- Talk to your healthcare provider before taking any supplements.
- Eat breakfast everyday.
- Eat high-fiber foods (fruits, vegetable, whole wheat bread, and high-fiber cereal) to prevent constipation.
- Avoid alcohol, raw fish, fish high in mercury, soft cheeses, and anything that is not food.
- Aim to exercise at least 30 minutes most days of the week. Talk to your healthcare provider before you begin.
- After you deliver, continue to eat well to return to a healthy weight.
- Slowly get back to your regular, moderate physical activity.
- Take pleasure in the miracles of pregnancy and birth.

What Is a Healthy Eating Plan?

- Vegetables: 3 to 5 servings (½ to 1 cup)
- Fruit: 2 to 4 servings (1 piece or ½ cup)
- Dairy: 2 to 3 servings (1 cup) of milk, yogurt, or cheese (2 oz)
- Protein or Equivalent: 2 to 3 servings of meat, poultry, fish, dry beans, eggs, or nuts. A serving is usually equal to 2 to 3 oz cooked meat, poultry, or fish; 2 eggs, 1 cup cooked beans, or 4 tablespoons or ⅔ cup nuts
- Bread, Cereal, Rice, or Pasta: A serving is usually 1 slice of bread or ½ cup rice or pasta.
- Drink plenty of fluids, drink when thirsty
- Folic Acid: Folic acid from a vitamin pill, fortified cereal, fortified bread, orange juice and strawberries is extremely important before, during and after pregnancy. Folic acid prevents birth defects.

How Many Calories Do I Need?

You do not need to increase your calorie intake until your third month of pregnancy. Women of normal weight should add 300 calories extra starting in the second trimester. Total calorie intake should be about 1,900 to 2,500 calories per day, depending on height and activity. Women who are very young or underweight need to eat at the higher calorie level.

To add 300 calories, include one of the following:

- 1 cup of yogurt and a piece of fruit
- 1 slice of whole wheat toast with 2 tablespoons peanut butter
- 1 cup of beef and bean chili with ½ oz cheese
- 1 cup raisin bran cereal with ½ cup milk and sliced banana
- 1 flour tortilla (7-inch), ½ cup refried beans, ½ cup cooked vegetables

How Much Weight Should I Gain?

Gaining the right amount of weight (not too much and not too little) can help you have a safe and healthy pregnancy.

- If you are underweight, you should gain about 27 to 40 pounds.
- If you are normal weight, you should gain about 25 to 35 pounds.
- If you are overweight, you should gain about 15 to 25 pounds.
- If you are obese, you should gain about 15 pounds or less.

Can I Continue a Vegetarian Diet During Pregnancy?

Yes, you can continue a vegetarian diet. If you do not eat animal foods, you need to make sure you are getting enough protein, iron, vitamin B_{12}, and vitamin D. You may want to ask to speak to a registered dietitian to learn how to obtain these nutrients in your diet.

What Food Should I Avoid While Pregnant?

- Alcohol
- Fish that may have a high level of methylmercury
- Soft cheeses (e.g., feta, Brie, and goat cheese), ready-to eat luncheon meats, hot dogs, and deli meats. These may contain listeria, which can be harmful to unborn babies.
- Raw fish
- Large amounts of caffeine
- Anything that is not food. Some women crave nonfood items, such as ice and laundry starch. This can be a sign of a nutrient deficiency and must be discussed with your healthcare provider.

Reprinted from Fit for Two: Tips for Pregnancy. NIDDK Weight-control Information Network available at: www.niddk.nih.gov/health/nutrit/pubs/fit4two/fitfortwo.htm

Where Can I Get More Information?

American College of Obstetrics and Gynecologists (ACOG) available at: www.acog.org or 1-800-762-2264.

March of Dimes available at: www.modimes.org or 1-888-663-4637.

U.S. Government's Food Safety Web Site available at: www.foodsafety.gov.

To find a nutrition professional in your area, contact www.eatright.org and click Find a Nutrition Professional or call the American Dietetic Association at 1-800-366-1655.

RECOMMENDED READING

- *Eating Expectantly* by Bridget Swinney
- *No More Morning Sickness* by Miriam Erick
- *The Pregnancy Diet* by Eileen Behan
- *When You're Expecting Twins, Triplets or Quads: A Complete Resource* by Barbara Luke & Tamara Eberlein

What You Need To Know About Mercury in Fish and Shellfish

Fish and shellfish are an important part of a healthy diet. Fish and shellfish contain high-quality protein and other essential nutrients; they are low in saturated fats and contain omega-3 fatty acids. A well-balanced diet that includes a variety of fish and shellfish can contribute to heart health and a child's proper growth and development. Women and young children, in particular, should include fish or shellfish in their diets because of their many nutritional benefits.

Nearly all fish and shellfish, however, contain traces of mercury. For most people, the risk from mercury by eating fish and shellfish is not a health concern. Yet, some fish and shellfish contain higher levels of mercury that may harm an unborn baby or young child's developing nervous system. The risks from mercury in fish and shellfish depend on the amount of fish and shellfish eaten and the levels of mercury in the fish and shellfish.

Women who may become pregnant, pregnant women, nursing mothers, and young children should avoid certain fish and shellfish and follow these recommendations:

1. Do not eat shark, swordfish, king mackerel, or tilefish because they contain high levels of mercury.

2. Eat up to 12 oz (2 average meals) a week of a variety of fish and shellfish that are lower in mercury. Five of the most commonly eaten fish that are low in mercury are shrimp, canned light tuna, salmon, pollock, and catfish. Another commonly eaten fish, albacore (white) tuna, has more mercury than canned light tuna. When choosing your two meals of fish and shellfish, you may eat up to 6 oz (one average meal) of albacore tuna per week.

Follow these same recommendations when feeding your young child, but serve smaller portions.

The full report is available at: www.cfsan.fda.gov/~dms/admehg3.html.

MERCURY LEVELS IN COMMERCIAL FISH AND SHELLFISH (U.S. DEPARTMENT OF HEALTH AND HUMAN SERVICES AND U.S. ENVIRONMENTAL PROTECTION AGENCY)

Fish and Shellfish with Highest Levels of Mercury

King mackerel

Shark

Swordfish

Tilefish (Gulf of Mexico)

Fish and Shellfish with Lower Levels of Mercury

Anchovies	Mullet
Butterfish	Oysters
Catfish	Perch (ocean)
Clams	Pickeral
Cod	Pollock
Crab (includes blue king and snow)	Salmon (canned, fresh, or frozen)
Crawfish	Sardine
Croaker (Atlantic)	Scallops
Flatfish (flounder, plaice, sole)	Shad (American)
Haddock	Shrimp
Hake	Squid
Herring	Tilapia
Jacksmelt	Trout (freshwater)
Lobster (spiny)	Tuna (canned, light)
Mackerel (North Atlantic)	Whitefish
Mackerel chub (Pacific)	Whiting

Where Can I Get More Information?

This list and the mercury level of specific fish species are available at: www.cfsan.fda.gov/~frf/sea-mehg.html.

What to Eat While Breastfeeding

Breastfeeding is the ideal way for women to feed their baby. Breastfeeding mothers do require more calories while nursing, but those extra calories should come from nutrient-rich food.

WHAT TO EAT

- Women should consume 3 or more calcium-rich foods (e.g., milk or yogurt) daily. If you do not eat dairy products, ask your healthcare provider for a list of nondairy foods rich in calcium.

- Drink plenty of fluids when thirsty.

- Eat a wide variety of colorful vegetables and fruit.

- Include in your diet some canola oil, flaxseed, walnuts, or fish (shrimp, canned light tuna, salmon, pollock, and catfish), which are sources of healthy omega-3 fatty acids.

- Include a variety of breads and cereal. Try to eat some whole grain foods daily.

- Eat meat or another protein rich food every day.

- Although breastfeeding women are advised to avoid diets that promote rapid weight loss, in general, weight loss of 4.5 pounds per month after the first month postpartum is a suggested weight loss guide.

WHAT NOT TO EAT

- Avoid drinking alcohol because it can pass through milk to the baby. If you do drink alcohol, drink just after you nurse.

- Limit caffeine from coffee and cola drinks; it can accumulate in the mothers body, potentially causing sleep disturbances, irritability, and poor feeding for mom and baby.

- Avoid "gassy" foods only if you notice they affect the baby or if the baby has symptoms every time you eat a certain food.

- If you are worried about food allergies because you have a family history of such, discuss the benefits of limiting common allergenic foods in your diet with your healthcare provider

- Discuss the use of medications with your healthcare provider before taking them. If you do take medications, take them after you nurse.

SUGGESTED MENU WHILE BREASTFEEDING

Breakfast
100% fruit juice, 6 oz
Whole grain cereal (Total, Cheerios, oatmeal) with milk and fruit, ½ to 1 cup
Whole grain toast with margarine or jam, 1 to 2 slices
Decaffeinated tea

Lunch
  Vegetable soup, 1 cup
  Sandwich: 2 slices bread, roll, or soft tortilla
                      2 to 3 oz lean meat, poultry, or peanut butter
                      Lettuce, tomato, mustard, ketchup
  Fruit or fruit salad
  Yogurt or milk
Dinner
  Lean meat, poultry, fish, or meat substitute, 3 oz
  Rice, potato, or pasta, ½ to 1 cup
  Salad, 1 cup
  Cooked vegetable, ½ cup or more
  Milk, 1 cup
  Fruit, fruit salad, or fruit with yogurt
Snacks
Fruit, fruit salad, canned fruit in water, or fruit juice
Whole grain crackers, 1 slice toast, whole grain cereal
Milk, yogurt, low-fat cheese with calcium

Where Can I Get More Information?

American Academy of Pediatrics available at: www.aap.org.

WebMDHealth, which provides information on a wide range of health issues, is available at: www.webmd.com.

Food and Nutrition Information Center, a directory to credible, accurate resources about food and nutrition, is available at: www.nal.usda.gov/fnic.

American Foundation for Maternal and Child Health 212-759-5510

La Leche League International is available at: www.lalecheleague.org.

Maternal and Child Health Information Resource Center is available at: www.mchirc.net.

To find a nutrition professional in your area, contact www.eatright.org and click Find a Nutrition Professional or call the American Dietetic Association at 1-800-366-1655.

RECOMMENDED READING
- *American Academy of Pediatrics Guide to Your Child's Nutrition* by William H. Dietz and Loraine Stern
- *Child of Mine: Feeding with Love and Good Sense* by Ellyn Satter
- *Feeding Your Child for Lifelong Health: Birth Through Age Six* by Susan Roberts
- *Fit Kids: Raising Physically and Emotionally Strong Kids with Real Food* by Eileen Behan
- *The Nursing Mother's Companion* by Kathleen Huggins
- *Eat Well lose Weight While Breastfeeding* by Eileen Behan

What I Need To Know About Gestational Diabetes

WHAT IS GESTATIONAL DIABETES?

Gestational diabetes is diabetes that is found for the first time when a woman is pregnant. Of every 100 pregnant women in the United States, 3 to 8 get gestational diabetes. Diabetes means that your blood glucose (also called blood sugar) is too high. When pregnant, too much glucose is not good for the baby.

HOW WILL GESTATIONAL DIABETES AFFECT MY BABY?

Untreated or uncontrolled gestational diabetes can mean problems for your baby, such as:

Being born very large and with extra fat; this can make delivery difficult and more dangerous for your baby

Low blood glucose right after birth

Breathing problems

Untreated or uncontrolled gestational diabetes can mean problems for the mother, such as

- Increases the risk of high blood pressure during pregnancy
- Increases the risk of a large baby and the need for cesarean section at delivery

The good news is your gestational diabetes will probably go away after your baby is born. However, you are more likely to get type 2 diabetes later in life. You may also get gestational diabetes again if you get pregnant again.

HOW IS GESTATIONAL DIABETES TREATED?

Treating gestational diabetes means taking steps to keep your blood glucose levels in a target range. You will learn how to correct your blood glucose using

- A meal plan
- Physical activity
- Insulin (if needed)

MEAL PLAN

Talk with a dietitian or a diabetes educator who will design a meal plan to help you choose foods that are healthy for you and your baby. Using a meal plan will help keep your blood glucose in your target range. The plan will provide guidelines on which foods to eat, how much to eat, and when to eat. Choices, amounts, and timing are all important in keeping your blood glucose levels in your target range.

You may be advised to

- Eat 3 small meals and 1 to 3 snacks every day
- Limit sweets
- Be careful about when and how much carbohydrate-rich food you eat; your meal plan will tell you when to eat carbohydrates and how much to eat at each meal and snack.
- Include fiber in the form of fruits, vegetables, and whole-grain crackers, cereals, and bread in your meals.

PHYSICAL ACTIVITY

Physical activity, such as walking and swimming, can help you reach your blood glucose targets. Talk with your healthcare team about the type of activity that is best for you. If you are already active, tell your healthcare team what you do.

INSULIN

Some women with gestational diabetes need insulin, in addition to a meal plan and physical activity, to reach their blood glucose targets. If necessary, your healthcare team will show you how to give yourself insulin shots. Insulin is not harmful for your baby. It cannot move from your blood stream to the baby's.

Reprinted from What I Need To Know About Diabetes. National Diabetes Information Clearinghouse (NDIC). The full report can be accessed at: http://diabetes.niddk.nih.gov/dm/pubs/gestational/.

Where Can I Get More Information?

Diabetes teachers (nurses, dietitians, and other health professionals). To find a diabetes teacher near you call the American Association of Diabetes Educators at 1-800-832-6374 or go to www.diabeteseducator.org and click on Find a Diabetes Educator or to find a dietitian near you, click Find a Nutrition Professional.

For more information about diabetes, Contact the National Institute of Diabetes and Digestive and Kidney Disorders (NIDDK) available at: www.niddk.nih.gov.

Colic is an extreme of normal crying, often occurring in late evening. A child can be healthy and happy one minute, then draw up the legs, clench the fists, and repeatedly cry for what can be hours. Infantile colic develops in about one third of infants between age 3 weeks and 3 months. In many cases, the crying can last for 3 hours and no matter what a parent does, the child is generally not comforted. Although the crying does no harm to the baby, it is extremely upsetting to the parents or caregivers.

HOW DO YOU RECOGNIZE COLIC?

A physician will call your child's crying colic if it occurs frequently (usually three times per week) when your child cannot be comforted with diaper change, feeding, or other measures and your child is otherwise healthy and well fed. Most pediatricians believe colic has to do with an immature digestive tract that creates abdominal gas or it might result from an immature nervous system that cannot regulate the crying once it starts. With time, infants outgrow the condition.

Some parents wonder if the condition is caused by a food allergy. The association between colic and food allergy is not clear. Do not switch formulas without talking to your pediatrician. Breastfeeding mothers can temporarily reduce dairy products or eliminate caffeine, chocolate, or gassy food if they think it has an impact on the baby, but breastfeeding should not be stopped. Keep in mind that both breast-fed and bottle fed babies get colic.

Fever, vomiting, or blood in the stools is not symptomatic of colic. Persistent crying accompanied by any of these symptoms requires medical attention.

WHAT CAN YOU DO?

Because colic is not a disease and infants outgrow it, the best treatment is to offer comfort.

Keep a diary. A diary can help track your child's crying so you can be prepared for it and perhaps reduce activities or limit stimulation in anticipation of colic. A diary can also be reassuring when a pattern can be identified and the concern of a medical reason is alleviated.

Hold your baby or use a backpack or infant carrier to keep the baby close while you carry out household chores. Some parents try the football hold: support the baby in your forearm, stomach side down, head in your hand, and legs dangling. Some children who are carried will have fewer crying bouts.

Rock your child in a rocker; wear headphones if it helps you stay relaxed.

Take a car ride with the baby in the infant seat.

Try white noise or gentle music, but do not over stimulate with sound, toys, light, or color.

Avoid smoking or individuals who smoke.

Watch your diet. Some breastfeeding women find limiting garlic, onion, broccoli, and cabbage can be useful. Do not stop breastfeeding just because your child is colicky.

Try to keep your infant on a flexible but established feeding schedule.

Ask your pediatrician about the size of the hole on the bottle's nipple. A large hole can promote air swallowing, making colic worse.

Burp your baby after every feeding and when the baby starts to cry. Many infants with colic pass gas and appear to feel better and cry less after.

Try to stay relaxed and do not underestimate how stressful the crying can be. Ask for help when you need it. Just talking to other parents or your healthcare provider can help relieve your stress and might benefit the baby too.

Read about colic in parenting books or online resources suggested below.

Where Can I Get More Information?

The American Academy of Pediatrics is available at: www.aap.org.

National Digestive Diseases Clearinghouse available at: http://www.niddk.nih.gov.

WebMDHealth, which provides information on a wide range of health issues, is available at: www.webmd.com

Food and Nutrition Information Center, a directory to credible, accurate resources about food and nutrition is available at: www.nal.usda.gov/fnic.

To find a nutrition professional in your area, contact www.eatright.org and click Find a Nutrition Professional or call the American Dietetic Association at 1-800-366-1655.

RECOMMENDED READING

- *American Academy of Pediatrics Guide to Your Child's Nutrition* by William H. Dietz and Loraine Stern.
- *Child of Mine: Feeding with Love and Good Sense* by Ellyn Satter.
- *Feeding Your Child for Lifelong Health: Birth Through Age Six* by Susan Roberts.
- *Fit Kids: Raising Physically and Emotionally Strong Kids with Real Food* by Eileen Behan.

Constipation in Children

WHAT IS CONSTIPATION?

Constipation means that bowel movements are hard and dry, difficult or painful to pass, and less frequent than usual. It is a common problem for children, but it is usually temporary and no cause for parents to be concerned.

When a child does not get enough fiber, liquids, or exercise, constipation is more likely to occur. It also happens when children ignore the urge to have a bowel movement, which they often do out of either embarrassment to use a public bathroom, fear, or lack of confidence in the absence of a parent, or unwillingness to take a break from play. Sometimes, medicines or a disease can cause constipation.

SYMPTOMS OF CONSTIPATION

- No bowel movement for several days or daily bowel movements that are hard and dry
- Cramping abdominal pain
- Nausea
- Vomiting
- Weight loss
- Liquid or solid, clay-like stool in the child's underwear—a sign that stool is backed up in the rectum
- Constipation can make a bowel movement painful, so the child may try to prevent having one. Clenching buttocks, rocking up and down on toes, and turning red in the face are signs of trying to hold a bowel movement.

Treatment depends on the child's age and the severity of the problem. Often, eating more fiber (fruits, vegetables, whole grain cereal), drinking more liquids, and getting more exercise will solve the problem. Sometimes, a child may need an enema to remove the stool or a laxative to soften it or prevent a future episode. Laxatives can be dangerous to children and should be given only with a doctor's approval.

When Should You Call the Doctor?

Although constipation is usually harmless, it can be a sign or a cause of a more serious problem. A child should see a doctor if

- Episodes of constipation last longer than 3 weeks
- The child is unable to participate in normal activities
- Small, painful tears appear around the anus
- A small amount of the intestinal lining is pushed out of the anus (hemorrhoids)

- Normal pushing is not enough to expel stool
- Liquid or soft stool leaks out of the anus

To help your child

- Have your child sit on the toilet the same time each day
- Do not force toilet training; some children do not master this task until 4 years of age
- Ask your child if any issue is preventing the child from using the toilet; fear, filth, and lack of privacy can all be deterrents.
- Improve your child's diet: Have the child eat at least 2 servings of fruit each day (a serving equals 1 to 3 tablespoons for each year of life), at least 3 servings of vegetables (a serving is 1 to 3 tablespoons for each year of age). Include whole wheat bread (instead of white) or a high-fiber whole grain cereal (instead of a low-fiber cereal). Make sure your child drinks plenty of fluids such as water or water flavored with juice.

This information was reprinted from Constipation in Children from the National Digestive Disease Information Clearinghouse. The full report can be accessed at: http://digestive.niddk.nih.gov/ddiseases/pubs/constipationchild/index.htm.

Where Can I Get More Information?

American Academy of Pediatrics available at: www.aap.org.

International Foundation for Functional Gastrointestinal Disorders (IFFGD) available at: www.iffgd.org.

WebMDHealth, which provides information on a wide range of health issues, is available at: www.webmd.com.

Food and Nutrition Information Center, a directory to credible, accurate resources about food and nutrition, available at: www.nal.usda.gov/fnic.

To find a nutrition professional in your area, contact www.eatright.org and click Find a Nutrition Professional or call the American Dietetic Association at 1-800-366-1655.

RECOMMENDED READING

- *American Academy of Pediatrics Guide to Your Child's Nutrition* by William H. Dietz and Loraine Stern
- *Child of Mine: Feeding with Love and Good Sense* by Ellyn Satter
- *Feeding Your Child for Lifelong Health: Birth Through Age Six* by Susan Roberts
- *Fit Kids: Raising Physically and Emotionally Strong Kids with Real Food* by Eileen Behan
- *Healthy Foods, Healthy Kids* by Elizabeth Ward

5-9 Diarrhea in Children

Routine ailments, including teething, and ear and urinary tract infections, can cause diarrhea as can excessive fruit juice consumption. Some cases of diarrhea can be caused by viruses or bacteria. Diarrhea can last between 3 and 7 days and becomes a concern because it increases the risk for dehydration.

Signs of dehydration include

- Poor appetite
- Weight loss
- Irritability
- No wet diapers or no urinating
- Dry mouth
- Dark urine
- Sunken eyes
- No tears when crying
- Infants under 18 months may have a sunken soft spot
- Skin loses its usual springiness

To prevent dehydration, infants should stay on formula or breast milk. Offer weaned children water or other clear liquids, such as chicken broth, ginger-ale, white grape juice, sports drinks, herbal tea, Jell-O, water ice, or popsicles. Hold off on apple juice and pear juice; they contain a natural chemical called sorbitol, which when consumed in excess, causes diarrhea in some children. Avoid caffeine-containing drinks such as colas and black tea, because the caffeine could act like a diuretic.

WHAT ABOUT FOOD OR FORMULA?

According to the American Academy of Pediatrics (AAP), most diarrhea cases do not lead to dehydration; continuing age-appropriate feeding is the best and most effective therapy. Breast-fed and formula-fed babies should continue on their regular feedings. In mild cases of diarrhea, formula does not need to be diluted. If the doctor does advise diluted formula, do so for as short a period as possible to prevent a low calorie intake. Switch to lactose-free formula or milk only if diarrhea becomes worse after consuming milk-based food, milk, or formula. Older infants and children should eat their regular diet. Even during acute cases of diarrhea, a child will absorb at least 60% of the food eaten. Good foods to encourage include

- Complex carbohydrates (e.g., rice, wheat, and potatoes)
- Chicken and eggs are a good protein source

- Continue on usual infant feedings (breast milk, formula or cow's milk, if older) unless advised to do otherwise
- Avoid foods with a high sugar or high fat content

The BRATT diet (bananas, rice, applesauce, tea, and toast) is no longer recommended by the AAP as a treatment of diarrhea because it is low in calories and not well balanced.

Ask your doctor about giving your child oral rehydration solution (ORS). ORS solutions contain the right mix of salt, sugar, potassium, and other elements to replace lost fluids.

WASH YOUR HANDS

Some cases of diarrhea are caused by a virus found in feces. To reduce this risk, dispose of diapers properly and wash hands after changing diapers. Wash hands every time you handle raw meat, poultry, or shellfish and after you clean up after pets.

CHRONIC NONSPECIFIC DIARRHEA

Chronic nonspecific diarrhea is the most frequent form of persistent diarrhea. The typical patient is 1 to 3 years of age, and has two to five loose, mucous-like stools most days of the week. Despite the frequent bowel movements, children are usually healthy and well nourished. Spontaneously, usually after the third birthday, the condition resolves itself. It is not uncommon to find the condition among siblings.

If chronic nonspecific diarrhea affects your child, try the following:

- Avoid prune, pear, cherry, or apple juice because of their higher sorbitol content
- Limit total juice to 4 to 8 oz per day
- Offer your child regular scheduled meals; try to stay flexible, but stabilize a three-meal and a two-to-three snack routine
- Avoid milk only if it makes diarrhea worse
- Include all the food groups suggested for age in Handout 5-2. Strive for the child to eat some of each food group, but do not allow the child to under- or overconsume any one food group. Limit juice to 8 oz or less per day.

Where Can I Get More Information?

American Academy of Pediatrics is available at: www.aap.org.

WebMDHealth, which provides information on a wide range of health subjects, is available at: www.webmd.com.

Food and Nutrition Information Center, a directory to credible, accurate resources about food and nutrition, is available at: www.nal.usda.gov/fnic.

To find a nutrition professional in your area, contact www.eatright.org and click Find a Nutrition Professional or call the American Dietetic Association at 1-800-366-1655.

RECOMMENDED READING

- *American Academy of Pediatrics Guide to Your Child's Nutrition* by William H. Dietz and Loraine Stern
- *Child of Mine: Feeding with Love and Good Sense* by Ellyn Satter
- *Feeding Your Child for Lifelong Health: Birth Through Age Six* by Susan Roberts
- *Fit Kids: Raising Physically and Emotionally Strong Kids with Real Food* by Eileen Behan

WHAT IS A FOOD ALLERGY?

Food allergy occurs when the body's own immune system perceives a protein as foreign and makes antibodies to fight it. Symptoms can be immediate, including hives or difficulty breathing (anaphylaxis), or it can be chronic with symptoms that include asthma, skin rash, diarrhea, or stomachaches.

WHAT CAUSES FOOD ALLERGY?

Virtually any food can cause a food allergy; however, only a small number account for 90% of all cases. The foods most likely to cause a food allergy in children include milk, egg, peanuts, soy, wheat, tree nuts, fish, and shellfish. In adults, the common food allergens can include peanuts, tree nuts, shellfish, and fish. To determine if an individual has a true food allergy requires careful searching for the cause of the symptoms, including specific allergy tests and, in some cases, food challenges. Treatment includes elimination of the food and education about the seriousness of the condition and its treatment, including the use of epinephrine in the event of a serious reaction.

FOOD ALLERGIES AND INFANTS

It is estimated that in the first 3 years of life, two to three infants out of one hundred will be found to be allergic to cow's milk, the most common food allergen in American babies. It is believed that some cases of constipation and gastroesophageal reflux disease (GERD) can be attributed to cow's milk allergy in infants. Breast milk is an infant's best source of nutrition and the best way to avoid food allergies, but it does not prevent food allergies in individuals genetically predisposed to food allergy. If breastfeeding is not possible, infant formulas developed for allergy-sensitive infants may be recommended by the baby's healthcare provider. Early feeding of food other than breast milk or infant formula is thought to increase the development of food allergies in susceptible children. Withholding highly allergenic foods (milk, eggs, peanuts, tree nuts, and fish) from children at high risk of food allergy may be advised for the first 2 to 3 years of life. Goat's milk is not a substitute for breast milk or hypoallergenic and it lacks essential nutrients.

Should I Change My Diet if I'm Breastfeeding?

The protein in some foods (e.g., cow's milk, eggs, and peanuts) can pass from the diet to breast milk and cause sensitization to these foods. Some infants may not experience a reaction until they start on solid foods that include the allergenic food. Infants who are suspected of being allergic to foods in the mother's diet may benefit by the mother trying a 2-week elimination diet free of milk, eggs, peanuts, and soy to see if symptoms in their child improve. If symptoms improve, the foods can be added back one at a time while observing for symptoms. Women who eliminate cow's milk from their diet need to obtain calcium with vitamin D from a supplemental source. The protein in egg, peanuts, or soy foods can be provided in other nonallergenic protein foods. To prevent poor nutrition, consult a registered dietitian when entire food groups must be restricted.

DIAGNOSIS OF FOOD ALLERGY

The initial evaluation of a food allergy begins with a physical examination and history to rule out metabolic disorders and other causes. Allergic reactions to animal dander, mold, and dust must be considered too. Once a food allergy is indicated, confirmation can proceed but definitive diagnosis is not simple. Tests can include Skin testing immunoassay capture test (CAP-RAST). Radioallergosorbent test (RAST), enzyme-linked immunosorbent assay (ELISA), and (CAP-RAST). These tests are used by allergists to confirm or rule out food allergies. Cytotoxic, sublingual (extracts placed under the tongue), and kinesiology (subject's arm is extended holding the food to be tested) testing are not considered reliable.

TREATMENT

Treatment for a food allergy is elimination of the identified food; this is not easy and in fact can be quite tricky. Once a food allergy is diagnosed, treatment must be initiated. Individuals needing to eliminate multiple foods need to speak with a dietitian to find alternative foods. Read all labels, including medicine and topical lotions.

ANAPHYLAXIS

In addition to treatment, an emergency treatment plan must be in place and injectable epinephrine and oral histamine always available. Anaphylaxis refers to a potentially life-threatening reaction. If food-related, anaphylaxis appears to be more common in people with underlying asthma. The most common foods for food-induced anaphylaxis are peanuts, tree nuts (walnuts, almond, pecan, cashew, hazel nut, brazil nut), and shellfish, but any food can be a potential allergen. Anaphylaxis often occurs when individuals are unaware they are ingesting the incriminating food. Allergy experts advise all patients with food allergy to be prepared to treat an anaphylaxis attack. (See the patient education Handout 5–11.)

Where Can I Get More Information?

The Food Allergy Network is a lay organization with an expert medical advisory board. It is recognized as a superb resource to families and healthcare providers. It can be reached at 1-800-929-4040 or at: www.foodallergy.org.

American Academy of Allergy, Asthma, and Immunology is available at: www.aaaai.org.

American Academy of Pediatrics is available at: www.aap.org.

WebMDHealth, which provides health information, is available at: www.webmd.com.

Food and Nutrition Information Center, a directory to credible, accurate resources about food and nutrition, is available at: www.nal.usda.gov/fnic.

To find a nutrition professional in your area, contact www.eatright.org and click Find a Nutrition Professional or call the American Dietetic Association at 1-800-366-1655.

RECOMMENDED READING

- *Food Allergies* by the American Dietetic Association
- *The Food Allergy News Cookbook: A Collection of Recipes from Food Allergy News and Members of the Food Allergy Network* by Anne Munoz-Furlong
- *American Academy of Pediatrics Guide to Your Child's Nutrition* by William H. Dietz and Loraine Stern
- *Child of Mine: Feeding with Love and Good Sense* by Ellyn Satter
- *Feeding Your Child for Lifelong Health: Birth Through Age Six* by Susan Roberts

5-11 Emergency Health Care Plan for Food Allergies

For children with multiple food allergies, use one form for each food.

Allergy to: _____

_____ _____ _____

Student's name   date of birth   teacher

Asthmatic?   Yes*   No

Signs and symptoms of an allergic reaction†:

Mouth	Itching and swelling of the lips, tongue or inside of mouth
Throat‡	Itching and/or a sense of tightness in the throat, hoarseness and a hacking cough
Skin	Hives, itchy rash or swelling of the face or extremities
GI system	Nausea, abdominal cramps, vomiting or diarrhea
Lungs‡	Shortness of breath, repeated coughing or wheezing
Heart‡	Thready pulse, "passing out"

Action

1. If ingestion of a food allergen is suspected, give _____
   (Specify medication/dose/route)

   and_____immediately!
   (Specify medication/dose/route)

2. Call rescue squad _____
   (phone number)

3. Call mother_____ father_____ or emergency contacts below
   (Phone number)   (Phone number)

4. Call doctor _____ at _____
   (Name)   (Phone number)

_____

*High risk for severe reaction.
†The severity of symptoms can quickly change.
‡All of these symptoms can progress to a life-threatening situation!

253

Do not hesitate to administer medication or to call rescue squad even if parents or doctor cannot be reached!

_____   _____ _____ _____
       Parent's signature   Date   Physician's signature   Date

Emergency contacts

1. Name _____

    _____ _____
        (Relation)   (Phone number)

2. Name_____

    _____ _____
        (Relation)   (Phone number)

3. Name _____

    _____ _____
        (Relation)   (Phone number)

Trained staff members

1. Name _____ Room ____

2. Name _____ Room ____

3. Name _____ Room ____

5-12 Wheat Allergy Diet

The Wheat Allergy Diet is a modification of a normal diet with the elimination of wheat-containing foods and any foods containing any wheat ingredients. Wheat is found in almost all baked foods and may be used as an additive to thicken foods. The following allergy-specific list can help identify foods containing wheat. Offending ingredients can be hidden in unfamiliar forms—read labels carefully. This is not a complete list; read labels every time you shop. Total avoidance of a food allergen is the only treatment proved effective for a food allergy.

FOODS TO AVOID

Bulgur

Couscous

Farina

Flour: bread, cake, durham, enriched, gluten, graham, kamut, multigrain, soft wheat, white, whole wheat, winter

Gluten

Graham flour

High gluten flour

High-protein flour

Malted cereals

Puffed wheat

Red wheat flakes

Rolled wheat

Seitan

Semolina

Shredded wheat

Spelt

Triticale

Vital gluten

Wheat bran

Wheat bread

Wheat breadcrumbs

Wheat cereals

Wheat flakes

Wheat germ

Wheat gluten

Wheat meal

Wheat pasta

Wheat protein beverage

Wheat protein powder

Wheat starch

Wheat tempeh

Whole wheat berries

Ingredients that may contain wheat or how wheat may appear on a food label

- Cereal extract
- Gluten
- Gelatinized starch
- Hydrolyzed vegetable protein
- Modified food starch
- Starch
- Vegetable gum

- Vegetable starch
- Natural flavoring

Where Can I Get More Information?

For additional information about food allergy, including cookbooks, contact

Food Allergy and Anaphylaxis Network available at: www.foodallergy.org or 703-691-3179.

American Academy of Allergy, Asthma, and Immunology available at: http://www.aaaai.org.

American Academy of Pediatrics available at: www.aap.org.

WebMDHealth, which provides information on many health issues, including food allergy, available at: www.webmd.com.

Food and Nutrition Information Center, a directory to credible, accurate resources about food and nutrition, available at: www.nal.usda.gov/fnic.

To find a nutrition professional in your area, contact www.eatright.org and click Find a Nutrition Professional or call the American Dietetic Association at 1-800-366-1655.

RECOMMENDED READING

- *American Academy of Pediatrics Guide to Your Child's Nutrition* by William H. Dietz and Loraine Stern
- *Food Allergies* by the American Dietetic Association
- *The Food Allergy News Cookbook: A Collection of Recipes from Food Allergy News and Members of the Food Allergy Network* by Anne Munoz-Furlong

---

The Wheat Allergy Diet has been adapted from the following sources: Kendall, P. A. (1994). Managing food allergies and sensitivities. *Topics in Clinical Nutrition, 9*, 1–10.
Mahan, L. K., & Escott-Stump, S. (2004). *Krause's Food, Nutrition and Diet Therapy* (p. 785b). New York: Elsevier.

5-13 Peanut Allergy Diet

Total avoidance of a food allergen is the only proved treatment for a food allergy. The following allergy-specific list can help identify offending foods, but it is essential food labels be read carefully. Offending foods can be hidden in unfamiliar forms. This is not a complete list; read labels every time you shop.

FOODS TO AVOID

Beer nuts

Chopped nuts

Cold-pressed peanut oil

Defatted peanuts

Egg rolls

Fresh peanuts

Granulated peanuts

Groundnuts

Marzipan

Mixed nuts

Nougat

Peanut butter

Peanut flakes

Peanut flour

Peanut oil

Peanut soup

Peanuts, roasted

Peanuts, shelled

Peanuts, whole

How peanuts may appear on a label

- Expelled or expressed peanut oil
- High-protein foods
- Hydrolyzed plant protein
- Hydrolyzed vegetable protein
- Peanut flakes
- Peanut flour
- African, Chinese, and Thai dishes often include peanuts in traditional recipes

Additional products that may contain peanuts (contact manufacturers for ingredient information).

- Baked goods
- Candy
- Cheesecake crusts
- Chili
- Chocolate candy
- Hamster food

- Ice cream
- Livestock feed and pet food
- Piecrust
- Prepared sauces

Where Can I Get More Information?

For additional information about food allergy, including cookbooks, contact

Food Allergy and Anaphylaxis Network available at: www.foodallergy.org or 703-691-3179.

American Academy of Allergy, Asthma, and Immunology available at: http://www.aaaai.org.

American Academy of Pediatrics available at: www.aap.org.

WebMDHealth, which provides information on many health issues, including food allergy, available at: www.webmd.com.

Food and Nutrition Information Center, a directory to credible, accurate resources about food and nutrition, available at: www.nal.usda.gov/fnic.

To find a nutrition professional in your area, contact www.eatright.org and click Find a Nutrition Professional or call the American Dietetic Association at 1-800-366-1655.

RECOMMENDED READING

- *American Academy of Pediatrics Guide to Your Child's Nutrition* by William H. Dietz and Loraine Stern
- *Food Allergies* by the American Dietetic Association
- *The Food Allergy News Cookbook: A Collection of Recipes from Food Allergy News and Members of the Food Allergy Network* by Anne Munoz-Furlong

The Peanut Allergy Diet has been adapted from the following sources: Kendall, P. A. (1994). Managing food allergies and sensitivities. *Topics in Clinical Nutrition, 9*, 1–10.
Mahan, L. K., & Escott-Stump, S. (2004). *Krause's Food, Nutrition and Diet Therapy* (p. 783). New York: Elsevier.

5-14 Soy Allergy Diet

Total avoidance of a food allergen is the only proved treatment for a food allergy. The following allergy-specific list can help identify offending foods, but it is essential food labels be read carefully. This is not a complete list; offending foods can be hidden in unfamiliar forms.

FOODS TO AVOID

Fermented soybean paste

Fermented soybeans

Miso

Natto

Shoyu sauce

Soy flour

Soy grits

Soy protein shakes

Soy sauce

Soybean curd

Soybean milk

Soybean oil

Soybean sprouts

Tempeh

Textured soy protein

Textured vegetable protein (TVP)

Tofu

Whey-soy drink

How soy may appear on a label

- Soybean concentrate
- Soy protein isolates
- Soybean hydrolysates
- Soybean or soy lecithin (may be tolerated by some individuals who are soy-allergenic)
- Textured soy protein
- Textured vegetables protein
- Hydrolyzed plant protein
- Hydrolyzed soy protein
- Hydrolyzed vegetable protein
- Natural flavoring
- Vegetable broth
- Vegetable gum
- Vegetable starch
- Veggie burgers
- Luncheon meats
- Fish canned in oil

- Fried foods
- Prepared Asian foods

Where Can I Get More Information?

For additional information about food allergy, including cookbooks, contact

Food Allergy and Anaphylaxis Network available at: www.foodallergy.org or 703-691-3179.

American Academy of Allergy, Asthma, and Immunology available at: http://www.aaaai.org.

American Academy of Pediatrics available at: www.aap.org.

WebMDHealth, which provides information on many health issues, including food allergy, available at: www.webmd.com.

Food and Nutrition Information Center, a directory to credible, accurate resources about food and nutrition, available at: www.nal.usda.gov/fnic.

To find a nutrition professional in your area, contact www.eatright.org and click Find a Nutrition Professional or call the American Dietetic Association at 1-800-366-1655.

RECOMMENDED READING

- *American Academy of Pediatrics Guide to Your Child's Nutrition* by William H. Dietz and Loraine Stern
- *Food Allergies* by the American Dietetic Association
- *The Food Allergy News Cookbook: A Collection of Recipes from Food Allergy News and Members of the Food Allergy Network* by Anne Munoz-Furlong

---

The Soy Allergy Diet has been adapted from the following sources: Kendall, P. A. (1994). Managing food allergies and sensitivities. *Topics in Clinical Nutrition, 9*, 1–10.
Mahan, L. K., & Escott-Stump, S. (2004). *Krause's Food, Nutrition and Diet Therapy* (p. 784). New York: Elsevier.

Total avoidance of a food allergen is the only proved treatment for a food allergy. The following allergy-specific list can help identify offending foods, but it is essential food labels be read carefully. This is not a complete list; offending foods can be hidden in unfamiliar forms.

FOODS TO AVOID

Acidophilus milk	Half-and-half cream
Artificial butter flavor	Ice cream
Butter	Imitation milk
Butter fat	Light cream
Butter oil	Low-fat ice cream
Caramel candy	Malted milk
Carob candies	Milk chocolate
Cheese	Nougat
Chocolate milk	Milk, all types
Cottage cheese	Semisweet chocolate
Custard	Sherbet, most types
Creamed candies	Sour cream
Cultured buttermilk	Sour cream dressing
Dry milk (whole, low, and nonfat)	Sour cream solids
Eggnog	Sweetened condensed milk, whipping cream
Evaporated milk	Yogurt, frozen and regular
Ghee	Pudding

SPECIAL CONSIDERATIONS

Luncheon meat and hot dogs may be made with milk solids.

Goat's milk contains a protein similar to cow's milk, potentially causing a reaction in those with a cow's milk allergy.

How cow's milk might appear on a label

- Ammonium caseinate
- Calcium caseinate
- Casein
- Casein hydrolysate
- Curds
- Delactosed whey
- Lactalbumin
- Magnesium caseinate

- Potassium caseinate
- Lactoglobulin
- Lactose
- Lactulose
- Milk protein
- Milk protein hydrolysates
- Protein hydrolysate

- Sodium caseinate
- Rennet casein
- Sweet whey
- Whey
- Whey protein hydrolysate
- Whey protein concentrate

Many baked goods, including cake, cookies, and bread will contain cow's milk. Ingredients listed as "flavorings" may contain cow's milk as may prepared luncheon meats.

To replace cow's milk in recipes, try substituting clear fruit juice (e.g., apple or white grape), soymilk, or plain water. Find alternate calcium sources such as fortified fruit juice, soymilk, or calcium-fortified bread.

Where Can I Get More Information?

For additional information about food allergy, including cookbooks, contact

Food Allergy and Anaphylaxis Network available at: www.foodallergy.org or 703-691-3179.

American Academy of Allergy, Asthma, and Immunology available at: http://www.aaaai.org.

American Academy of Pediatrics available at: www.aap.org.

WebMDHealth, which provides information on many health issues, including food allergy, available at: www.webmd.com.

Food and Nutrition Information Center, a directory to credible, accurate resources about food and nutrition, available at: www.nal.usda.gov/fnic.

To find a nutrition professional in your area, contact www.eatright.org and click Find a Nutrition Professional or call the American Dietetic Association at 1-800-366-1655.

RECOMMENDED READING

- *American Academy of Pediatrics Guide to Your Child's Nutrition* by William H. Dietz and Loraine Stern
- *Food Allergies* by the American Dietetic Association
- *The Food Allergy News Cookbook: A Collection of Recipes from Food Allergy News and Members of the Food Allergy Network* by Anne Munoz-Furlong

The Cow's Milk Allergy Diet has been adapted from the following sources: Kendall, P. A. (1994). Managing food allergies and sensitivities. *Topics in Clinical Nutrition, 9*, 1–10.
Mahan, L. K., & Escott-Stump, S. (2004). *Krause's Food, Nutrition and Diet Therapy* (p. 782). New York: Elsevier.

Total avoidance of a food allergen is the only proved treatment for a food allergy. The following allergy-specific list can help identify offending foods, but it is essential food labels be read carefully. This is not a complete list; offending foods can be hidden in unfamiliar forms.

FOODS TO AVOID

All forms of eggs and foods made with eggs, including

- Béarnaise sauce
- Cake
- Cookies
- Custard
- Dried eggs
- Eggnog
- Eggs
- Egg substitute
- Egg white
- Egg yolk
- French toast
- Frozen eggs
- Hollandaise sauce
- Ice cream
- Imitation egg product
- Mayonnaise
- Meringue
- Powdered egg
- Simplesse (fat substitute)

How egg might appear on a food label (most baked goods are prepared with egg)

- Albumin
- Apovitellin
- Avidin
- Egg solids
- Flavoprotein
- Globulin
- Livetin

- Lysozyme
- Ovalbumin
- Ovogyprotein
- Ovomucin
- Ovomucoid
- Ovomuxoid

COOKING WITHOUT EGGS

Ener G Egg Replacer made by ENERG-G Foods, Inc., which is available in most health food stores, is a good replacement for eggs when baking. Just mix 1 tablespoon Egg Replacer powder with 1 ½ teaspoon water to equal one egg.

Where Can I Get More Information?

For additional information about food allergy, including cookbooks, contact

Food Allergy and Anaphylaxis Network available at: www.foodallergy.org or 703-691-3179.

American Academy of Allergy, Asthma, and Immunology available at: http://www.aaaai.org.

American Academy of Pediatrics available at: www.aap.org.

WebMDHealth, which provides information on many health issues, including food allergy, available at: www.webmd.com.

Food and Nutrition Information Center, a directory to credible, accurate resources about food and nutrition, available at: www.nal.usda.gov/fnic.

To find a nutrition professional in your area, contact www.eatright.org and click Find a Nutrition Professional or call the American Dietetic Association at 1-800-366-1655.

RECOMMENDED READING

- *American Academy of Pediatrics Guide to Your Child's Nutrition* by William H. Dietz and Loraine Stern
- *Food Allergies* by the American Dietetic Association
- *The Food Allergy News Cookbook: A Collection of Recipes from Food Allergy News and Members of the Food Allergy Network* by Anne Munoz-Furlong

---

The Egg Allergy Diet has been adapted from the following sources: Kendall, P. A. (1994). Managing food allergies and sensitivities. *Topics in Clinical Nutrition, 9*, 1–10.
Mahan, L. K., & Escott-Stump, S. (2004). *Krause's Food, Nutrition and Diet Therapy* (p. 781). New York: Elsevier.

5-17 Ten Steps to a Healthy Vegetarian Diet

1. Eat enough to meet your energy needs. A stable, healthy weight is one way to tell whether you are eating enough food.

2. Choose a wide variety of foods from all food groups. Do not get stuck in a food rut; for example, alternate between brown rice, barley, or quinoa; try different colored vegetables; and find ways to meet protein needs from a variety of sources, including nuts, beans, or tofu.

3. Include the recommended 3 to 4 servings of calcium-rich foods every day. See the milk and milk alternatives listed below.

4. Include two foods rich in omega-3 fatty acids on most days. A serving equals 1 teaspoon flaxseed oil, 3 teaspoons canola or soybean oil, 1 tablespoon ground flaxseed, or ¼ cup walnuts. Omega-3 fatty acids are also found in seafood.

5. Use olive oil or canola oil for cooking; they have a good balance of healthy fats.

6. Substitute nuts and seeds in place of fat from the fat group, from which you will get extra protein.

7. Get enough vitamin B_{12} every day. This recommendation is particularly important for individuals eating an unsupplemented vegan diet, because vitamin B_{12} is found in animal foods. A nonanimal source of vitamin B_{12} can include 1 tablespoon Red Star Vegetarian Support Formula nutritional yeast, 1 cup B_{12} fortified soymilk, 1 oz fortified breakfast cereal, 1½ oz of fortified meat analog. Animal products such as ½ cup cow's milk, ¾ cup yogurt, or 1 large egg also provide vitamin B_{12}. If you do not eat any of these foods regularly (at least 3 servings per day, 2 for children and adolescents, and 4 while pregnant or lactating), you will need a vitamin B_{12} supplement of 5 to 10 μg a day or 2000 μg per week.

8. Consume alcohol only in moderation. Moderation is defined as one drink for women and two for men. A serving is a 12 oz-beer, 5 oz of wine, or 1.5 oz liquor.

9. Limit sweets or foods high in calories and low in nutrition.

10. To be healthy include the following food groups:

    Milk and milk alternatives: 3 to 4 servings daily

    Each serving provides approximately 300 mg calcium, 8 g of protein, and 1 μg of vitamin B_{12}.

    Milk, yogurt, or fortified soymilk, and calcium-fortified cottage cheese, 1 cup

    Tofu, ½ cup

    Natural cheese, 1 ½ oz

    Beans, nut butters, green leafy vegetables, black strap molasses, dried seaweed, and fortified foods and juices are good sources of calcium, read labels for amounts.

    Protein sources: 2 to 3 servings daily

    (A serving should contain 16 to 24 g of protein)

The following foods provide approximately 7 g of protein:

- Egg, 1
- Egg whites, 2
- Fish, 1 oz
- Parmesan cheese, 3 tablespoons
- Hard Cheese, 1 oz
- Beans, ⅓ to ½ cup
- Soy flour, ¼ cup
- Tempeh, 4 oz
- Tofu, 3 oz
- Walnuts, cashews, peanuts, and sunflower or pumpkin seeds, ¼ cup
- Tahini (sesame butter), 1 ½ tablespoons
- Soymilk and cow's milk contain approximately 8 g of protein per 8 oz-serving

Grains and Starches: 6 to 11 serving daily

This food group is a small but significant source of protein because it makes up the foundation of most daily menus. The following serving sizes have about 2 g of protein per serving:

- Brown rice, bulgur, and wild rice, rolled oats, whole wheat cereal, and white rice, ½ cup
- Bread, 1 slice
- Bagel, ½
- English muffin, hamburger roll, 2-inch dinner roll, 6-inch pita, or tortilla
- Plain popcorn, 2 to 3 cups
- Rice cakes, 2
- Other grain-based product or baked good, 1 oz

Vegetables: 3 to 5 servings daily

A ½ cup portion of cooked vegetable or 1 cup chopped raw or leafy vegetable or ¾ cup vegetable juice has approximately 1 to 2 g of protein. This food group is a rich source of fiber, vitamin A, vitamin C, potassium, and even some calcium.

All vegetables including fresh, frozen, or canned are included in this group.

Fruit: 2 to 4 servings daily

This food group provides mostly carbohydrate, vitamins A, vitamin C, fiber, and potassium.

A serving size is 1 piece medium fresh fruit, ¾ cup fruit juice, or ½ cup canned or cooked fruit.

Fats and Oils: 3 or more servings daily

This food group can be a source of healthy vegetable fats.

A serving size is usually 1 teaspoon vegetable oil, 1 tablespoon salad dressing, 4 walnuts, or 10 almonds.

Where Can I Get More Information?

American Academy of Pediatrics available at: www.aap.org.

WebMDHealth, which provides health information, available at: www.webmd.com.

Food and Nutrition Information Center, a directory to credible, accurate resources about food and nutrition, available at: www.nal.usda.gov/fnic.

To find a nutrition professional in your area, contact www.eatright.org and click Find a Nutrition Professional or call the American Dietetic Association at 1-800-366-1655.

RECOMMENDED READING

- *Becoming Vegan* by Vesanto Melina and Brenda Davis
- *Being Vegetarian for Dummies* by Suzanne Havala
- *The Teen's Vegetarian Cookbook* by Judy Krizmanic
- *Vegetarian Cooking for Everyone* by Deborah Madison
- *American Academy of Pediatrics Guide to Your Child's Nutrition* by William H. Dietz and Loraine Stern
- *Child of Mine: Feeding with Love and Good Sense* by Ellyn Satter
- *Feeding Your Child for Lifelong Health: Birth Through Age Six* by Susan Roberts
- *Fit Kids: Raising Physically and Emotionally Strong Kids with Real Food* by Eileen Behan

Iron deficiency is the most common nutritional deficiency in the United States. Untreated iron deficiency can affect intellect, behavior, and motor function. The condition is most common during rapid growth and has an impact on older infants, young children, and women of childbearing age.

WHAT IS IRON DEFICIENCY ANEMIA?

Iron deficiency anemia means the blood has smaller blood cells than is normal. Iron is needed to make hemoglobin, the part of red blood cells that carries oxygen in the body. An iron deficiency can occur when not enough iron is included in the diet to make a normal amount of hemoglobin to prevent anemia.

HOW CAN IRON DEFICIENCY ANEMIA BE PREVENTED?

For infants and toddlers, the most important factor is a good diet adequate in iron. In infants the greatest risk factor for the condition is the addition of cow's milk (which is low in iron and can increase the need for iron) in the first 12 months of life. Therefore, strictly avoid giving your child cow's milk for the first 12 months. Breastfeeding is an ideal way to feed infants because, although breast milk is low in total iron, the iron it does contain is absorbed very efficiently.

The American Academy of Pediatrics suggests the following dietary recommendations for infants and children younger than 3 years:

Healthy, full-term breast-fed infants: Starting at 4 to 6 months of age introduce iron-fortified infant cereal and meats. After your infant is 6 months of age, your baby's doctor may recommend an infant iron supplement. When and if formula is added, only iron-fortified formula should be used for weaning or supplementing breast milk.

Formula-fed infants: Use only iron-fortified formula in the first year of life, and supplement with iron only when recommended by the baby's doctor.

Introducing solid foods: When the child is developmentally able to sit up and swallow (about 4 to 6 months of age), food sources of iron can be added. Ask your baby's doctor when to add solid foods and what type. Iron-fortified cereals, breads, and grains are good sources of iron but the iron from animal foods (e.g., beef and chicken) is better absorbed. Serving small amounts of meat or chicken with grains, beans, or vegetables significantly boosts the iron that is absorbed. Vitamin C improves iron absorption too.

Your baby and child can get vitamin C from a small glass of orange juice, a slice of citrus fruit, or berries served with the meal.

IRON CONTENT OF SELECTED FOODS (mg)

Bagel, 1	2.83
White bread, 1 slice	1.08

Whole wheat bread, 1 slice	1.30
Corn chips, 1 oz	0.37
Chex mix, 1 oz	6.92
Fruit leather (Fruit Roll-up), 1 each	0.549
Cream cheese, low-fat, 1 tablespoon	0.252
Egg, large, boiled, 1	0.59
Raisins, 2/3 cup	2.08
Cheerios, 1 cup	8.10
Total, ¾ cup	18.0
Shredded wheat, 1 cup	1.44
Wheaties, 1 cup	8.10
Cream of Wheat, ¾ cup	9.05
Infant beef, 2.8 oz jar	1.11
Infant chicken, 2.8 oz jar	1.26
Mixed nuts, 1 cup	5.08
Peanut butter, 2 tablespoons	0.61
Garbanzo (chickpea), 1 cup	3.24
Soybean tofu, raw, firm, ½ cup	13.19

MILK

Avoid the use of cow, goat, or soymilk before age 12 months.

Milk is a great source of calcium, but not iron; 24 oz per day is enough to meet the calcium needs of children age 1 to 5. Drinking a lot more milk can cause iron deficiency anemia in some children, because it replaces foods rich in iron.

Young Children: Even after infancy, the risk of iron deficiency is present. If your baby's doctor recommends an iron supplement be sure to take it and choose some of the iron-rich foods listed above every day.

WHAT TO DO

- Ask your healthcare provider for advice.
- Give your child an iron supplement if advised by the healthcare provider.
- Breastfeed or use iron-fortified infant formula for the first 12 months.
- Do not serve cow's milk until after the first birthday. Then keep it to approximately 24 oz per day
- Once your child starts solids, serve iron-rich foods such as iron-fortified bread, cereal, pasta, or rice (these products will list iron on the nutrition facts panel) or animal-based foods such as beef, poultry, or fish.

- Serve a good source of vitamin C with every meal; chopped, fresh or minimally cooked fruits and vegetables are very good choices.
- Go to the resources suggested below for more help.

Where Can I Get More Information?

www.fda.gov

www.healthfinder.gov Family Food and Nutrition Resources:

American Academy of Pediatrics available at: www.aap.org

WebMDHealth, which provides health information, available at: www.webmd.com.

Food and Nutrition Information Center, a directory to credible, accurate resources about food and nutrition, available at: www.nal.usda.gov/fnic.

To find a nutrition professional in your area, contact www.eatright.org and click Find a Nutrition Professional or call the American Dietetic Association at 1-800-366-1655.

RECOMMENDED READING

- *American Academy of Pediatrics Guide to Your Child's Nutrition* by William H. Dietz and Loraine Stern
- *Child of Mine: Feeding with Love and Good Sense* by Ellyn Satter
- *Feeding Your Child for Lifelong Health: Birth Through Age Six* by Susan Roberts
- *Fit Kids: Raising Physically and Emotionally Strong Kids with Real Food* by Eileen Behan

5-19 Stomachache

Nearly one of four school-aged children complains of chronic stomach pain. No physical cause is found for most of these complaints. Many things can cause a stomachache, including a food intolerance, early sign of illness, indigestion, overeating, stress, constipation, and serious illness that requires medical treatment.

Do not ignore a stomachache, particularly if it is accompanied by fever, vomiting, diarrhea, or an injury near or at the stomach area. Contact your healthcare provider when your child has a persistent, unexplained stomachache. If no medical explanation exists, look at your child's diet and stress level. A stomachache caused by stress or emotions does not mean the pain is imaginary. An emotionally induced stomach pain requires treatment too. Ask your child about what is bothering him or her. Talk to your child's teacher about stress at school. Also, consult the resources listed at the end of this handout.

If you suspect diet is a factor, review what your youngster has been eating. The dietary factors to consider can include lack of fiber and fluids, irregular meals, or overconsumption of certain foods. When your healthcare provider has ruled out any medical explanations, get your child on a menu that includes all the essential foods and adequate fluids, and time eat, chew, and relax. Provide your child with food and opportunity that will promote good digestion. Consider the following:

- Offer three meals per day. Allow enough time (at least 15 minutes) to eat.
- Is your child eating at least 5 servings of fruits and vegetables per day? A serving is about 1 tablespoon for each year of life or one small serving.
- Try serving whole grain foods (e.g., brown rice or whole wheat bread) to add fiber.
- If your child drinks a lot of juices, try serving whole fruit instead. For example, sliced oranges instead of orange juice.
- Your child might be swallowing air while chewing gum, sucking on candy, or drinking carbonated beverages.
- Broccoli, cauliflower, brussel sprouts and baked beans can cause gas when consumed in excess. Do not eliminate these; just serve them in lesser amounts.
- Try keeping a food diary to identify a pattern of food consumption linked to the stomachache.
- Some fruit juices, fruit drinks, and desserts and candies sweetened with artificial sweeteners can cause stomach pain.
- Milk shakes, large servings of ice cream, and other foods with a lot of sugar can provide your child with a large dose of sweet carbohydrate that can be hard to handle all at once.
- Do not start a milk-free diet unless advised to do so by your healthcare provider. A short-term, milk-free diet will not have an impact on the child's calcium needs, but if told to follow a milk-free diet permanently, alternate calcium sources will need to be found.

If stress is a suspected factor, try to relieve it with a little exercise such as a walk with your child or dancing to a favorite song. Teach your child the deep breathing techniques used in childbirth classes. Deep breathing used before meals or when a stomachache occurs might help relieve a stomachache. Discuss the role anxiety and depression can have on your child's health with your healthcare provider.

Where Can I Get More Information?

American Academy of Pediatrics available at: www.aap.org.

American Academy of Family Physicians available at: www.aafp.org.

National Digestive Diseases Information Clearinghouse available at: www.niddk.nih.gov/.

WebMDHealth, which provides health information, available at: www.webmd.com.

Food and Nutrition Information Center, a directory to credible, accurate resources about food and nutrition, available at: www.nal.usda.gov/fnic.

To find a nutrition professional in your area, contact www.eatright.org and click Find a Nutrition Professional or call the American Dietetic Association at 1-800-366-1655.

RECOMMENDED READING

- *American Academy of Pediatrics Guide to Your Child's Nutrition* by William H. Dietz and Loraine Stern
- *Child of Mine: Feeding with Love and Good Sense* by Ellyn Satter
- *Feeding Your Child for Lifelong Health: Birth Through Age Six* by Susan Roberts
- *Fit Kids: Raising Physically and Emotionally Strong Kids with Real Food* by Eileen Behan

Snacks have a place in a child's diet, but make sure they provide the nutrition a child actually needs. Parents need to protect their children from highly advertised products that are marketed in kid-pleasing containers and often use vague nutrition claims like "made with real fruit" to sell them to parents.

Many children need more fiber and calcium, not more sugar and salt!

CALCIUM CHOICES

A good calcium choice should contain approximately 30% of the daily calcium requirement. Look for the calcium percentage on the food label.

Choose skim and low-fat milk, low-fat yogurt, homemade fruit smoothie made with low-fat milk or yogurt, and low-fat cheese.

FRUIT CHOICES

A serving of fruit is a good source of fiber, vitamins A and C, and potassium. Whole fruit is filling and recommended over fruit juice for most children. When you do serve juice, serve apple juice with vitamin C added, and orange, pineapple, or grapefruit juice.

Choose, apples, applesauce, bananas, berries, cantaloupe, cherries, dates, figs, grapefruit, grapes, honeydew melon, kiwi fruit, mandarin oranges, mangoes, nectarines, oranges, papayas, peaches, pears, pineapple, plums, raisins, watermelon, canned fruit packed in fruit juice, and frozen fruit without added sugar.

Avoid fruit bars and fruit rollups, unless served as a dessert.

VEGETABLE CHOICES

Vegetables are a great source of fiber, vitamins A and C, and potassium. Most children do not eat enough vegetables at meals, so do offer them as a snack. When serving vegetables as a snack, include a low-fat dressing for a dip. Salsa, a favorite with many children, is a great choice when served with green pepper slices, carrot sticks, or low-fat tortilla chips.

Choose carrot sticks, cucumber slices, pea pods, all types of peppers, radishes, mixed vegetable salad, and tomato slices.

GRAIN, CEREAL, AND BREAD CHOICES

The best snack foods in this group are made with whole grains and whole grain flour. Whole grains are less likely to lead to overeating. The next best foods are those with a low sugar content. Granola bars and cereal bars are really cookies, and should be served only as often as you think your child should eat dessert. Read labels on snack foods. Avoid buying foods with a high salt or sugar content because they will be hard for a child to resist and puts the child at risk of overeating.

Choose whole wheat bread, flat bread, rice cakes, whole grain crackers, air popped popcorn, dry cereals high in fiber and low in sugar, including bran cereals, Cheerios, Fruit Wheats (Nabisco), Multigrain Cheerios, Oatmeal Squares, Raisin Bran, and Shredded Wheat squares.

Next best choices for snacks include animal crackers, bagel chips, graham crackers, whole grain homemade muffins or whole grain muffins from a mix, pretzels, saltine-type crackers, and zwieback.

Where Can I Get More Information?

American Academy of Pediatrics available at: www.aap.org.

WebMDHealth, which provides information on a wide range of health issues, is available at: www.webmd.com.

Food and Nutrition Information Center, a directory to credible, accurate resources about food and nutrition, available at: www.nal.usda.gov/fnic.

5 A Day Fruits and Vegetables available at: www.5aday.gov

To find a nutrition professional in your area, contact www.eatright.org and click Find a Nutrition Professional or call the American Dietetic Association at 1-800-366-1655.

RECOMMENDED READING

- *American Academy of Pediatrics Guide to Your Child's Nutrition* by William H. Dietz and Loraine Stern
- *Child of Mine: Feeding with Love and Good Sense* by Ellyn Satter
- *Feeding Your Child for Lifelong Health: Birth Through Age Six* by Susan Roberts
- *Fit Kids: Raising Physically and Emotionally Strong Kids with Real Food* by Eileen Behan

Ten Ways To Create Healthy Family Food Habits

1. **Have a regularly scheduled mealtime**. A regular meal schedule can help your child feel secure. Young children thrive on routines, and it will help a child better self-regulate food intake.

2. **Eat meals together that last 15 minutes**. Families tend to eat better and include more variety when they eat together. Rushed meals can promote excessive calorie intake.

3. **Avoid making family members "clean their plate."** Telling a child to clean the plate when full is teaching the child to overeat. Instead, tell the child to try one bite of a new food, which encourages variety and trying new things.

4. **Have a thought-out list of appropriate snacks to eat between meals**. You can avoid food battles and poor snack choices if you are proactive in this area. Talk to your children about what they would like to eat between meals. Come up with a list that suits both of you.

5. **Eat only in designated areas (kitchen, dining room)**. Eating in one or two areas, such as the kitchen or the dining room, is an effective way to promote conscious eating and awareness of what is being consumed.

6. **Snack only when hungry and not to ease boredom or soothe emotions**. If you suspect your child is eating emotionally ask if the child is really hungry. If so, the child should eat from a wholesome list of snacks. If the child is not truly hungry, try an alternate activity (e.g., exercise or working on a hobby) to ease emotional tension. Try to help your child see the difference between eating when hungry and eating when bored.

7. **Avoid phrases such as "that will make you fat," "I need to go on a diet,"and "we are a fat family."** The words you use to describe your family and its eating habits will be prophetic. Make sure the words you say are actually sending the message you want.

8. **Eat five fruits and vegetables each day**. To prevent obesity, heart disease, and cancer, everyone in the family should eat fruits and vegetables. If you have trouble getting your child to eat vegetables, then offer four fruits and one vegetable and try to offer as much variety as possible.

9. **Treat soda as if it were liquid candy**. Nothing is wrong with a can of soda, just as nothing is wrong with a candy bar. Keep soda in its place. As with having ice cream or a candy bar, soda should not be an everyday food item. Any drink with 25 g of sugar per 100-calorie portion is a liquid candy. This includes most sports drinks and fruit drinks.

10. **Know what your child needs to eat to have a "balanced diet."** Your child will learn very little in the way of meaningful information about food from teachers or the doctor. If your child does not learn about food from you, the child will learn about it from food advertisers. Who do you want to teach your child about a balanced diet?

Adapted from *Fit Kids: How To Raise Physically and Emotionally Strong Kids with Real Food* by Eileen Behan. 2001. New York: Pocket Books.

Where Can I Get More Information?

American Academy of Pediatrics available at: www.aap.org.

WebMDHealth, which provides information on a wide range of health issues, is available at: www.webmd.com.

Food and Nutrition Information Center, a directory to credible, accurate resources about food and nutrition, available at: www.nal.usda.gov/fnic

To find a nutrition professional in your area, contact www.eatright.org and click Find a Nutrition Professional or call the American Dietetic Association at 1-800-366-1655.

RECOMMENDED READING

- *American Academy of Pediatrics Guide to Your Child's Nutrition* by William H. Dietz and Loraine Stern
- *Child of Mine: Feeding with Love and Good Sense* by Ellyn Satter
- *Feeding Your Child for Lifelong Health: Birth Through Age Six* by Susan Roberts
- *Fit Kids: Raising Physically and Emotionally Strong Kids with Real Food* by Eileen Behan

What You Should Know About Eating Disorders

WHAT ARE EATING DISORDERS?

Eating disorders are real illnesses that can affect how we eat and how we feel about food. Sometimes a person eats so little, or nothing at all, and they begin to starve (called anorexia nervosa). A person can also eat an extreme amount of food all at once and then rid the body of food by vomiting and other measures (called bulimia nervosa). And, a person may not be able to control the need to overeat, often keeping it a secret (called binge eating disorder). Eating disorders affect people of all ages, races, and income levels, but they affect women much more than they do men. These disorders increase the risk for *osteoporosis* (thinning of the bones) and heart problems. People who have these disorders can also be depressed and anxious, and may turn to alcohol and drugs for relief.

WHAT CAUSES EATING DISORDERS?

No one knows what causes eating disorders. It is thought that these disorders cannot be willed or wished away, but require treatment. If you or someone you know has an eating disorder, get help immediately. Talk with a healthcare provider right away.

HOW CAN YOU TELL IF SOMEONE HAS AN EATING DISORDER?

Because many people with eating disorders keep them a secret, their condition can go unnoticed for long periods of time. With anorexia, extreme weight loss is easy to see. Bulimics who can stay at their normal body weight may be better able to hide their illness. Family members and friends may notice some of the warning signs of an eating disorder.

A person with anorexia may

- Eat only "safe" foods, low in calories and fat
- Have odd rituals, such as cutting food into small pieces or measuring food
- Spend more time playing with food than eating it
- Cook meals for others, without eating
- Exercise to excess
- Dress in layers to hide weight loss
- Spend less time with family and friends
- Become withdrawn and secretive

A person with bulimia may

- Become very secretive about food
- Spend a lot of time thinking about and planning the next eating binge

■ Keep making trips to the bathroom after eating

■ Steal food or hoard it in strange places

■ Eat to excess

A person with binge-eating disorder may

■ Become very secretive about food

■ Spend a lot of time planning the next eating binge

■ Start eating alone most of the time

■ Steal food or hoard it in strange places

■ Eat to excess

■ Become overweight

■ Become withdrawn, not wanting to go out or see family and friends

If you or someone you know has any of these warning signs, see a healthcare provider right away. Help is available for people with these disorders. With help, they can lead a healthy full life.

Reprinted from Frequently Asked Questions About Eating Disorders available at: www.4woman.gov/faq/eatingdi.htm. The National Health Women's Information Center, A project of the U.S. Department of Health and Human Services, Office of Women's Health.

Where Can I Get More Information?

The National Women's Health Information Center at: 800-994-9662 or www.4woman.gov.

Body Wise Packet: Eating disorders information for school personnel and healthcare providers available at: http://www.4women.gov/bodyimage/bodywise/bodywise.htm.

National Institute of Mental Health available at: http://www.nimh.nih.gov.

Weight Control Information Network available at: www.niddk.nih.gov/health/nutrit/win.htm.

National Mental Health Information Center available at: www.mentalhealth.org.

Academy for Eating Disorders available at: www.aedweb.org.

Harvard Eating Disorders Center available at: www.hedc.org.

To find a nutrition professional in your area, contact www.eatright.org and click Find a Nutrition Professional or call the American Dietetic Association at 1-800-366-1655.

Recommended Books, Newsletters, and Web Pages

CHILDREN'S NUTRITION

Recommended Reading

- *ADA Guide to Healthy Eating for Kids: How Your Children Can Eat Smart From 5 to 12* by Jodie Shield and Mary Catherine Mullen. American Dietetic Association, 2002.
- *American Academy of Pediatrics Guide to Your Child's Nutrition* by William Dietz & Loraine Stern. American Academy of Pediatrics, 1999.
- *How to Get Your Child to Eat But Not Too Much* by Ellen Satter
- *Child of Mine: Feeding with Love and Good Sense* by Ellen Satter. Bull Publishing, 2000.
- *Fit Kids: Raising Physically and Emotionally Strong Kids With Real Food* by Eileen Behan. Pocket Books, 2001.
- *Healthy Foods, Healthy Kids* by Elizabeth Ward. Adams Media Corporation, 2002.
- *Feeding Your Child for Lifelong Health: Birth Through Age Six* by Susan Roberts, Melvin B. Heyman, & Lisa Tracy. Bantam Publishers, 1999.

Resources

American Academy of Pediatrics www.aap.org.
American School Food Service Association www.asfsa.org.
American Academy of Family Physicians
   www.aafp.org.
National Child Care Information Center
   http://nccic.org.
National Clearinghouse on Families and Youth
   www.ncfy.com.
National Dissemination Center for Children with Disabilities
   www.nichcy.org.
National Institute of Child Health and Human Development Resource Center
   www.nichd.nih.gov/default.htm.

FOOD AND COOKING

Recommended Reading

- *The New Joy of Cooking*, Revised Ed. by Marion Rombauer Becker, Irma S. Rombauer, & Ethan Becker. Scribner, 1997.
- *Cooking Light Annual 2004 Recipes* by the editors of Cooking Light. Oxmoor House, 2003.
- *The New Basics Cookbook* by Julie Russo & Sheila Leukin. Workman Publishers, 1989.

- *How To Cook Everything: Simple Recipes for Great Food* by Mark Bittman. John Wiley & Sons, 1998.
- *The Good Food Book* by Jane Brody. WW Norton & Co., 1985.

Resources

5 A Day Fruits and Vegetables
   www.5aday.gov
Recipe Finder
   www.epicurious.com
FDA's Food Information and Seafood Hotline
   888-723-3366

CANCER
Recommended Reading

- *A Dietitian's Cancer Story* by Dina Dyer. Swan Press, 2002.

Resources

American Cancer Society
   www.cancer.org
American Institute for Cancer Research
   www.aicr.org
National Cancer Institute
   www.nci.nih.gov

DIABETES
Recommended Reading

- *The American Dietetics Association Guide to Eating Right When You Have Diabetes* by Maggie Powers. American Diabetes Association, 2003.
- *The American Diabetes Guide to Healthy Restaurant Eating* by Hope Warshaw. American Diabetes Association, 2002.
- *The Diabetes Carbohydrate and Fat Gram Guide* by Lea Ann Holzmeister. American Diabetes Association and The American Dietetics Association, 2000.
- *The Diabetes Food and Nutrition Bible: A Complete Guide to Planning, Shopping, Cooking and Eating* by Hope Warshaw & Robyn Webb. American Diabetes Association, 2001.
- *Month of Meals: Classic Cooking & Quick & Easy Menus for People with Diabetes* by the American Diabetes Association, 2002.
- *No-Fuss Diabetes Recipes for 1 or 2* by Jackie Boucher, Marcia Hayes, & Jane Stephson. Wiley, 1999.

Resources

American Diabetes Association
   www.diabetes.org
Joslin Diabetes Center
   www.joslin.org
Juvenile Diabetes Foundation International
   http://www.jdf.org
National Diabetes Information Clearinghouse
   http://diabetes.niddk.nih.gov/

FITNESS AND SPORTS NUTRITION

Recommended Reading

- *Weight Training for Dummies, 2nd ed.,* by Liz Neporant & Suzanne Schlossberg. 2000: Hungry Minds Publisher

- *Nancy Clark's Sports Nutrition Guidebook*, 3rd ed., by Nancy Clark. Human Kinetics Publishers, 2003.

- *Nancy Clark's Food Guide for Marathoners* by Nancy Clark. Sports Nutrition Publishers, 2003.

Resources

American College of Sports Medicine
   www.acsm.org
President's Council on Physical Fitness and Sports
   www.surgeongeneral.gov/

FOOD SENSITIVITIES

Recommended Reading

- *Food Allergies* by the American Dietetic Association. Wiley, 1998.

- *Gluten-free Gourmet: Cooks Fast and Healthy: Wheat-free and Gluten-free with Less Fuss and Less Fat* by Bette Hagman. Owl Books, 2000.

- *Celiac Disease Nutrition Guide* by Tricia Thompson & Merri Lou Dobler. American Dietetic Association, 2003.

- *Lactose Intolerance Nutrition Guide* by Merri Lou Dobler. American Dietetic Association, 2003.

- *The Food Allergy News Cookbook: A Collection of Recipes From Food Allergy News and Members of the Food Allergy Network* by Anne Munoz-Furlong (editor). Chromed Publishing, 1998.

Resources

American Academy of Allergy, asthma, and Immunology
   www.aaaai.org
American Celiac Society
   973-325-8837
Celiac Sprue Association/USA
   www.csaceliacs.org

HEART HEALTH
Recommended Reading

- *American Heart Association Low-Salt Cookbook: A Complete Guide To Reducing Sodium and Fat in Your Diet* by the American Heart Association. Crown Publishing Group, 2001.
- *The DASH diet for Hypertension: Lower Your Blood Pressure in 14 Days Without Drugs* by Thomas Moore, Njeri Karanja, Laura P. Svetkey, & Mark Jenkins. Simon and Schuster, 2001.

Resources

American Heart Association
   www.americanheart.org
Heart Information Network
   www.heartinfo.org/
National Cholesterol Education Program Adult Treatment Panel Guidelines
   www.nhlbi.nih.gov/guidelines/cholesterol/atp_iii.htm

BASIC NUTRITION
Recommended Reading

- *The American Dietetic Association's Complete Food and Nutrition Guide* by Roberta Larson Duyff. Wiley, 2002.
- *Eating on the Run* by Evelyn Tribole & P. J. Skerrett. Freepress, 2002.
- *Eat Drink and Be Healthy* by Walter Willett. Simon and Schuster, 2001.
- *Vitamins, Herbs, Minerals and Supplements: The Complete Guide, revised ed.,* by H. Winter, M.D. Griffith. Perseus Publisher, 2000.
- *Monthly Nutrition Companion: 31 Ways to a Healthier Lifestyle* by Paul Insel, Don Ross, & R. Elaine Turner. Jones and Bartlett, 2003.

Resources

U.S. Department of Agricultural, Food, Nutrition and Consumer Services
   www.fns.usda.gov/fncs
U.S Department of Health and Human Services
   www.hhs.gov
U.S. Government Food Safety
   www.foodsafety.gov

PREGNANCY AND BREASTFEEDING
Recommended Reading

- *Eating Expectantly* by Bridget Swinney. Simon and Schuster, 2000.
- *No More Morning Sickness* by Miriam Erick. Plume Books, 1993.
- *The Pregnancy Diet* by Eileen Behan. Pocket Books, 1999.

Resources

American Foundation for Maternal and Child Health
  212-759-5510
La Leche League International
  www.lalecheleague.org
Maternal and Child Health Information Resource Center
  www.mchirc.net

OSTEOPOROSIS

Recommended Reading

■ *Strong Women, Strong Bones* by Miriam Nelson. Perigree Books, 2001.

Resources

Menopause and Osteoporosis
  www.menopause.org/
National Osteoporosis Foundation
  www.nof.org/
Tufts University Nutrition
  www.navigator.tufts.edu
American Association of Retired Persons
  www/aarp.org
National Institute on Aging Information Office
  www.nih.gov.nia

VEGETARIANISM

Recommended Reading

■ *Becoming Vegan* by Vesanto Melina & Brenda Davis. The Book Publishing Company, 2000.

■ *Being Vegetarian for Dummies* by Suzanne Havala. Wiley, 2001.

■ *The Teen's Vegetarian Cookbook* by Judy Krizmanic. Viking Press, 1999.

Resources

North American Vegetarian Society
  www.navs-online.org
Vegetarian Resource Group
  www.vrg.org

WEIGHT LOSS

Recommended Reading

■ *Diet Simple* by Katherine Tallmadge. Lifeline Press, 2002.

■ *Dieting for Dummies* by Jane Kirby. IDG Books Worldwide, 1998.

- *Strong Women Stay Slim* by Miriam Nelson. Bantam, 1999.
- *Thin for Life: 10 keys to Success From People Who Have Lost Weight and Kept It Off.* Anne Fletcher & Jane Brody. Houghton Mifflin, 2003.
- *Volumetrics Weight Control Plan: Feel Full on Fewer Calories* by Barbara Rolls & Robert Barnett. Perrenial Current, 2000.

Resources

Healthy Weight Network
    www.healthyweight.net
Overeaters Anonymous
    www.overeatersanonymous.org
Environmental Nutrition
    www.environmentalnutrition.com
Mayo Clinic Health Letter
    www.mayohealth.org
Tufts University, Health and Nutrition Letter
    www.healthletter.tufts.edu
University of California, Berkley Wellness Letter
    1-800-829-9080
Center for Science in the Public Interest Nutrition Action Health Letter
    www.cspinet.org

REFERENCES

American Dietetic Association. *Manual of clinical dietetics* (6th ed.) Chicago, IL: American Dietetic Association.

Barker, D.J. (1999). Early growth and cardiovascular disease. *Archive of Disease in Childhood, 80*:305–307. http://www. fetalneonatal.com/cgi/content/full/archdischild:80/ 4/305.

Czeizel, A.E., & Dudas I. (1992). Prevention of the first occurrence of neural-tube defects by periconceptional vitamin supplementation. *New England Journal of Medicine, 327*(26):1832–1835.

Keppel, K.G., & Taffel, S.M. (1993). Pregnancy-related weight gain and retention: implications of the 1990 Institute of Medicine Guidelines. *American Journal of Public Health, 83*:1100–1103.

Food and Nutrition Board, Institute of Medicine. *Dietary reference intakes for thiamin, riboflavin, niacin, vitamin B6, folate, vitamin B12, pantothenic acid, biotin, and choline.* Washington, DC: National Academy Press.

Institute of Medicine, Subcommittee on Nutrition During Lactation. (1991). *Nutrition during lactation.* Washington, DC: National Academy Press.

Lovelady, C.A., Garner, K.E., Moreno, K.L., & Williams, J.P. (2000). The effect of weight loss in overweight lactating women on the growth of their infants. *New England Journal of Medicine 342*:449–453.

Messina, V., Melina, V., & Mangels, R. (2003). A new food guide for North American vegetarians. *Journal of the American Dietetic Association, 103*(6):771–775.

Munoz, K.A., Krebs-Smith, S.M., Ballard-Barbash, R., & Cleveland, L.E. (1997). Food intakes of U.S. children and adolescents compared with recommendations. *Pediatrics, 101*(5):952–953.

National Institute of Allergy and Infectious Diseases, National Institutes of Health, U.S. Department of Health and Human Services (2002). *Facts and figures: Allergy statistics, January 2002.* www.naid.nih.gov/factsheets/allergystat. htm. Accessed June, 2004.

Polhamus, B., Dalenius, K., Thompson D., Scanlon K., Borland E., Smith B., & Grummer-Strawn. L. (2001). *Pediatric nutrition surveillance 2001 report.* Atlanta: U.S. Department of Health and Human Services, Centers for Disease Control and Prevention.

Sicherer, S.H. (1999). Manifestations of food allergy: Evaluation and treatment. *American Family Physician,* January 15, 1999. www.aafp.org/afp/990115ap/415.html. Accessed December 9, 2003.

Somvanshi, N.P. (2002). Preventing postpartum weight retention (editorial). *American Family Physician,* August 1, 2002. www.aafp.org/afp/20020801/editorials.html. Accessed January 21, 2004.

Turok, D.K., Ratcliffe, S.D., & Baxley, E.G. (2003). Management of gestational diabetes mellitus. *American Family Physician, 68*:1767–1772. www.aafp.org.afp/20031101/ 1767.html. Accessed January 21, 2004.

Woodside, D.B. (1995). A review of anorexia nervosa and bulimia nervosa. *Current Problems in Pediatrics, 25*:67.

Weight Control, Obesity Treatment and Prevention

Obesity and overweight continues to rise in the United States. According to the third National Health and Nutrition Examination survey, 97 million Americans are overweight or obese, and obesity costs approximately $100 billion dollars per year in health-related costs.

To assist primary care providers, the National Heart, Lung, and Blood Institute (NHLBI), in cooperation with the National Institute of Diabetes and Digestive and Kidney Diseases (NIDDK), published *Clinical Guidelines on the Identification, Evaluation, and Treatment of Overweight and Obesity in Adults.* These guidelines are intended to help healthcare providers improve their understanding and emphasize the importance of weight management in patient care. The guidelines are based on a review of published scientific literature. A brief overview of the important treatment goals and assessment tools are provided in this section. Most of the patient education handouts in this section have been reprinted from this report. The full report can be found at www.nhlbi.nih.gov./nhlbi/cardio/obes /prof/guidelns /ob_home.htm.

Strong evidence indicates that weight loss will improve blood pressure, reduce triglycerides, increase high-density lipoprotein (HDL) cholesterol, lower low-density (LDL) lipoprotein, and reduces blood glucose. Adults age 18 and older with a body mass index (BMI) ≥25 are considered at risk of developing comorbidity, including hypertension, high blood cholesterol, type 2 diabetes, coronary artery disease, and other disease. Healthcare providers can offer sound, reasonable guidance and support small weight loss goals, which can lead to major health improvements. The following ten steps offer a simple plan of action.

TEN STEPS TO TREATING OVERWEIGHT AND OBESITY IN THE PRIMARY CARE SETTING

These ten steps have been adapted from the NHLBI Obesity Education Initiative: *The Practical Guide to the Identification, Evaluation, and Treatment of Overweight and Obesity in Adults* NIH publication no. 02-4084.

1. Measure height and weight; estimate BMI. See Box 6-1 and assess status using Box 6-2.
2. Measure waist circumference (Box 6-3).
3. Assess any comorbidity (Box 6-4).
4. Using information gathered from above, assess the need for treatment.
5. Assess if the patient is ready and motivated to lose weight. Review past weight loss attempts, explain how this treatment will be different, offer encouragement and hope, but be realistic. The recommended 6-month weight loss goal for most individuals is 10% of total body weight.
6. Recommend a diet. A low-calorie diet, limited in total calories and designed to create a deficit of 500 to 1,000 calories per day, should lead to a weight loss of 1 to 2 pounds per week. The NHLBI guidelines suggest 1,000 to 1,200 calories per day for most women and 1,200 to 1,600 calories per day for most men and women who weigh 165 pounds or more or who exercise regularly. A referral to a registered dietitian should be considered for an individualized diet and ongoing support.
7. Discuss a physical activity goal. Initially, encourage moderate levels of exercise three to five

BOX 6-1 ■ Calculating Body Mass Index (BMI)

$$BMI = \frac{Weight\ (pounds)\ \times\ 703}{Height\ (inches)^2}$$

A person who weighs 164 pounds and is 68 inches tall has a BMI of 25

$$BMI = \frac{Weight\ (164)}{Height\ (68)^2} \times 703 = \frac{164}{4624} \times 703 = 25$$

BOX 6-2 ■ Classification of Overweight and Obesity by Body Mass Index

	BMI
Underweight	<18.5
Normal	18.5–24.9
Overweight	25.0–29.9
Obesity (class I)	30.0–34.9
(class II)	35.0–39.9
Extreme obesity (class III)	≥ 40

BOX 6-3 ■ Determining Waist Circumference

Measure waist just above the hipbone while standing. Excess abdominal fat can increase disease risk even if body mass index (BMI) is normal.

High Risk Weight Circumference
Men > 102 cm (>40 inches)
Women > 88 cm (>35 inches)

BOX 6-4 ■ Evaluating Risk Status

The presence of the following conditions heightens the need for weight reduction in obese persons:

Established coronary artery disease
Type 2 diabetes
Sleep apnea
Gynecologic abnormalities
Osteoarthritis
Gallstones
Stress incontinence
Cigarette smoking
Hypertension
High-density lipoprotein (HDL) cholesterol
Low-density lipoprotein (LDL) cholesterol
Physical inactivity
High triglycerides

BOX 6-5 ■ *Pharmacotherapy*

Weight loss drugs approved by the U.S. Food and Drug Administration (FDA) may be a useful adjunct to diet and exercise. Drugs can be used as adjunctive therapy in patients with a body mass index (BMI) ≥ 30 or ≥ 27 with other risk factors or diseases.

Weight Loss Drugs

Sibutramine (Meridia)

Dose: 5, 10, 15 mg. 10 mg po qd to start; may be increased to 15 mg or decreased to 5 mg
Action: Norepinephrine, dopamine, and serotonin reuptake inhibitor
Adverse effects: Increase in heart rate and blood pressure.

Orlistat (Xenical)

Dose: 120 mg po tid before meals.
Action: Inhibits pancreatic lipase, decreases fat absorption
Adverse effects: Decrease in absorption of fat-soluble vitamins, soft stools, and anal leakage.

"Ephedrine plus caffeine, and fluoxetine have also been tested for weight loss but are not approved for use in the treatment of obesity. Mazindol, diethylpropion, phentermine, benzphetamine, and phendimetrazine are approved for only short-term use for the treatment of obesity. Herbal preparations are not recommended as part of a weight loss program. These preparations have unpredictable amounts of active ingredients and unpredictable, and potentially harmful, effects."

Reprinted from *The Practical Guide Identification, Evaluation, and Treatment of Overweight and Obesity in Adults.* NIH Publication no. 02-4048, p. 36.
www.nhlbi.nih.gov./nhlbi/cardio/obes/prof/guidelns/ob_home.htm.

---

times a week for 30 to 45 minutes. Three 10-minute daily walks may be a realistic goal for many. Activity is an important part of weight maintenance and risk reduction (Box 6-5).

8. Provide the patient with educational materials about activity, behavior change, and food diary forms.
9. Review the weekly food and activity diary with the patient. Do not focus solely on weight lost; the healthcare provider can track improvement in blood sugar, lipids, and blood pressure.
10. Keep track of goals set with the patient by recording them and schedule the patient for follow-up in 2 to 4 weeks.

Resources

Obesity and Cancer: Questions and Answers
  http://cis.nci.nih.gov/fact/3_70.htm
Medline Plus topic: Obesity
  http://www.nlm.nih.gov/medlineplus/obesity.html
Weight-control Information Network
  www.niddk.nih.gov/health/nutrit/nutrit.htm

DIET BOOKS AND COMMERCIAL WEIGHT LOSS PROGRAMS

Obesity, a growing problem in America, is a major concern among adults. To address this concern, the diet book industry publishes many new titles annually. A search of Amazon.com with the words "diet books" will reveal over 72,000 titles. Most current best-selling diet books have been published since 1999 and the top sellers seem to promote carbohydrate restriction (Freedman, 2001).

Because of this proliferation of diet books and our obesity problem, almost every health-care provider will be asked about popular diets. Three principal components can be used to answer patient's questions (Cautioning Patients, 2001).

1. What is the quality of the proposed eating plan? In general, an adequate diet should include a variety of foods; whole food groups should not be eliminated.
2. What quantity of food is to be consumed? Both exercise and portion control should be considered.

3. How safe are the foods recommended as part of the diet? Foods can be considered safe if they are prepared using sanitary practices, such as pasteurization.

When talking to patients, ask them to consider the following six points to identify a sound weight loss program (National Cancer Institute):

- Does the diet include a variety of readily available low-fat, complex carbohydrate foods?
- The diet should not rely exclusively on single foods or food groups, prepackaged foods, or vitamin and mineral supplements.
- The diet should not exclude any food groups.
- The diet should include at least 1,200 calories per day.
- The diet should emphasize exercise as a weight control strategy along with moderate calorie restriction.
- The program addresses behavior changes, teaches skills to maintain weight loss, and provides relapse prevention strategies.

What About Low-Carbohydrate Diets?

Low carbohydrate diets have reemerged as the dominant weight loss tool. The first low- carbohydrate diet was written in 1860 by Dr. William Banting. The most popular-low carbohydrate diet today is *Atkins New Diet Revolution* by Robert Atkins, a book that has been on the *New York Times* bestsellers list for more than 5 years. In early 2004, the top selling diet book at Amazon.com was *The South Beach Diet* by Arthur Agastson, also a low-carbohydrate diet.

When researchers conducted a systematic review of efficacy and safety of low-carbohydrate diets, they found "insufficient evidence to make recommendations for or against the use of low-carbohydrate diets. . . "(Bravata et al., 2003). The authors included 107 articles in their review, reporting data for 3,268 participants. Ultimately, the authors concluded weight loss within the studies occurred because of decreased caloric intake and duration of diet, not reduced carbohydrate content. Two additional reports find weight loss does occur, but at a much more modest rate than publicity and anecdotes might suggest. Another study of obese men and women with an average weight of 215 pounds found that they had lost 9 pounds over 12 months (15 pounds in the first 6 months followed by a 6 pound regain) (Foster et al., 2003). And, of 132 individuals with an average weight of 288 pounds, found that they had lost 12 pounds at 6 months (Samaha et al., 2003). A total weight loss of 9 and 12 pounds will improve health, but many dieters expect to do much better, potentially perpetuating the cycle of dieting (Box 6-6).

BOX 6-6 ■ *Battle of the Diet Books*

None of the diet books have been studied long term and no claims about their efficacy can be made.

Title	Is the Diet Healthy?
South Beach Diet Arthur Agatston	Mostly healthy foods
The Ultimate Weight Solution Phil McGraw	Mostly healthy foods
Dr. Atkins' New Diet Revolution Robert C. Atkins	High in red meat; may raise risk of colon or prostate cancer Lacks fiber, vegetables, and fruit; may increase risk of heart disease, stroke, cancer, diverticulosis, and chronic constipation
Good Carbs, Bad Carbs Joanna Burani & Linda Rao	Mostly healthy foods Sponge cake, chips, chocolate have a low-glycemic-index, but may be unhealthy
Eat Right for Your Type Peter J D'Adamo & Catherine Whitney	Diet varies by blood type; no one menu to evaluate
Weight Watchers New Complete Cookbook	Mostly healthy foods

BOX 6-6 ■ *Continued*

The New Glucose Revolution Jennie Brand-Miller, Thomas Wolever, Kaye Foster-Powell & Stephen Colagiuri	Mostly healthy foods
Enter the Zone Barry Sears	Mostly healthy foods
The Fat Flush Plan Ann Louise Gittleman	Mostly healthy foods; too much red meat and eggs
Eat More, Weigh Less Dean Ornish	Mostly healthy foods

Source: Liebman, B. *Nutrition Action Health Letter, January/February,* 2004. A brief look at popular diets can also be accessed at the Center for Science web page http://www.cspinet.org/nah/5_00/diet.htm.

CALCIUM AND WEIGHT LOSS

The dairy industry is promoting the role of calcium in the treatment of obesity. One study found a diet rich in calcium may promote a healthy body weight and produce a greater weight and fat loss while on a low calorie diet (Zemel, 2002). The role of calcium in weight loss is being marketed aggressively, but the Center for Science in the Public Interest states that the lead researcher of this study has a patent on treating obesity with a high calcium diet (Liebman, 2004). Calcium is an essential nutrient and healthcare providers should encourage adequate consumption. Whether it is the key to weight loss requires further study. Use the patient education Handout 6-05 to educate your patients about calcium-rich food sources.

THE GLYCEMIC INDEX

The glycemic index (GI) has been around since 1981 (Jenkins, 1981), but it took the low-carbohydrate diet craze of this century to make it a household word. Many weight-loss diets use it to justify their eating plans, but most of these diet books oversimplify how GI works. The GI is determined by measuring blood glucose after a single food is consumed. The rise in blood glucose is compared with the rise caused from a control food such as white bread or sugar. The average change in blood glucose levels relative to the control food becomes the food's GI.

Many factors will affect GI when eaten as part of a real meal and not as an individual test food. How the food is processed, stored, ripened, cooked, and even chopped or pureed have an impact the GI of a food. The fat and fiber content in a given food will alter digestion and raise the level in blood glucose and the GI. When cereal is mixed with milk, or bread topped with peanut butter, the GI of the whole meal will be different from that of the individual foods. Even the amount of total food, usually 50 g in a test meal, but often larger at a real meal, is likely to also have an impact on GI. All these variables make it difficult to apply the GI to daily food selection.

The GI does hold promise for helping people lose weight. David Ludwig at Children's Hospital in Boston has found that when obese teenage boys were fed a high-GI meal, they had greater serum insulin levels and ate more food than after eating a medium or low-GI menu (Ludwig, 1999). The GI, however, is often simplified into good carbs and bad carbs. Whole grain foods are generally thought to have a low GI and are considered "good," whereas foods made with white flour have a higher GI and are "bad." Look at the GI content of the food listed below (Box 6-7) and see the numbers that appear contradictory. When the GI leads people to avoid bananas, kiwi, and papaya because they are a high GI fruit, that is not advantageous.

Glycemic load (GL) is another tool that helps researchers measure the quantity and quality of a food's effect on insulin and blood glucose. The GL is determined by multiplying a food's GI by the carbohydrate content of the food. Meal plans based on the glycemic load of food have not yet been made, making its practical application speculative. Refer patients to Handout 6-18 (Box 6-7).

POLYOLS: SUGAR ALCOHOLS

Sugar alcohols are neither a sugar nor an alcohol but they taste sweet and have fewer calories than sugar. They are often used to replace sugar or combined with non-caloric sweeteners (e.g., aspartame) to sweetened food without adding a lot of calories. They are gaining in popularity and healthcare providers are likely to be

BOX 6-7 ■ *Glycemic Index (GI) and Glycemic Load (GL) of Selected Foods*

Glucose = 100

Breakfast Cereal	GI	GL
Kellogg's All Bran	30	4
Kellogg's cocoa Puffs	77	20
Kellogg's Cornflakes	92	24
Old-fashioned oatmeal	42	9

Grains and Pasta		
Brown rice	50	16
Instant rice	87	36
Spaghetti	38	18

Bread		
Bagel	72	35
White bread	70	10
Whole wheat bread	77	9

Cookies and Cakes		
Oatmeal	55	12
Milk arrowroot	69	12
Chocolate, frosted, Betty Crocker	38	20
Oatbran muffin	69	24
Waffles	76	10

Vegetables		
Beet, canned	64	5
Carrots	47	3
Peas, green	48	3
Potato, new	57	12

Fruit and Juice		
Apple	38	6
Banana	51	13
Grapefruit	25	3
Kiwi	53	6
Watermelon	72	4
Apple juice	40	12
Orange juice	52	12

Milk		
Whole	27	3
Skim	32	4
Chocolate	42	13
Yogurt, low-fat	33	10

Source from Mahan, L. K., & Escott-Stump, S. (2004). *Krauses' Food, Nutrition, & Diet Therapy*. Philadelphia: WB Saunders, Appendix 54, p. 1271.
More information about the GI of food can be found in Foster-Powell, K., & Brand Miller, J. (1995). International tables of glycemic index *American Journal of Clinical Nutrition, 871S–890S.*

BOX 6-8 ■ *Polyols: How They Appear on the Label*

Sugar alcohols include erythritol, hydrogenated starch hydrolysates (polyglycitol, polyglucitol), isomalt, lactitol, maltitol, mannitol, sorbitol, and xylitol.

asked about their use and limitations. Polyols do not promote tooth decay and they can be used by people with diabetes as a "free" food if the total carbohydrate in a serving is <10 g. For some individuals, consuming 50 g of polyols can result in a laxative effect. For more information go to www.caloriecontrol.org and search "sugar alcohols" (Box 6-8).

EXERCISE

Physical activity should be part of a comprehensive weight-loss program and may confer the following benefits:

1. Modestly contributes to weight loss in overweight and obese adults
2. May decrease abdominal fat
3. Increases cardiorespiratory fitness
4. May help with maintenance of weight loss

The National Heart, Lung, and Blood Institute (NHLBI) recommends that physical activity be part of weight-loss therapy and weight maintenance. Initially, encourage moderate levels of activity for 30 to 45 minutes, 3 to 5 days per week. Define moderate activity with patients using the patient education handouts 6-13 and 6-14. Many patients find a step pedometer to be very helpful when increasing activity. Patients are asked to wear a pedometer and measure their steps for 1 day and set goals to increase the number until they reach 10,000 steps most days of the week. Obtaining 10,000 steps is a level of exercise equal to 30 minutes of moderate activity for most individuals. Inactive and very overweight individuals may need to set goals well below 10,000. A tool for recording steps is found in Handout 6-15.

What Really Works

It is a popularly cited (and possibly incorrect) statistic that the rate of permanent weight loss is <10% (Cautioning Patients, 2001). James Hill, PhD at the University of Colorado Health Sciences in Denver Colorado (Wing & Hill, 2001) (National Weight Control Registry, 2004) has created a weight-loss registry (The National Weight Loss Registry) that includes more than 3,000 successful losers. These are

people who kept an average weight loss of 66 pounds off for 5.5 years.

How they do it:

■ Three-quarters of the registry members weigh themselves once per week
■ Some members keep food diaries
■ Most eat five small meals each day
■ Breakfast is never skipped
■ Less than 1% ate a low-carbohydrate diet for maintenance
■ Most eat a low-fat, high-carbohydrate diet
■ Losers tend to exercise about an hour a day, or walk 12,000 steps (5 to 6 miles) per day
■ Many of the successful losers have tried and failed diets several times

The National Weight Loss Registry offers inspiration and hope to those who want to lose weight. It proves that long-term commitment to exercise and healthy eating do lead to weight loss. Individuals who have maintained a weight loss of 30 pounds for a minimum of 1 year are eligible to join the registry. For more information call 1-800-606-NWCR.

TREATMENT OF OVERWEIGHT CHILDREN AND ADOLESCENTS

Since 1980, obesity rates have doubled among American children and tripled among adolescents (CDC, 2004). About 9 million American young people are considered overweight. In the *Surgeon General's Call to Action To Prevent and Decrease Overweight and Obesity* (USDHHS, 2002), the health factors associated with overweight in children include high cholesterol, high blood pressure, and increased risk for type 2 diabetes and some form of cancer. Social discrimination, low self-esteem, and depression are also factors. Overweight adolescents have a 70% chance of becoming overweight or obese adults and this increases to 80% if one or more parents are overweight.

To combat the problem of childhood obesity, the Maternal and Child Health Bureau, Health Resources and Services Administration, the Department of Health and Human Service convened a committee of pediatric obesity experts to make recommendations for physicians, nurse practitioners, and nutritionists to guide the evaluation and treatment of overweight children and adolescents (Barlow & Deitz, 1998).

The committee made the following recommendations for healthcare providers working with children and adolescents. The full article can be accessed at: http://www.pediatrics.org/cgi/content/full/102/3/e29.

- Children with health complications and a body mass index (BMI) ≥85th percentile or those with or without complications with a BMI ≥95th percentile should undergo evaluation and possible treatment.
- Clinicians should be alert to rare causes of obesity, including genetic syndromes, endocrinologic diseases, and psychological disorders.
- Clinicians should screen for hypertension, dyslipidemia, orthopedic conditions, sleep disorders, gall bladder disease, and insulin resistance.
- Consult with a pediatric obesity specialist when the following conditions are present: pseudotumor cerebri, obesity-related sleep disorder, orthopedic problems, massive obesity, and obesity in children <2 years.

Recommendations for treatment include the following:

- Assess patient and family readiness to change.

"A practical way to address readiness is to ask all members of the family how concerned they are about the patient's weight, whether they believe weight loss is possible, and what practices need to be changed" (Barlow & Deitz, 1998).

- Assess diet and physical activity habits. Ask the family to keep a food and activity record and assess it.
- Begin treatment early; involve the whole family and make permanent changes slowly. Use a food and activity record to identify a positive goal, such as better snack choices, and including more fruits and vegetables.

Specific parenting skills to promote (Barlow, 1998)

- Find reasons to praise the child's behavior
- Never use food as a reward
- Establish daily meal and snack times
- Parents are to determine what and when food is to be served and the child can decide whether to eat
- Offer healthy food options
- Remove temptations
- Be a role model
- Be consistent

The primary goals for treatment include the following:

- Healthy eating and activity
- Weight maintenance versus weight loss (depending on age and BMI).

Body Mass Index for Children

Body mass index is used differently with children than it is with adults. BMI provides a guideline based on weight and height to determine underweight and overweight. In boys and girls, BMI is plotted according to sex and age because boys and girls mature differently in their body fatness with age. To determine BMI, measure height and weight and refer to Box 6-1.

Plot BMI using the BMI for age percentiles for boys, 2 to 20 years and BMIndex for age percentiles for girls, 2 to 20 years. These charts can be downloaded at www.cdc.gov/nchs/data/nhanes/growthcharts/set1/all.pdf (page 15 and 16).

To interpret BMI for age in children and adolescents, establish cut-off points to identify underweight and overweight. The extremes in BMI for age established by the Centers for Disease Control and Prevention that raise concern in children age 2 to 20 years of age are as follows:

Underweight	BMI for age <5th percentile
At risk for overweight	BMI for age ≥85th percentile to <95th percentile
Overweight	BMI for age ≥95th percentile

More information about the correct use and interpretation of BMI for age can be found at the Centers for Disease Control web site BMI for Children and Teens (also referred to as BMI for age): www.cdc.gov/nccdphp/dnpa/bmi/bmi-for-age.htm.

RESOURCES

Weight programs for Children
Shapedown: A 10-week Program for Parents and Child
www.shapedown.com
KidShape
A family-Based Pediatric Weight Management Program
888-600-6444
www.kidshape.com
American Dietetic Association
www.eatright.org
American Heart Association
www.americanheart.org; click Healthy Lifestyle
USDA Center for Nutrition Policy and Promotion
www.usda.gov/cnpp
Weight Loss Information Network
www.niddk.nih.gov/health/nutrit/win.htm

PATIENT EDUCATION HANDOUTS

The following handouts are intended to assist primary care providers in helping their patients eat well and exercise more. Most are reprinted from the National Institutes of Health and National Heart, Lung, and Blood Institute *Clinical Guidelines on the Identification, Evaluation, and Treatment of Overweight and Obesity in Adults: The Evidence Report*. All reports, including the *Full Report*, *Executive Summary*, and *Practical Guide* can be accessed at www.nhlbi.nih.gov./guidelines/obesity/ob_home.htm

6-1   Body Mass Index

BMI measures your weight in relation to your height, and is closely associated with measures of body fat. You can calculate your BMI using this formula:

$$\text{BMI} = \frac{\text{weight (pounds)} \times 703}{\text{height squared (inches}^2)}$$

For example, for someone who is 5 feet, 7 inches tall and weighs 220 pounds, the calculation would look like this:

$$\text{BMI} = \frac{220 \text{ pounds} \times 703}{67 \text{ inches} \times 67 \text{ inches}} = \frac{154660}{4489} = 34.45$$

A BMI of 18.5 to 24.9 is considered healthy. A person with a BMI of 25 to 29.9 is considered overweight, and a person with a BMI of 30 or more is considered obese.

Because BMI does not show the difference between fat and muscle, it does not always accurately predict when weight could lead to health problems. For example, someone with a lot of muscle (such as a body builder) may have a BMI in the unhealthy range, but still be healthy and have little risk of developing diabetes or having a heart attack.

BMI also may not accurately reflect body fat in people who are very short (under 5 feet) and in older people, who tend to lose muscle mass as they age. But for most people, BMI is a reliable way to tell if your weight is putting your health at risk.

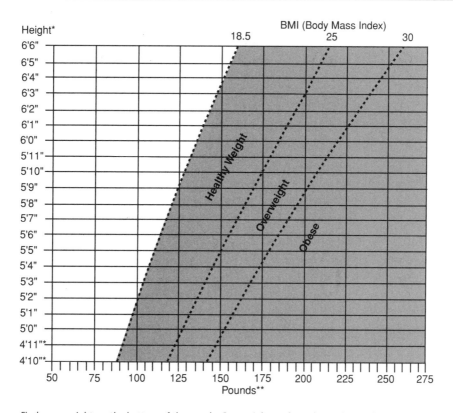

Find your weight on the bottom of the graph. Go straight up from that point until you come to the line that matches your height. Then look to find your weight group. The higher your BMI is over 25, the greater chance you may have of developing health problems.

* Without shoes.   **Without clothes.

Source: Weight-control Information Network www.niddk.nih.gov/ health/nutrit/nutrit.htm

A LOW-CALORIE SHOPPING LIST

Make a shopping list. Include the items you need for your menus and any low-calorie basics you need to restock in your kitchen.

Dairy Foods

Low-fat (1%, 0) or fat-free (skim) milk

Low-fat or reduced-fat cottage cheese

Low-fat cheeses

Low-fat or nonfat yogurt

Light or diet margarine (tub, squeeze, or spray)

Reduced-fat or fat-free sour cream

Eggs or egg substitute

Other_____

Breads, Muffins, Rolls

Choose whole grain foods as often as possible. Look for the word "whole" in the ingredients list and compare fiber content on the nutrition facts panel to find products that are made from whole grains.

Bread, bagels, pita bread

English muffins

Yeast breads (whole wheat, rye, pumpernickel, multigrain, raisin)

Corn tortillas (not fried)

Low-fat flour tortillas

Fat-free biscuit mix

Rice crackers

Challah

Other_____

Cereals, Crackers, Rice, Noodles, and Pasta

Plain cereal, dry or cooked

Saltines, soda crackers (low sodium or unsalted tops)

Graham crackers

Other low-fat crackers_____

_____

Rice (brown, white, etc.)

Pasta (noodles, spaghetti)

Bulgur, couscous, kasha

Potato mixes (made without fat)

Rice mixes (made without fat)

Wheat mixes

Tabouli grain salad

Hominy

Polenta

Polvillo

Hominy grits

Quinoa

Millet

Amaranth

Oatmeal

Other_____

Meat and Other Protein

White meat chicken and turkey (skin off)

Fish (not in batter)

Beef, round or sirloin

Extra lean ground beef (e.g., ground round)

Pork tenderloin

95% fat-free lunch meats or low-fat deli meats

Meat equivalents:

Tofu or bean curd

Beans (see list)

Eggs/egg substitute (see dairy list)

Other_____

Fruit (Fresh, Canned, and Frozen)

Apples	Pears
Bananas	Grapes
Peaches	Grapefruit
Oranges	Apricots

Dried fruits	Lemons
Cherries	Limes
Plums	Plantains
Melons	Mangoes

Other_____

Exotic Fresh Fruits

Kiwi	Guanabana
Olives	Mamey
Figs	Zapote
Quinces	Guava
Currants	Starfruit
Persimmons	Ugli fruit
Pomegranates	Dried pickle plums
Anon	Litchee nuts
Caimito	Winter melon
Cherimoya	Papayas

Other_____

Canned Fruit in Juice or Water

Canned pineapple

Applesauce

Other canned fruits (mixed or plain)

Frozen fruits

Frozen blueberries

Frozen raspberries

Frozen 100% fruit juice

Other_____

Dried Fruits

Raisins or dried fruit (these tend to be higher in calories than fresh fruit)

Vegetables

Fresh

Broccoli	Cucumber
Peas	Asparagus
Corn	Mushrooms
Cauliflower	Carrots or celery
Squash	Onions
Green beans	Potatoes
Green leafy vegetables	Tomatoes
Spinach	Green peppers
Lettuce	Chilies
Cabbage	Tomatillos
Artichokes	

Other_____

Canned (Low Sodium or No Salt Added)

Canned tomatoes

Tomato sauce or pasta

Other canned vegetables

Canned vegetable soup (reduced sodium)

Frozen (Without Added Fats)

Broccoli

Spinach

Mixed medley, and so forth

Yucca

Other_____

Exotic Fresh Vegetables

Okra	Boniato
Dandelions	Chayote
Eggplant	Borenjena
Grape leaves	Plantain
Mustard greens	Cassava
Kale	Prickly pear cactus
Leeks	Bamboo shoots

Chinese celery

Bean sprouts

Water chestnuts

Amaranth

Bok choy

Choy sum

Burdock root

Calabacita

Napa cabbage

Sea vegetables

Taro

Rhubarb

Seaweed

Other_____

Beans and Legumes (If Canned, Choose No Salt Added)

Lentils

Black beans

Red beans (kidney beans)

Navy beans

Black beans

Pinto beans

Blackeyed peas

Fava beans

Mung beans

Italian white beans

Great white northern beans

Chickpeas (garbanzo beans)

Dried beans, peas, and lentils (without flavoring packets)

Canned bean soup

Baking Items

Flour

Sugar

Imitation butter (flakes or buds)

Nonstick cooking spray

Canned evaporated milk, fat free (skim) or low fat (1%)

Nonfat dry milk powder

Cocoa powder, unsweetened

Baking powder

Baking soda

Cornstarch

Unflavored gelatin

Gelatin, any flavor (reduced calorie)

Pudding mixes (reduced calorie)

Angel food cake mix

Other low-fat mixes

Other_____

Frozen Foods

Frozen fish fillets (unbreaded)

Egg substitute

Frozen 100% fruit juice (no sugar added)

Frozen fruits (no sugar added)

Frozen vegetables (plain)

Vegetarian burgers

Frozen whole grain waffles

Frozen ravioli

Frozen potato pierogi

Frozen tortellini

Other_____

Condiments, Sauces, Seasonings, and Spreads

Salad dressing

Mustard

Catsup

Barbecue sauce

Jam

Jelly

Spices

Flavored vinegars

Hoisin sauce, plum sauce

Salsa or picante sauce

Canned green chilies

Soy sauce (low sodium)

Bouillon cubes or granules (low sodium)

Other_____

Beverages

No-calorie drink mixes

Unsweetened iced tea

Carbonated water

Water

These low-calorie alternatives provide new ideas for old favorites. When making a food choice, remember to consider vitamins and minerals. Some foods provide most of their calories from sugar and fat, but have few if any vitamins and minerals. This guide is not meant to be an exhaustive list. Read labels to find out just how many calories are in the specific products you decide to buy.

Higher-Fat Foods	Lower-Fat Foods
Dairy	
Evaporated whole milk	Evaporated fat-free (skim) or reduced-fat (2%) milk
Whole milk	Low-fat (1%), or fat-free (skim) milk
Ice cream	Sorbet, sherbet, low-fat or fat-free frozen yogurt, or ice
Milk	(check label for calorie content)
Whipping cream	Imitation whipped cream (made with fat-free [skim] milk) or low-fat vanilla yogurt
Sour cream	Plain low-fat yogurt
Cream cheese	Neufchatel or "light" cream cheese or fat-free cream cheese
Cheese (cheddar, Swiss, Monterey jack)	Reduced-calorie cheese, low-calorie processed cheeses, and so forth
American cheese	Fat-free cheese
Regular (4%) cottage cheese	Low-fat (1%) or reduced-fat (2%) cottage cheese
Whole milk mozzarella	Part skim milk, low-moisture mozzarella cheese
Whole milk ricotta cheese	Part skim milk ricotta cheese
Coffee cream or nondairy creamer (liquid, powder)	Low-fat (1%) or reduced-fat (2%) milk or nonfat dry milk powder
Cereals, Grains, and Pasta	
Raman noodles	Rice or noodles (spaghetti, macaroni, and so forth)
Pasta with white sauce (alfredo)	Pasta with red sauce (marinara)
Pasta with cheese sauce	Pasta with vegetables (primavera)
Granola	Bran flakes, crispy rice, cooked grits, oatmeal, reduced-fat granola
Meat, Fish, Poultry	
Cold cuts or luncheon meats (bologna, salami, and so forth)	Low-fat cold cuts (95% to 97% fat-free lunch meats, low-fat pressed meats)

Reprinted from Clinical Guidelines on the Identification, Evaluation, and Treatment of Overweight and Obesity in Adults. The full report can be accessed at http://www.nhlbi.nih.gov/guidelines/obesity/ob_gdlns.htm.

Hot dogs (regular)	Lower-fat hot dogs
Bacon or sausage	Canadian bacon or lean ham
Regular ground beef	Extra lean ground beef or ground turkey
Chicken or turkey with skin. Duck or goose	Chicken or turkey without skin (white meat)
Oil-packed tuna	Water-packed tuna (rinse to reduce sodium)
Beef (chuck, rib, brisket)	Beef (round, loin) trimmed of external fat (choose select grades)
Pork (spareribs, untrimmed loin)	Pork tenderloin or trimmed, lean smoked ham
Frozen breaded fish or fried Fish or fried fish (homemade or commercial)	Fish or shellfish, not breaded (fresh, frozen, canned in water)
Frozen TV dinners (containing >13g of fat per serving)	Frozen TV dinners (containing <13 g of fat and lower in sodium)
Chorizo sausage	Turkey sausage, drained well (read label) or vegetarian sausage (made with tofu)

Baked Goods

Croissants, brioches, etc.	Hard French rolls or soft brown and serve rolls
Donuts, sweet rolls, muffins, scones, or pastries	English muffins, bagels, reduced-fat muffins or scones
Party crackers	Low-fat crackers (choose lower in sodium), saltine or soda crackers
Cake (pound, chocolate, yellow)	Cake (angel food, white, gingerbread)
Cookies	Graham crackers, ginger snaps, fig bars (compare calorie level)

Snacks and Sweets

Nuts	Popcorn (air-popped or light microwave) fruits, vegetable sticks
Ice cream cone or bar	Frozen yogurt, frozen fruit or chocolate pudding bars
Custards or puddings (made with whole milk)	Pudding (made with skim milk)

Fats, Oils, and Salad Dressings

Regular margarine or butter	Light spread margarine, diet margarine, or whipped butter, tub or squeeze bottle
Regular mayonnaise	Mustard
Regular salad dressing	Lemon juice, or plain or herb flavored or wine vinegar
Butter or margarine on toast or bread	Jelly, jam, or honey on bread or toast

Solid shortening or lard	Nonstick cooking spray
	As a substitute for shortening, use applesauce or prune puree in baked goods

Miscellaneous

Canned cream soups	Canned broth-based soups
Canned beans and franks	Canned baked beans in tomato sauce
Gravy (homemade with fat or milk)	Gravy mixes made with water or homemade with fat skimmed off and fat-free milk
Fudge sauce	Chocolate sauce
Refried beans with lard	Salsa

Fat-free Versus Regular: Calorie Comparison

A calorie is a calorie is a calorie . . . whether it comes from fat or carbohydrate. Anything eaten in excess can lead to weight gain. Lose weight by eating fewer calories and increasing your physical activity. Reduce the amount of fat and saturated fat to limit overall calorie intake. Eating fat-free or reduced-fat foods is not always the answer to weight loss. For example, if twice as many fat-free cookies as regular cookies are eaten, overall calorie intake is not reduced. The following list of foods and their fat-free varieties will show that just because a product is fat-free, does not mean that it is "calorie-free." And calories do count!

Fat-free or Reduced Fat	Calories	Regular	Calories
Reduced-fat peanut butter, 2 tablespoons	190	Regular peanut butter 2 tablespoons	190
Cookies		Cookies	
Reduced-fat chocolate chip cookie 1 cookie	128	Regular chocolate chip cookie 1 cookie	136
Fat-free fig cookie 1 cookie	70	Fig cookie 1 cookie	50
Ice cream		Ice cream	
Premium nonfat frozen yogurt ½ cup	190	Regular ice cream ½ cup	180
Premium reduced-fat ice cream ½ cup	190	Butterscotch caramel topping 2 tablespoons	130
Fat-free caramel topping, 2 tablespoons	130	Regular granola cereal ¼ cup	130
Reduced-fat granola cereal ¼ cup	110	Regular croissant roll 1 roll	130
Reduced-fat croissant roll 1 roll	110	Regular tortilla chips 1 oz	130
Baked tortilla chips 1 oz	110	Breakfast bar 1 bar	130
Reduced-fat breakfast bar 1 bar	140		

Reprinted from *Clinical Guidelines on the Identification, Evaluation, and Treatment of Overweight and Obesity in Adults.* The full report can be accessed at http://www.nhlbi.nih.gov/guidelines/obesity/ob_gdlns.htm

Good Sources of Calcium

Calcium is not just for growing children. It is an important mineral that adults need to keep their bones and teeth strong and their muscles functioning. Many people do not get enough calcium every day. Following is a list of good sources of calcium and tips on how to include more calcium in your diet everyday.

Source	Calcium (mg)	Source	Calcium (mg)
Milk (1 cup)		**Ice Cream**	
Whole	300	Regular, ½ cup	90
2% reduced fat	300	Lowfat, ½ cup	100
1% lowfat*	300		
Fat-free*	300	**Frozen Yogurt**	
		Lowfat, ½ cup	100
Yogurt* (1 cup)			
Plain, lowfat	415	**Miscellaneous**	
Flavored, lowfat	315	Beans, dried cooked, 1 cup	90
Plain, fat-free	315	Salmon, with bones, 3 oz	205
		Tofu, processed with calcium sulfate, ½ cup	435
Cheese (1 oz)		Spinach, fresh cooked	94
Reduced-fat Cheddar*	120	Turnip greens, fresh cooked, 1 cup	100
American	175	Kale, fresh cooked	94
Swiss cheese	270	Broccoli, fresh cooked	75
Mozzarella, part-skim	185	Waffle, 7-in diameter	180
		Pancakes, (2) 4-in diameter	115
Cottage Cheese (½ cup)		Pizza, with vegetables, ¼ 12-in pie	180
2% reduced-fat	75		
Calcium-fortified cottage cheese	300		

CALCIUM REQUIREMENTS

Age	Women (mg)	Men (mg)
19–24	1,200	1,200
25–50	1,000	800

Reprinted from *Clinical Guidelines on the Identification, Evaluation, and Treatment of Overweight and Obesity in Adults*. The full report can be accessed at http://www.nhlbi.nih.gov/guidelines/obesity/ob_gdlns.htm

TIPS FOR FITTING IN CALCIUM

- Eat cereal with fat-free milk; add fresh fruit.
- Drink an extra glass of milk every day; try calcium-fortified milk.
- Spread calcium-fortified cottage cheese* on crackers or bagel; add fresh fruit.
- Drink calcium-fortified orange juice*.
- Blend a yogurt smoothie with lowfat or fat-free yogurt and milk and fresh or frozen fruit.
- Make instant pudding with lowfat or fat-free milk.
- Choose frozen yogurt for dessert instead of cake or cookies.
- Add a slice of lowfat or fat-free cheese to sandwiches.
- Substitute calcium-fortified tofu for chicken, shrimp, or beef in stir-fries.
- Sauté greens (kale, bok choy, collard greens) in cooking spray with lemon juice and herbs.

---

* Lowfat and non-fat dairy foods are still good sources of calcium. Read food labels for products with added calcium.

LOW-CALORIE, LOW-FAT COOKING

Serving Methods

Cooking low-calorie, low-fat dishes may not take a long time, but best intentions can be lost with the addition of butter or other added fats at the table. It is important to learn how certain ingredients can add unwanted calories and fat to low-fat dishes, making them no longer lower in fat! The following list provides examples of lower fat cooking methods and tips on how to serve your lowfat dishes.

LOWFAT COOKING METHODS

These cooking methods tend to be lower in fat

- Bake
- Broil
- Microwave
- Roast: vegetables and chicken without skin
- Steam
- Lightly stir-fry or sauté in cooking spray, small amounts of vegetable oil, or reduced sodium broth
- Grill seafood, chicken, or vegetables

HOW TO SAVE CALORIES AND FAT

Look at the following examples on how to save calories and fat when preparing and serving foods. You might be surprised at how easy it is!

- Two tablespoons of butter on a baked potato can add an extra 200 calories and 22 g of fat! However, ¼ cup salsa only adds 18 calories and no fat!
- Two tablespoons of regular clear Italian salad dressing will add an extra 136 calories and 14g of fat. Reduced fat Italian dressing only adds 30 calories and 2 g of fat!

Try these low-fat flavorings during preparation or at the table

- Herbs: oregano, basil, cilantro, thyme, parsley, sage, or rosemary.
- Spices: cinnamon, nutmeg, pepper, or paprika
- Reduced-fat or fat-free salad dressing
- Mustard

Reprinted from *Clinical Guidelines on the Identification, Evaluation, and Treatment of Overweight and Obesity in Adults.* The full report can be accessed at http://www.nhlbi.nih.gov/guidelines/obesity/ob_gdlns.htm

- Catsup
- Fat-free or reduced-fat mayonnaise
- Fat-free or reduced-fat sour cream
- Fat-free or reduced-fat yogurt
- Reduced sodium soy sauce
- Salsa
- Lemon or lime juice
- Vinegar
- Horseradish
- Fresh ginger
- Sprinkle of butter flavor (not made with real butter)
- Red pepper flakes
- Sprinkle of parmesan cheese (stronger flavor than most cheese)
- Sodium-free salt substitute
- Jelly or fruit preserves on toast or bagels

GENERAL TIPS FOR HEALTHY DINING OUT

Whether or not you are trying to lose weight, you can eat healthy when dining out or bringing in food, if you know how. The following tips will help you move toward healthier eating as you limit your calories, fat, saturated fat, cholesterol, and sodium when eating out. You are the customer:

- Ask for what you want! Most restaurants will honor your requests.
- Ask questions! Don't be intimidated by the menu; your server can tell you how foods are prepared or suggest substitutes on the menu.
- If you wish to reduce portion sizes, order appetizers as your main meal.

Limiting your calories and fat can be easy when you know what to order. Try asking questions when you call ahead or before you order. Ask the restaurant "Do you or would you on request . . .":

- Serve margarine (rather than butter) with the meal?
- Serve fat-free (skim) milk rather than whole milk or cream?
- Use less oil when cooking?
- Trim visible fat off poultry or meat?
- Leave all butter, gravy, or sauces off a side dish or entrée?
- Serve salad dressing on the side?
- Accommodate special requests if made in advance by telephone or in person?
- Above all else, do not get discouraged. Several healthy choices are usually available at most restaurants.

READING THE MENU

- Choose lower calorie, low-fat cooking methods. Look for terms such as steamed, in its own juice (au jus), garden fresh, broiled, baked, roasted, poached, tomato juice, dry boiled (in wine or lemon juice), and lightly sautéed or stir-fried.
- Be aware of foods high in calories, fat, and saturated fat. Watch for terms such as butter sauce, fried, crispy, creamed, in cream or cheese sauce, au gratin, au fromage, escalloped, parmesan, hollandaise, béarnaise, marinated (in oil), stewed, basted, sautéed, stir-fried, casserole, hash, prime, pot pie, and pastry crust.

SPECIFIC TIPS FOR HEALTHY CHOICES

Breakfast

- Fresh fruit or small glass of citrus juice
- Whole grain bread, bagel, or English muffin with jelly or honey

---

Reprinted from *Clinical Guidelines on the Identification, Evaluation, and Treatment of Overweight and Obesity in Adults*. The full report can be accessed at http://www.nhlbi.nih.gov/guidelines/obesity/ob_gdlns.htm.

- Whole grain cereal with lowfat (1%) or fat-free milk
- Oatmeal with fat-free milk topped with fruit
- Omelet made with egg whites or egg substitute
- Multigrain pancakes without butter on top
- Nonfat yogurt (try adding cereal or fresh fruit)

BEVERAGES

- Water with lemon
- Flavored sparkling water (noncaloric)
- Juice spritzer (half fruit juice and half sparkling water)
- Iced tea
- Tomato juice (reduced sodium)

BREAD

Most bread and breadsticks are low in calories and in fat. The calories add up when you add butter, margarine, or olive oil to the bread. Also, eating a lot of bread in addition to your meal will fill you up with extra, unwanted calories and not leave enough room for fruits and vegetables.

APPETIZERS

- Steamed seafood
- Shrimp cocktail (limit cocktail sauce; it is high in sodium)
- Melons or fresh fruit
- Bean soups
- Salad with reduced fat dressing (or add lemon juice or vinegar)

ENTRÉES

- Poultry, fish, shellfish, and vegetable dishes are healthy choices.
- Pasta with red sauce or with vegetables (primavera) is a good choice.
- Look for terms such as baked, broiled, steamed, poached, lightly sautéed, or stir-fried.
- Ask for sauces and dressings on the side.
- Limit the amount of butter, margarine, and salt you use at the table.

SALAD AND SALAD BARS

- Fresh greens: lettuce and spinach
- Fresh vegetables: tomato, mushroom, carrots, cucumber, peppers, onion, radishes, and broccoli
- Beans, chick peas, and kidney beans

- Skip the nonvegetable choices: deli meats, bacon, egg, cheese, croutons
- Choose lower-calorie, reduced-fat or fat-free dressing, lemon juice, or vinegar

SIDE DISH

- Plain vegetables and starches (rice, potato, noodles) make good additions to meals and can also be combined for a low-calorie alternative to high-calorie entrées.
- Ask for side dishes without butter or margarine.
- Ask for mustard, salsa, or low-fat yogurt instead of sour cream.

DESSERT AND COFFEE

- Fresh fruit
- Nonfat frozen yogurt
- Sherbert or fruit sorbet (these are usually fat free, but check the calorie content)
- Share a dessert
- Ask for low-fat milk for your coffee (instead of cream or half-n-half)

TIPS FOR ETHNIC RESTAURANTS

If you are dining out or bringing in, it is easy to find healthy foods. Knowing about American food terms, as well as other ethnic cuisine, can help make your dining experience healthy and enjoyable! The following list includes healthy food choices (lower in calories and fat) and terms to look for when making your selection.

Chinese

Choose more often:

- Steamed
- Jum (poached)/chu (boiled)
- Kow (roasted)
- Shu (barbecued)
- Hoison sauce with assorted Chinese vegetables: broccoli, mushroom, onion, cabbage, snow peas, scallions, bamboo shoots, water chestnuts, asparagus
- Oyster sauce (made from seafood)
- Lightly stir-fried in mild sauce
- Cooked in light wine sauce
- Hot and spicy tomato sauce
- Sweet and sour sauce
- Hot mustard sauce
- Reduced sodium soy sauce
- Dishes without monosodium glutamate (MSG) added

- Garnished with spinach or broccoli
- Fresh fish fillets, shrimp, scallops
- Chicken, without skin
- Lean beef
- Bean curd (tofu)
- Moo sho vegetable, chicken or shrimp
- Steamed rice
- Lychee fruit

French

Choose more often:

- Dinner salad with vinegar or lemon juice dressing
- Crusty bread without butter
- Fresh fish, shrimp, scallops, steamed mussels (without sauces)
- Chicken breast, without skin
- Rice and noodles without cream or added butter or other fat
- Fresh fruit for dessert

Italian

Choose more often:

- Lightly sautéed with onions
- Shallots
- Peppers and mushrooms
- Artichoke hearts
- Sun-dried tomatoes
- Red sauces: spicy marinara sauce (arrabiata), marinara sauce, or cacciatore
- Light red sauce or light red or white wine sauce
- Light mushroom sauce
- Red clam sauce
- Primavera (no cream sauce)
- Lemon sauce
- Capers
- Herbs and spices: garlic and oregano
- Crushed tomatoes and spices
- Florentine (spinach)
- Grilled (often fish or vegetables)
- Piccata (lemon)
- Manzanne (eggplant)

Middle Eastern

Choose more often:

- Lemon dressing, lemon juice
- Blended or seasoned with Middle Eastern spices
- Herbs and spices
- Mashed chickpeas
- Fava beans
- Smoked eggplant
- With tomatoes, onions, green peppers, and cucumbers
- Spiced ground meat
- Basted with tomato sauce
- Garlic
- Chopped parsley and onion
- Couscous (grain)
- Rice or bulgur (cracked wheat)
- Stuffed with rice and imported spices
- Grilled on a skewer
- Marinated and barbecued
- Baked
- Charboiled or charcoal broiled
- Fresh fruit

Japanese

Choose more often:

- House salad with fresh ginger and cellophane (clear rice) noodles
- Rice
- Nabemono
- Chicken, fish, or shrimp teriyaki, broiled in sauce
- Menrui or soba noodles, often used in soups
- Yakimono (broiled)
- Tofu or bean curd
- Grilled vegetables

Indian

Choose more often:

- Tikka (pan roasted)
- Cooked with or marinated in yogurt
- Cooked with green vegetables, onions, tomatoes, peppers, and mushrooms

- With spinach (saag)
- Baked leavened bread
- Masala
- Tandoori
- Paneer
- Cooked with curry, marinated in spices
- Lentils, chick beans, garbanzo beans, beans
- Garnished with dried fruit
- Chickpeas (garbanzo) and potatoes
- Basmati rice (pullao)
- Marta (peas)
- Chicken or shrimp kebab

Mexican

Choose more often:

- Shredded spicy chicken
- Rice and black beans
- Rice
- Ceviche (fish marinated in lime juice and mixed with spices)
- Served with salsa (hot red tomato sauce)
- Served with salsa verde (green chili sauce)
- Covered with enchilada sauce
- Topped with shredded lettuce, diced tomatoes, and onions
- Served with or wrapped in a corn or wheat flour (soft) tortilla
- Grilled
- Marinated
- Picante sauce
- Simmered with chili vegetarian tomato sauce

Thai

Choose more often:

- Barbecued, sautéed, broiled, boiled, or steamed, braised, marinated
- Charbroiled
- Basil sauce, basil, or sweet basil leaves
- Lime sauce or lime juice
- Chili sauce or crushed dried chili flakes
- Thai spices
- Served in hollowed-out pineapple

- Fish sauce
- Hot sauce
- Napa, bamboo shoots, black mushrooms, ginger, garlic
- Bed of mixed vegetables
- Scallions, onions

Steakhouses

Choose more often:

- Lean broiled beef (no more than 6 oz), London broil, filet mignon, round and flank steaks
- Baked potato without added butter, margarine, or sour cream; top with low-fat yogurt or mustard
- Green salad with reduced fat dressing
- Steamed vegetables without added butter or margarine; try lemon juice and herbs
- Seafood dishes (usually indicated as "surf" on menus).

Fast Foods

Choose more often:

- Grilled chicken breast sandwich without mayonnaise
- Single hamburger without cheese
- Grilled chicken with reduced-fat dressing
- Garden salad with a small portion of dressing
- Low-fat or nonfat yogurt
- Cereal with low-fat milk
- Pancakes without butter or margarine

Deli or Sandwich Shop

Choose more often:

- Fresh sliced vegetables in pita bread with a small serving of salad dressing, yogurt, or mustard
- Cup of bean soup (lentil, minestrone)
- Turkey breast sandwich with mustard, lettuce, tomato
- Sandwich made with 2 slices of bread instead of sub roll or bulky roll
- Fresh fruit

Sample Menu: Traditional American Cuisine, Reduced Calorie

CALORIES	1,600	1,200
Breakfast		
Whole wheat bread	1 slice	1 slice
Jelly, regular	2 tsp	2 tsp
Cereal, Shredded Wheat	1 cup	½ cup
Milk, 1% low-fat	1 cup	1 cup
Orange juice	¾ cup	¾ cup
Coffee, regular	1 cup	1 cup
Milk, 1% low-fat	1 oz	—
Lunch		
Roast beef sandwich		
Whole wheat bread	2 slices	2 slices
Lean roast beef, unseasoned	2 oz	2 oz
American cheese, low-fat, low sodium	1 slice (¾ oz)	—
Lettuce	1 leaf	1 leaf
Tomato	3 slices	3 slices
Mayonnaise, low-calorie	2 teaspoons	1 teaspoon
Apple	1 medium	1 medium
Water	1 cup	1 cup
Dinner		
Salmon	3 oz	2 oz
Vegetable oil	1½ teaspoons	1½ teaspoons
Baked potato	¾ medium	¾ medium
Margarine	1 teaspoon	1 teaspoon
Carrots with 1 teaspoon margarine	½ cup	½ cup
Green beans with 1 teaspoon margarine	½ cup	½ cup
White dinner roll	1 medium	1 small

Reprinted from *Clinical Guidelines on the Identification, Evaluation, and Treatment of Overweight and Obesity in Adults.*
The full report can be accessed at http://www.nhlbi.nih.gov/guidelines/obesity/ob_gdlns.htm.

Ice milk	½ cup	—
Iced Tea, unsweetened	1 cup	1 cup
Water	2 cups	2 cups

Snack

Popcorn, air popped	2 ½ cups	2 ½ cups
Margarine	1 ½ teaspoons	¾ teaspoon

Calories	1,613	1,247
*Sodium	1,341	1,043
Cholesterol (mg)	142	96

---

*No salt added in recipe preparation or as seasoning. Consume at least 32 oz water.

Sample Menu: Asian-American Cuisine, Reduced Calorie

CALORIES	1,600	1,200
Breakfast		
Banana	1 small	1 small
Whole wheat bread	2 slices	1 slice
Margarine	1 tsp	1 tsp
Orange juice	¾ cup	¾ cup
Milk, 1% low-fat	¾ cup	¾ cup
Lunch		
Beef noodle soup, canned, low-sodium	½ cup	½ cup
Chinese noodle and beef salad		
Beef roast	3 oz	2 oz
Peanut oil	1½ teaspoons	1 teaspoon
Soy sauce, low sodium	1 teaspoon	1 teaspoon
Carrots	½ cup	½ cup
Zucchini	½ cup	½ cup
Onion	¼ cup	¼ cup
Apple	1 medium	1 medium
Tea, unsweetened	1 cup	1 cup
Dinner		
Pork stir-fry with vegetable		
Pork cutlet	2 oz	2 oz
Peanut oil	1 teaspoon	1 teaspoon
Soy sauce, low-sodium	1 teaspoon	1 teaspoon
Broccoli	½ cup	½ cup
Carrots	1 cup	½ cup
Mushrooms	¼ cup	½ cup
Steamed white rice	1 cup	½ cup
Tea, unsweetened	1 cup	1 cup

Reprinted from *Clinical Guidelines on the Identification, Evaluation, and Treatment of Overweight and Obesity in Adults*. The full report can be accessed at http://www.nhlbi.nih.gov/guidelines/obesity/ob_gdlns.htm.

Snack

Almond cookies	2 cookies	
Milk, 1% low-fat	¾ cup	¾ cup
Calories	1,609	1,220
*Sodium (mg)	1,296	1,043
Cholesterol (mg)	148	117

*No salt added in recipe preparation or as seasoning. Consume at least 32 oz water.

6-10 Sample Menu: Southern Cuisine, Reduced Calorie

CALORIES	1,600	1,200
Breakfast		
Oatmeal, prepared with 1% low-fat milk	½ cup	½ cup
Milk, 1% low-fat	½ cup	½ cup
English muffin	1 medium	—
Cream cheese, light,	1 tablespoon	—
Orange juice	¾ cup	½ cup
Coffee	1 cup	1 cup
Milk, 1 % low-fat	1 oz	1 oz
Lunch		
Baked chicken, without skin	2 oz	2 oz
Vegetable-oil	1 teaspoon	½ teaspoon
Salad		
Lettuce	½ cup	½ cup
Tomato	½ cup	½ cup
Cucumber	½ cup	½ cup
Oil and vinegar dressing	2 teaspoons	1 teaspoon
White rice, with ½ teaspoon diet margarine	½ cup	¼ cup
Baking powder biscuit prepared with vegetable oil	1 small	½ small
Margarine	1 teaspoon	1 teaspoon
Water	1 cup	1 cup
Dinner		
Lean roast beef	3 oz	2 oz
Onion	¾ cup	¼ cup
Beef gravy, water-based	1 tablespoon	1 tablespoon
Turnip greens, with ½ teaspoon diet margarine	½ cup	½ cup
Sweet potato, baked	1 small	1 small

Reprinted from *Clinical Guidelines on the Identification, Evaluation, and Treatment of Overweight and Obesity in Adults*. The full report can be accessed at http://www.nhlbi.nih.gov/guidelines/obesity/ob_gdlns.htm.

Margarine, diet	½ teaspoon	¼ teaspoon
Ground cinnamon	1 teaspoon	1 teaspoon
Brown sugar	1 teaspoon	1 teaspoon
Cornbread prepared with diet margarine	½ medium slice	½ medium slice
Honeydew melon	¼ medium	⅛ medium
Iced tea, sweetened with sugar	1 cup	1 cup

Snack

Saltine crackers, unsalted tops	4	4
Mozzarella cheese, part skim, low-sodium	1 oz	1 oz

Calories	1,653	1,225
*Sodium (mg)	1,231	867
Cholesterol (mg)	172	142

*No salt added in recipe preparation or as seasoning. Consume at least 32 oz water.

Sample Menu: Mexican-American Cuisine, Reduced Calorie

CALORIES	1,600	1,200
Breakfast		
Cantaloupe	1 cup	½ cup
Farina w/1% low-fat milk	½ cup	½ cup
White bread	1 slice	1 slice
Margarine	1 teaspoon	1 teaspoon
Jelly	1 teaspoon	1 teaspoon
Orange juice	1½ cup	¾ cup
Milk, 1% low-fat	½ cup	½ cup
Lunch		
Beef enchilada		
Tortilla, corn	2	2
Lean roast beef	2 ½ oz	2 oz
Vegetable oil	⅔ teaspoon	⅔ teaspoon
Onion	1 tablespoon	1 tablespoon
Tomato	4 tablespoons	4 tablespoons
Chili peppers	2 teaspoons	2 teaspoons
Refried beans, prepared with vegetable oil	¼ cup	¼ cup
Carrots	5 sticks	5 sticks
Milk, 1% low-fat	½ cup	—
Dinner		
Chicken taco		
Tortilla, corn	1	1
Chicken breast, w/out skin	2 oz	1 oz
Vegetable oil	⅔ teaspoon	⅔ teaspoon
Cheddar cheese, low-fat, low-sodium	1 oz	½ oz
Guacamole	2 tablespoons	1 tablespoon
Salsa	1 tablespoon	1 tablespoon

Reprinted from *Clinical Guidelines on the Identification, Evaluation, and Treatment of Overweight and Obesity in Adults.* The full report can be accessed at http://www.nhlbi.nih.gov/guidelines/obesity/ob_gdlns.htm.

Corn, seasoned	½ cup	½ cup
with margarine	½ tsp	—
Spanish rice without meat,	½ cup	½ cup
seasoned without margarine		
Banana	1 large	½ large
Coffee	1 cup	1 cup
Milk, 1%	1 oz	1 oz
Calories	1,638	1,239
*Sodium (mg)	1,616	1,364
Cholesterol (mg)	143	91

_____

*No salt added in recipe or as seasoning. Consume at least 32 oz water.

Sample Menu: Lacto-Ovo Vegetarian Cuisine, Reduced Calorie

CALORIES	1,600	1,200
Breakfast		
Orange	1 medium	1 medium
Pancakes, made with 1% low-fat milk, egg whites	3 4-in circles	2 4-in circles
Pancake syrup	2 tablespoons	1 tablespoon
Margarine, diet	1½ teaspoons	1½ teaspoons
Milk, 1% low-fat	1 cup	½ cup
Coffee	1 cup	1 cup
Milk, 1%	1 oz	1 oz
Lunch		
Vegetable soup, canned low sodium	1 cup	½ cup
Bagel	1 medium	½ medium
Processed American cheese, low-fat, low-sodium	¾ oz	—
Spinach salad		
Spinach	1 cup	1 cup
Mushrooms	⅛ cup	⅛ cup
Salad dressing, regular calorie	2 teaspoons	2 teaspoons
Apple	1 medium	1 medium
Iced tea, unsweetened	1 cup	1 cup
Dinner		
Omelet		
Egg whites	4 large eggs	4 large eggs
Green pepper	2 tablespoons	2 tablespoons
Onion	2 tablespoons	2 tablespoons
Mozzarella cheese, made from part skim milk, low-sodium	1½ oz	1 oz
Vegetable oil	1 tablespoons	½ tablespoons

Reprinted from *Clinical Guidelines on the Identification, Evaluation, and Treatment of Overweight and Obesity in Adults.* The full report can be accessed at http://www.nhlbi.nih.gov/guidelines/obesity/ob_gdlns.htm.

Brown rice, seasoned with	½ cup	½ cup
Margarine, diet	½ teaspoon	½ teaspoon
Fig bar cookie	1 bar	1 bar
Tea	1 cup	1 cup
Honey	1 teaspoon	1 teaspoon

Snack

Milk, 1% low-fat	¾ cup	¾ cup

Calories	1,650	1,205
*Sodium (mg)	1,829	1,335
Cholesterol (mg)	82	44

---

*No salt added in recipe preparation or as seasoning. Consume at least 32 oz water.

Examples of Moderate Amounts of Activity

A moderate amount of activity is approximately equivalent to physical activity that uses approximately 150 calories of energy per day or 1,000 calories per week. Some activities can be performed at various intensities; the suggested durations correspond to expected intensity of effort.

Less vigorous, more time

↑

Washing and waxing a car for 45–60 minutes

Washing windows or floors for 45–60 minutes

Playing volleyball for 45 minutes

Playing touch football for 30–45 minutes

Gardening for 30–45 minutes

Wheeling self in wheelchair for 30–45 minutes

Walking 1¾ miles in 35 minutes (20 min/mile)

Basketball (shooting baskets) for 30 minutes

Bicycling 5 miles in 30 minutes

Dancing fast (social) for 30 minutes

Pushing a stroller 1½ miles in 30 minutes

Raking leaves for 30 minutes

Walking 2 miles in 30 minutes (15 min/mile)

Water aerobics for 30 minutes

Swimming laps for 20 minutes

Wheelchair basketball for 20 minutes

Basketball (playing a game) for 15–20 minutes

Bicycling 4 miles in 15 minutes

Jumping rope for 15 minutes

Running 1½ miles in 15 minutes (10 min/mile)

Shoveling snow for 15 minutes

Stair walking for 15 minutes

↓

More vigorous, less time

Reprinted from *Clinical Guidelines on the Identification, Evaluation, and Treatment of Overweight and Obesity in Adults.* The full report can be accessed at http://www.nhlbi.nih.gov/guidelines/obesity/ob_gdlns.htm.

6-14

Duration of Various Activities for an Average 154-Pound Adult to Expend 150 Calories

Intensity	Activity	Approximate Duration (minutes)
Moderate	Volleyball, noncompetitive	43
Moderate	Walking, moderate pace (3 mph, 20 min/mile)	37
Moderate	Walking, brisk pace (4 mph, 15 min/mile)	32
Moderate	Table tennis	32
Moderate	Raking leaves	32
Moderate	Social dancing	29
Moderate	Lawn mowing (powered push mower)	29
Hard	Jogging (5 mph, 12 min/mile)	18
Hard	Field hockey	16
Very hard	Running (6 mph, 10 min/mile)	13

Reprinted from *Clinical Guidelines on the Identification, Evaluation, and Treatment of Overweight and Obesity in Adults.* The full report can be accessed at http://www.nhlbi.nih.gov/guidelines/obesity/ob_gdlns.htm.

The average adult walks approximately 3,000 steps every day. By increasing the number of steps you walk daily to 10,000, you reach a level of activity that can reduce your risk of disease and help you lead a longer, healthier life. To keep track of the steps you walk, you need a pedometer that counts steps. Most sports stores will carry pedometers. Not everyone needs to start at 10,000 steps. You can begin by taking a baseline reading of your walking for 1 week. Then, increase those steps by 10% or 20% until you eventually reach the recommended level of 10,000 steps.

Keep track of the steps by using the log below or writing it in a calendar or other convenient location. Remember to reset your pedometer each morning.

Date	Total steps

The full publication can be seen at www.niddk.nih.gov/health/nutrit/pubs/parentips/tipsforparents.htm. Click *How Can I Help My Overweight Child,* pages 6 and 7.

- Do not put your child on a weight-loss diet unless instructed to do so by your healthcare provider. Limiting what children eat may interfere with their growth.

- Involve the whole family in building healthy eating and physical activity habits. It benefits everyone and does not single out the child who is overweight.

- Accept and love your child at any weight. It will boost his or her self-esteem.

- Help your child find ways other than food to handle setbacks or successes.

- Talk with your healthcare provider if you are concerned about your child's eating habits or weight.

Remember, you play the biggest role in your child's life. You can help your children learn healthy eating and physical activity habits that they can follow for the rest of their lives.

TIPS FOR PARENTS

- Make sure your child eats breakfast. Breakfast provides children with the energy they need to listen and learn in school.

- Offer your child a wide variety of foods, such as grains, vegetables and fruits, low-fat dairy products, and lean meat or beans.

- Cook with less fat; bake, roast, or poach foods instead of frying.

- Limit the amount of added sugar in your child's diet. Serve water or low-fat milk more often than sugar-sweetened soda and fruit-flavored drinks.

- Involve your child in planning and preparing meals. Children may be more willing to eat the dishes they help fix.

- Be a role model for your children. If they see you being physically active and having fun, they are more likely to be active and stay active throughout their lives.

- Encourage your child to be active everyday.

- Involve the whole family in activities such as hiking, biking, dancing, basketball, or roller-skating.

ADDITIONAL READING

Guide to Your Child's Nutrition by William Dietz. American Academy of Pediatrics, 1999.

Fit Kids: Raising Physically and Emotionally Strong Kids with Real Food by Eileen Behan. Pocket Books, 2001.

Child of Mine by Ellen Satter. Bull Publishing Co., 2000.

WHAT IS GLYCEMIC INDEX?

Glycemic index (GI) is a measure of how carbohydrate-containing foods affect blood glucose levels. All foods that contain carbohydrates (e.g., starchy vegetables [potatoes and corn], desserts, fruits, bread, pasta, and rice) can be tested for how they affect blood sugar levels after being eaten.

HOW IS GI DETERMINED?

Glycemic index is assessed by having one or more people eat a specific food, after which the change in blood sugar is measured and compared with a control food (often white bread). The average change in blood sugar relative to the levels after consumption of the control food is the food's GI.

WHAT AFFECTS THE GI OF A FOOD?

Foods high in fat and fiber usually have a lower GI than low-fat, high-fiber foods because fat and fiber delay digestion and slow blood sugar rise. The ripeness of a fruit affects GI and so can the food it is eaten with. For example, when cereal is eaten with milk, bread with peanut butter, or butter on vegetables, the GI of the meal will be different from that of either food alone.

HOW CAN I USE THE GI?

Right now GI is used most often as a research tool than for planning menus. It is difficult to use GI to plan meals because of the wide variability of GI, depending on ripeness, cooking methods, and how the food is chopped and served.

Creating a diet based solely on GI may be too difficult and result in an eating plan that excludes nutrient-rich foods.

Where Can I Get More Information?

National Diabetes Information Clearinghouse http://diabetes.niddk.nih.gov/

To find a dietitian in your area, go to www.eatright.org and click Find a Nutrition Professional.

Reprinted from the International Food Information Council Foundation publication *Questions and Answers about Glycemic Index,* September 2002. The complete source can be read at http://ific.org/publications/qa/glycemicqa.cfm.

REFERENCES

Barlow, S. E. & Dietz, W. H. (1998). Electronic article: Obesity Evaluation and Treatment: Expert Committee Recommendations. *Pediatrics, 102*, no. 3. URL: http://www.pediatrics.org/cgi/content/full/102/3/e29.

Bravata, D. M., Sanders, L., Huang, J., Krumholz, H. M., Olkin, I., Gardner, C. D., & Bravata, D. M. (2003). Efficacy and Safety of low-carbohydrate diets: A systematic Review. *Journal American Medical Association, 289*, 1837–1850.

Barnard, N. D., Eckal, R. H., & Garza, C. Cautioning patients about extreme diets: diet and nutrition in your practice. (2001). *Journal of Patient Care*, August 15, 28–46 vol. 35.

Centers for Disease Control. Chronic disease prevention fact sheet: preventing obesity and chronic diseases through good nutrition and physical activity http://www.cdc.gov/nccdphp/pe_pa.htm. Accessed January 21, 2004.

Freedman, M. J., King, J., & Kennedy, E. (2001). Popular diets: a scientific review executive summary. *Obesity Research, 9* (suppl. 1), 1S–15S. http://www.obesityresearch.org.

Foster, G. D., Wyatt, H. R., Hill, J. O., McGuckin, B. G., Brill, C., Mohammed, B. S., Szapary, P. O., Rader, D. J., Edman, J. S., & Klein, S. (2003). A randomized trial of a low-carbohydrate diet for obesity. *New England Journal of Medicine, 348*, 2082, 2136.

Jenkins, D. J. A. (1981). Glycemic index of food: a physiological basis for carbohydrate exchange. *American Journal of Clinical Nutrition, 34*, 362.

Liebman, B. (2004). Weighing the diet books. *Nutrition Action Heath Letter, 31*, 1, 3–7.

Liebman, B., & Schardt, D. (2004). Mad about fads. *Nutrition Action Health Letter, 31*, 8–9.

Ludwig, D. S., Majzoub, J. A., Al-Zahrani, A., Dallal, G. E., Blanco, I., & Roberts, S. B. (1999). Electronic article: *High glycemic index foods, overeating, and obesity. Pediatrics, 103*, e26. www.pediatrics.org/cgi/content/full/103/3/e26.

How to help your patients improve their eating habits. *Nutrition in Primary Care* NIH Publication No. 94-3855 NCI 9000. National Cancer Institute, Rockville Pike, Bethesda, MD 20892.

National Weight Control Registry http://www.uchsc.edu/nutrition/WyattJortberg/nwcr.htm. Accessed May 12, 2004.

Samaha, F. F., Iqbal, N., Seshadri, P., Chicano, K. L., Daily, D. A., McGrory, J., Williams, T., Williams, M., Gracely, E. J., & Stern, L. (2003). A low-carbohydrate as compared with a low-fat diet in severe obesity. *New England Journal of Medicine, 348*, 2074.

United States Department of Health and Human Services. http://www.surgeongeneral.gov/topics/obesity/calltoaction/fact_adolescents.htm. Accessed January 2, 2002.

Wing, R. R., & Hill, J. O. (2001). Successful weight loss maintenance. *Annual Review Nutrition, 21*, 323–341.

Zemel, M. (2002). Dietary calcium and dairy products accelerate weight and fat loss during energy restriction in obese adults. *American Journal of Clinical Nutrition, 275* (suppl.), 342s–343s.

Calories, Fast Food, and Caffeine

CALORIES COUNT

Food labels provide an accurate and reliable calorie reference, but a list of the calorie content in food can be useful to healthcare providers in a medical office when food labels are not available. This section can be helpful for individuals keeping food records and counting calories or it can be used by providers to assist patients in accurately counting the calories they consume at a meal or in a day.

Resources

A partial list of fast food items and restaurant meals is included in this section, but complete nutrition information can be obtained at the following web pages:

Arby's
    www.arbys.com
Baskin Robbins
    www.baskinrobbins.com
Burger King
    www.burgerking.com
Carl's Jr.
    www.carlsjr.com
Dairy Queen
    www.dairyqueen.com
Domino's Pizza
    www.dominos.com

Dunkin' Donuts
    www.dunkindonuts.com
Einstein Brothers Bagels
    www.einsteinbros.com
Jack in the Box
    www.jackinthebox.com
Jamba Juice
    www.jambajuice.com
Kentucky Fried Chicken
    www.kfc.com
Krispy Kreme Doughnuts
    www.krispykreme.com
McDonald's
    www.mcdonalds.com
Panda Express
    www.pandaexpress.com
Pizza Hut
    www.pizzahut.com
Starbucks
    www.starbucks.com
Subway
    www.subway.com
Taco Bell
    www.tacobell.com
Wendy's
    www.wendys.com

CALORIE CONTENT OF SELECTED FOODS PER COMMON MEASURE, LISTED ALPHABETICALLY

Alcoholic beverage: Beer light	12 oz	99
Beer, regular	12 oz	146
Daiquiri, prepared from recipe, 2 oz		117

Distilled, all (gin, rum, vodka, whiskey)

80 proof 1.5 oz	97
86 proof 1.5 oz	105
90 proof 1.5 oz	110
Liqueur, coffee 1.5 oz	175
Piña colada, prepared from mix, 4.5 oz	245
Wine, dessert dry, 3.5 oz	157
Wine, table red, 3.5 oz	74
Wine, table white, 3.5 oz	70
Apples, dried, 5 rings	78
Apple, raw, 1 medium	72
Applesauce, canned unsweetened, 1 cup	105
Apricots, dried, 10 halves	84
Apricot, raw, 1	17
Artichoke, cooked, 1 medium	60
Asparagus, cooked 4 spears	13
Avocado, raw, California, 1 oz	47
Bagel, plain 4 inch	245
Bamboo shoots, canned, 1 cup	25
Banana, raw, 1	105
Barley, pearled, cooked, 1 cup	193
Beans, baked, 1 cup	236
Beans, baked canned with franks, 1 cup	368
Beans, kidney cooked, 1 cup	258
Beef stew, canned, 1 cup	218
Beef chuck, blade roast, 3 oz	293
Beef, ground, 75% lean, 3 oz	236
80% lean 3 oz	230
85% lean 3 oz	212
Beet greens, 1 cup	39
Beets, cooked, 1 cup	75
Biscuit, 4 inch	358
Blackberries, raw, 1 cup	62
Blueberries, raw, 1 cup	83
Bologna, 2 slices	172
Bread stuffing, ½ cup	178
Bread: French, ½-inch slice	68
Italian, 1 slice	54
Oatmeal, 1 slice	73
Pita, 4 inch slice	77
Pumpernickel, 1 slice	80
Raisin, 1 slice	71
Rye, 1 slice	83
Wheat, 1 slice	65
White, 1 slice	67
Whole wheat, 1 slice	69
Broccoli, cooked, 1 cup	55
Brussel sprouts, cooked, 1 cup	56
Bulgur, cooked, 1 cup	151
Butter, 1 tablespoon	101
Cabbage, cooked, 1 cup	33
Cake: Angel food, 1 piece 1 oz	72
Boston cream pie, 1 piece 3 oz	232
Chocolate with chocolate frosting, 1 piece 2 oz	235
Fruitcake, 1 piece 1½ oz	140
Gingerbread, 1 piece 2½ oz	263

	Pound, 1 piece 1 oz	109
	Short-cake, biscuit type, 1 shortcake 2 oz	225
Candy:	Kit Kat, 1.5 oz bar	217
	Milky Way, 2.15 oz bar	258
	Snickers, 2 oz bar	273
	Starburst, 1 piece	20
	Marshmallow, 1 cup	159
	Milk chocolate, 1.55 oz bar	235
	Mr. Good bar, 1.75 oz bar	263
	Reese's Peanut Butter Cups, 2 cups	232
	Semisweet chocolate, 1 cup	805
Carambola, star fruit, 1 fruit		30
Carbonated beverage, club soda, 12 oz		0
	Cola, 12 oz	155
	Ginger ale, 12 oz	124
	Grape soda, 12 oz	160
	Lemon-lime, 12 oz	147
	Orange, 12 oz	179
	Pepper-type 12 oz	151
	Root beer, 12 oz	152
Carrot juice, 1 cup		94
Carrot, raw, 1		30
Catsup, 1 tablespoon		14
Cauliflower, cooked, 1 cup		29
Celery, raw, 1 stalk		6
Cereals:	Apple Cinnamon Cheerios, ¾ cup	118
	Basic 4, 1 cup	202
	Berry Berry Kix, ¾ cup	118
	Cheerios, 1 cup	111
	Cinnamon Toast, ¾ cup	127
	Cocoa Puffs, 1 cup	117
	Corn Chex, 1 cup	112
	Frosted Wheaties, ¾ cup	112
	Golden Grahams, ¾ cup	112
	Honey Nut Cheerios, 1 cup	112
	Kix, 1⅓ cup	113
	Lucky Charms, 1 cup	114
	Reese's Puffs, ¾ cup	128
	Total Cornflakes, 1⅓ cup	112
	Total Raisin Bran 1 cup	171
	Trix, 1 cup	117
	Wheaties, 1cup	107
	Quaker Cap'n Crunch, ¾ cup	108
	Rice, puffed, 1 cup	56
	Wheat germ, 1 tablespoon	27
Cooked cereal:	Cream of Wheat, 1 cup	129
	Oats, plain, 1 packet	97
	Oats, maple brown sugar, 1 packet	157
	Wheatena, 1 cup	136
Cheese:	Blue, 1 oz	100
	Cheddar, 1 oz	114
	Cottage, creamed with fruit, 1 cup	219
	Cottage, low-fat 1%, 1 cup	163
	Cream, 1 tablespoon	51
	Cream, fat-free, 1 tablespoon	15
	Feta, 1 oz	75

	Mozzarella, part skim milk, 1 oz	86
	Muenster, 1 oz	104
	Neufchatel, 1 oz	74
	Parmesan, grated, 1 tablespoon	22
	Processed American, 1 oz	106
	Provolone, 1 oz	100
	Ricotta, part skim, 1 cup	339
	Ricotta, whole milk, 1 cup	428
	Swiss, 1 oz	108
Cheesecake, 1 piece 2½ cup		256
Cherries, 10		43
Chicken potpie, 1 small		484
Chicken, roasted, ½ breast		142
Chickpeas, 1 cup		286
Chili con carne, 1 cup		253
Chocolate syrup, 1 tablespoon		52
Coffeecake, cinnamon with crumb topping, 1 piece 2 oz		263
Coleslaw, 1 cup		83
Collards, cooked, 1 cup		61
Cookies:	Brownie, 2 oz piece	227
	Butter, 1 cookie	23
	Chocolate chip, 1 cookie	48
	Chocolate cream-filled sandwich, 1 sandwich	47
	Fig bar, 1 bar	57
	Graham cracker, 2 squares	59
	Molasses, 1 medium	65
	Oatmeal, 1 soft cookie	61
	Oatmeal with raisins, 1 cookie	65
	Peanut butter, 1 cookie	72
	Shortbread, 1 cookie	40
	Sugar, 1cookie	71
	Vanilla sandwich with cream filling, 1 sandwich	72
	Vanilla wafers, lower fat, 1 cookie	18
Corn, 1 ear		83
Corn, 1 cup		184
Cornmeal, 1 cup		505
Cornstarch, 1 tablespoon		31
Couscous cooked, 1 cup		176
Cowpeas (black-eyed), 1 cup		200
Crackers:	Cheese, 10	50
	Cheese, sandwich-type with peanut butter filling, 1 sandwich	35
	Matzo, 1 matzo	112
	Melba toast, 4 pieces	78
	Rye wafers, 1 wafer	37
	Saltines, 4	52
	Wheat, 4	38
	Whole wheat, 4	71
Cranberry juice cocktail, 8 oz		144
Cranberry sauce, 2 oz slice		86
Cream substitute, powdered, 1 teaspoon		11
Cream, light, 1 tablespoon		29
	Heavy, whipping, 1 tablespoon	44
Cream sour, 1 tablespoon		26
Croissant, butter, 2 oz		231
Croutons, 1 cup		186
Crustacean: Crab, 3 oz		87
	Lobster, 3 oz	83

	Shrimp, 3 oz	102
	Shrimp, breaded and fried, 3 oz	205
Cucumber, 1 cup		14
Dandelion greens, cooked, 1 cup		34
Danish pastry, cheese, 2.5 oz piece		266
Danish pastry, with fruit, 2.5 oz piece		263
Dates, 5 dates		117
Doughnut, cake-type, old-fashioned plain, 1 medium		198
Doughnut, glazed, 1 medium		242
Duck, meat only, ½ duck		444
Éclair, 1		262
Egg substitute, ¼ cup		53
Egg white, raw, 1 large		17
Egg, whole, raw, 1 large		74
Egg yolk, raw, 1 large		53
Eggnog, 1 cup		343
English muffin, 1		133
Entrees:	Fish fillet, fried, 1 fillet	211
	Pizza with cheese, 1 slice	141
	Pizza with pepperoni, 1 slice	181
Figs, dried, 2 figs		94
Fish:	Catfish, fried, 3 oz	195
	Cod, 3 oz	89
	Fish stick, 1 oz sticks	76
	Flatfish (flounder and sole), 3 oz	99
	Haddock, 3 oz	95
	Halibut, 3 oz	119
	Herring, 3 oz	223
	Ocean perch, 3 oz	103
	Pollock, 3 oz	96
	Rockfish, 3 oz	103
	Roughy, orange, 3 oz	76
	Salmon, smoked, 3 oz	100
	Salmon canned, 3 oz	118
	Sardine, in oil, 3 oz	177
	Swordfish, 3 oz	132
	Trout, 3 oz	144
	Tuna salad, 1 cup	383
	Tuna, light, canned in oil, 3 oz,	168
	Tuna, light, canned in water, 3 oz	109
	Tuna, cooked, 3 oz	118
Frankfurt, beef, 1 frank		149
Frankfurt, chicken, 1 frank		116
Frozen yogurt, chocolate, ½ cup		115
Frozen yogurt, vanilla, ½ cup		117
Fruit butter, apple, 1 tablespoon		29
Fruit cocktail, canned heavy syrup, 1 cup		181
Fruit cocktail canned, light syrup, 1 cup		109
Fruit punch drink, 1 cup		117
Garlic, raw, 1 clove		4
Gelatin dessert, ½ cup		84
Grape drink, 1 cup		113
Grape juice, 1 cup		128
Grapefruit juice, 1 cup		96
Grapes, red or green, 10 grapes		35
Gravy, beef, ¼ cup		31
Gravy, chicken, ¼ cup		47

Ham, sliced, 2 oz 92
Hearts of palm, canned, 1 piece 9
Honey, 1 tablespoon 64
Horseradish, prepared, 1 tsp 2
Hummus, 1 tablespoon 23
Ice cream: Chocolate, ½ cup 143
　　　　　 Vanilla, ½ cup 133
Jam and preserves, 1 tablespoon 56
Jellies, 1 tablespoon 51
Jerusalem artichokes, 1 cup 114
Kale, cooked, 1 cup 36
Kiwi fruit, 1 medium 46
Kohlrabi, cooked, 1 cup 48
Lamb, cooked, 3 oz 219
Lard, 1 tablespoon 115
Leeks, cooked, 1 cup 32
Lemon juice, 1 tablespoon 3
Lemonade, 1 cup 131
Lemon, 1 raw 17
Lentils, cooked, 1 cup 230
Lettuce, cos or romaine, 1 cup 10
Lettuce, iceberg, 1 cup 6
Lima beans, cooked, 1 cup 189
Lime juice, 1 tablespoon 3
Macaroni and cheese, 1 cup 199
Mango, raw, 1 cup 107
Margarine, 1 tablespoon 101
Melon, cantaloupe, 1 cup 54
Melon, honeydew, 1 cup 61
Milkshake, chocolate or vanilla, 11 oz 355
Milk:　　 Buttermilk, 1 cup 98
　　　　　Canned, condensed, sweetened, 1 cup 982
　　　　　Canned, evaporated, nonfat, 1 cup 200
　　　　　Canned, evaporated, 1 cup 338
　　　　　Chocolate, 1 cup 207
　　　　　Chocolate, low-fat, 1 cup 158
　　　　　Chocolate, reduced fat, 1 cup 180
Dry, nonfat instant powder, ⅓ cup 82
Low-fat (1%), 1 cup 102
Nonfat (fat-free, skim), 1 cup 83
Reduced fat (2%), 1 cup 122
Whole (3.2%), 1 cup 146
Miso, 1 cup 142
Molasses, blackstrap, 1 tablespoon 47
Mollusks:　 Clams, 3 oz 63
　　　　　Oysters, (6 medium), 3 oz 57
　　　　　Scallops, fried, 3 oz 200
Muffin:　 Blueberry, 2 oz 158
　　　　　Corn, 2 oz 178
　　　　　Oat bran, 2 oz 154
　　　　　Wheat bran, toaster type, 1 muffin 106
Mung beans, sprouted, 1 cup 31
Mushrooms, canned, 1 cup 39
　　　　　Shitake, cooked, 1 cup 80
　　　　　Mustard greens, cooked, 1 cup 21
Mustard, 1 teaspoon 3

Nectarines, 1 60
Noodles, Chinese, chow mein, 1 cup 237
Noodles, egg, cooked, 1 cup 212
Nuts: Almonds, (24 nuts), 1 oz 164
          Brazil nuts, (6–8 nuts), 1 oz 186
          Cashew, (18 nuts), 1 oz 165
          Coconut meat, 1 cup 350
          Hazelnuts or filberts, 1 oz 178
          Macadamia, (10–12 nuts), 1 oz 203
          Mixed, 1 oz 175
          Pecans, (20 halves), 1 oz 196
          Pine nuts, 1 oz 191
          Pistachio, (47 nuts), 1 oz 161
          Walnuts, English (14 halves) 185
Oat bran, cooked, 1 cup 88
Oil: Olive, 1 tablespoon 119
          Peanut, 1 tablespoon 119
          Sesame, 1 tablespoon 120
          Soybean, 1 tablespoon 120
          Vegetable, corn, 1 tablespoon 120
Safflower, 1 tablespoon 120
Sunflower, 1 tablespoon 120
Okra, cooked, 1 cup 35
Olives, large, 5 25
Onion rings, fried, 10 rings 244
Onion, raw, 1 cup 67
Onions, scallions, 1 cup 32
Orange juice, 1 cup 112
Oranges, 1 orange 62
Pancakes, 1 pancake (~1 oz) 74
Papaya, raw, 1 cup 55
Parsley, 10 sprigs 4
Parsnips, cooked, 1 cup 110
Pasta, with meatballs, canned entrée, 1 cup 260
Peaches, canned in heavy syrup, 1 cup 194
Peaches, canned in juice, 1 cup 109
Peaches, dried, 3 pieces 93
Peanut butter, chunk style, 1 tablespoon 94
Peanut butter, smooth style, 1 tablespoon 96
Peanuts, all types (28 nuts), 1 oz 166
Pears, Asian, 1 pear 51
Pears, canned heavy syrup, 1 cup 197
Pears, canned in juice, 1 cup 124
Pear, raw, 1 96
Peas, edible pods, cooked, 1 cup 67
Peas, green, canned, 1 cup 117
Peas, green, frozen, 1 cup 125
Peas, split, cooked, 1 cup 231
Peppers, hot chili, 1 18
          Sweet green, 1 24
          Sweet red, 1 31
Pickle relish, sweet, 1 tablespoon 20
Pickles, dill, 1 12
Piecrust, graham cracker, baked, 1 piecrust 1181
Piecrust, frozen, ready-to-bake, 1 piecrust 648
Pie filling: Apple canned, 1/8 of 21 oz can 75

	French, 1 tablespoon	71
	French, reduced fat, 1 tablespoon	38
	Italian, 1 tablespoon	43
	Italian, reduced fat, 1 tablespoon	11
	Mayonnaise, 1 tablespoon	99
	Russian, 1 tablespoon	76
	Russian, low-calorie, 1 tablespoon	23
	Thousand island, 1 tablespoon	31
	Thousand island, reduced-fat, 1 tablespoon	31
	Salami, 2 oz	142
	Salt	0
Sauce:	Barbecue, 1 tablespoon	12
	Cheese, ready-to-serve, ¼ cup	110
	Hoisin, 1 tablespoon	35
	Homemade, white, 1 cup	368
	Nacho cheese sauce, ready-to-serve, ¼ cup	119
	Pasta, spaghetti or marinara, 1 cup	143
	Ready-to-serve hot sauce, 1 tablespoon	15
	Teriyaki, 1 tablespoon	15
Sauerkraut, canned, 1 cup		45
Seaweed, kelp, 2 tablespoon		4
Seaweed, spirulina, dried, 1 tablespoon		3
Seeds:	Sesame, 1 tablespoon	47
	Sunflower, ¼ cup	186
Shake, fast food, chocolate, 16 oz		423
Shake, fast food vanilla, 16 oz		370
Shallots, raw, 1 tablespoon		7
Sherbet, orange, ½ cup		106
Shortening, 1 tablespoon		113
Snacks:	Beef jerky, 1 large piece	81
	Chex mix, (⅔ cup), 1 oz	120
	Corn chips, 1 oz	157
	Fruit leather, 1 oz	100
	Granola bar, 1	120–140
	Oriental mix, rice-based, ¼ cup	143
	Popcorn, air popped, 1 cup	31
	Popcorn, cake, 1	38
	Popcorn, caramel-coated with peanuts, 1 cup	168
	Popcorn, caramel-coated without peanuts, 1 cup	151
	Popcorn, cheese flavored, 1 cup	58
	Popcorn, oil-popped, 1 cup	55
	Pork skins, 1 oz	155
	Potato chips barbecue flavor, 1 oz	139
	Potato chips, plain, 1 oz	152
	Pretzels, 2 oz	229
	Rice cake, brown rice, 1	35
	Tortilla chips, 1 oz	141
	Trail mix, with chocolate chips, nuts, and seeds, 1 cup	706
	Trail mix, tropical, 1 cup	570
Soup:	Bean with ham, 1 cup	230
	Beef broth or bouillon, 1 cup	29
	Beef noodle, 1 cup	83
	Chicken noodle, chunky, 1 cup	176
	Chicken noodle, 1 cup	75
	Chicken vegetable, 1 cup	166
	Chicken with rice, 1 cup	60

Turkey patty, fried, 2 oz	181
Turkey, dark meat, 3 oz	157
Turkey, light meat, 3 oz	132
Turnip greens, 1 cup	29
Vanilla extract, 1 teaspoon	12
Veal, 3 oz	179
Vegetable juice cocktail, 1 cup	46
Vegetable oil, canola, 1 tablespoon	124
Vegetables mixed, frozen, cooked, 1 cup	118
Vinegar, cider, 1 tablespoon	2
Waffle, plain frozen, 1	87
Water, municipal, 8 oz	0.0
Water chestnuts, 1 cup	70
Watermelon, raw, 1 cup	46
Wheat flour, white, 1 cup	442
Wheat flour, whole grain, 1 cup	407
Wild rice, cooked, 1 cup	166
Yogurt: Fruit, low-fat, 10 g protein per 8 oz	232
Plain, low-fat, 12 g protein per 8 oz	143
Plain skim milk, 13 g protein per 8 oz	127
Plain whole milk, 8 g per 8 oz	138

Resources

For more nutrient data access the web page at www.nal.usda.gov/fnic/foodcomp/Data/SR16-1/wtrank/wt_rank.html.

CALORIE CONTENT OF SELECTED FAST FOOD ITEMS

Hardee's

Baked beans, 5 oz	170
Big cookie, 2 oz	280
Big country breakfast with bacon	820
Ultimate omelet, 1 biscuit	570
Burger, Frisco	720
Burger, the Works	530
Cheeseburger	310
Chicken fillet sandwich	480
Chicken, fried, 1 breast	370
Chicken, grilled sandwich	350
Coleslaw, 4 oz	240
Cone, vanilla	170
Fish fillet sandwich	560
French fries, large	430
French fries, small	240
Hamburger	270
Roast beef sandwich	460
Roast beef sandwich, big	460
Shake, vanilla	350
Sundae, hot fudge	290

Jack-In-The Box

Breakfast Jack sandwich	300
Burger, ¼ pound sandwich	510
Carrot cake	370
Cheeseburger	320
Cheeseburger, double	450
Cheeseburger, ultimate	1030
Chicken caesar sandwich	520
Chicken fajita pita	290
Chicken fillet, grilled sandwich	520
Chicken strips, 4 breaded pieces	290
Chicken teriyaki bowl	580
Curley fries	360
Egg rolls, 3 pieces	440
French fries, jumbo	400
French fries, small	220
Jalapenos, stuffed, 7 pieces	420
Jumbo Jack sandwich	560
Pancake platter	400
Salsa, 1 oz	10
Sausage croissant	620
Shake, vanilla	610
Taco	190
Taco, monster	283

Kentucky Fried Chicken

Chicken, Extra Tasty Crispy breast 470
Chicken, Hot & Spicy breast 530
Chicken, Original Recipe, breast 400
Chicken sandwich, BBQ 256
Coleslaw, 5 oz 180
Colonel's Crispy Strips, 3 261
Cornbread, 2 oz 228
Garden rice, 4.4 oz 120
Hot Wings, 6 pieces 471
Kentucky nuggets, 3.4 oz 284
Potatoes, mashed with gravy, 4.8 oz 120
Red beans & rice, 4.5 oz 130

McDonald's

Big Mac 560
Biscuit, 1 260
Biscuit with sausage 440
Cheeseburger 310
Chicken McNugget sauce 65
Chicken McNuggets 290
Cookies, McDonaldland 290
Egg McMuffin 290
English muffin with butter 170
Fillet-O-Fish sandwich 440
French fries, large 400
French fries, small 220
Hamburger 260
Hash brown potatoes 130
Hotcakes with butter and syrup 410
McChicken sandwich 490
Pie, apple 260
Quarter pounder 410
Quarter pounder with cheese 520
Sausage McMuffin 370
Sausage McMuffin with egg 440
Shake, low-fat vanilla 290

Pizza Hut

Bigfoot, cheese, 3 oz slice 186
Hand tossed pizza, cheese 4 oz slice 235
Pan pizza, cheese, 4 oz slice 261
Thin'n Crispy, cheese, 3 oz 205

Taco Bell

Burrito, bean 373
Burrito Supreme 449
Fajita, chicken 461
Fajita, Supreme chicken 505
Fajita, Supreme, vegetable 466
Mexican pizza 565
Nachos 322

Soft taco 226
Taco 183
Taco salad with salsa and shell 856
Tostada with red sauce 292

Wendy's

Breadstick, soft, 1.6 oz 130
Cheeseburger, junior 320
Chicken breaded sandwich 440
Chicken club sandwich 470
Chicken grilled sandwich 310
Chicken nugget with 1 oz BBQ sauce 50
Chicken nuggets, 5 pieces 210
Chili, large 310
Chili, small 210
Cookie chocolate chip 270
French fries, biggie 460
French fries, small 260
Frosty dairy dessert, large 570
Frosty dairy dessert, small 340
Big Bacon Classic burger 570
Hot chocolate, 6 oz 80
Potato baked 310
Potato baked with bacon and cheese 540
Potato salad, 2 tablespoons 80
Pudding, chocolate or vanilla, ¼ cup 70
Salad caesar, side 110
Seafood salad, ¼ cup 70
Stuffed pita, chicken caesar 490
Stuffed pita, garden veggie 390

CAFFEINE

Caffeine is a naturally occurring alkaloid found in tea, Kola nuts, coffee, and chocolate. In small amounts, it is a mild stimulant. In high doses, it can be toxic, causing heart palpitations, sleeplessness, high blood pressure, vomiting, and convulsions. Pregnant women are advised to limit caffeine during pregnancy (Pennington, 1998).

APPROXIMATE CAFFEINE CONTENT IN MILLIGRAMS IN COMMON FOODS

Coffee

Brewed, 6 oz 103
Ground, 1 tablespoon 59
Instant, 6 oz 57
Instant cappuccino flavor, 2 teaspoons 73
Instant decaf 2
Instant mocha flavored, 2 teaspoons 33

Tea

Black 36
Iced, 8 oz from instant powder 31

Carbonated Beverages

Cherry cola, 8 oz 31
Cherry RC, 12 oz 12
Coca-Cola, classic 8 oz 35
Mellow Yellow, 8 oz 35
Mountain Dew 55
Pepsi 37

Candy, Chocolate, and Dessert

Baby Ruth, 1 oz bar 2
Chocolate, semisweet, 1 oz 17
Milk chocolate, 1 oz 7
Reese's Peanut Butter Cup, 1.8 oz 6
Twix, 2 oz 2

Chocolate ice cream, ½ cup 2
Chocolate syrup, 2 tablespoons 5
Baking chocolate, unsweetened, 1 oz 57
Baking cocoa, unsweetened dry
    powder, 1 tablespoon 12

MILK DRINKS

Chocolate malted milk, 8 oz 8
Chocolate milk, 8 oz 8
Hot chocolate, mix, prepared with water 4

REFERENCES

Pennington, J. A. (1998). *Bowes & Church's Food Values of Portions Commonly Used* (17th ed., 383–384). Philadelphia: Lippincott Williams & Wilkins.

United States Department of Agriculture. National Nutrient Database for Standard Reference, Release 16-1. www.nal.usda.gov/fnic/foodcomp/Data/SR16.1/wtrunk/wt_rank.html

INDEX

Page numbers followed by letters *f* or *b* indicate figures and boxes, respectively.

1789

1789